This LifeBook belongs to:

· · · · · · · ·

· · · · · · · ·

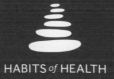

HABITS *of* HEALTH

CONTENTS

INTRODUCTION:
YOUR LIFEBOOK

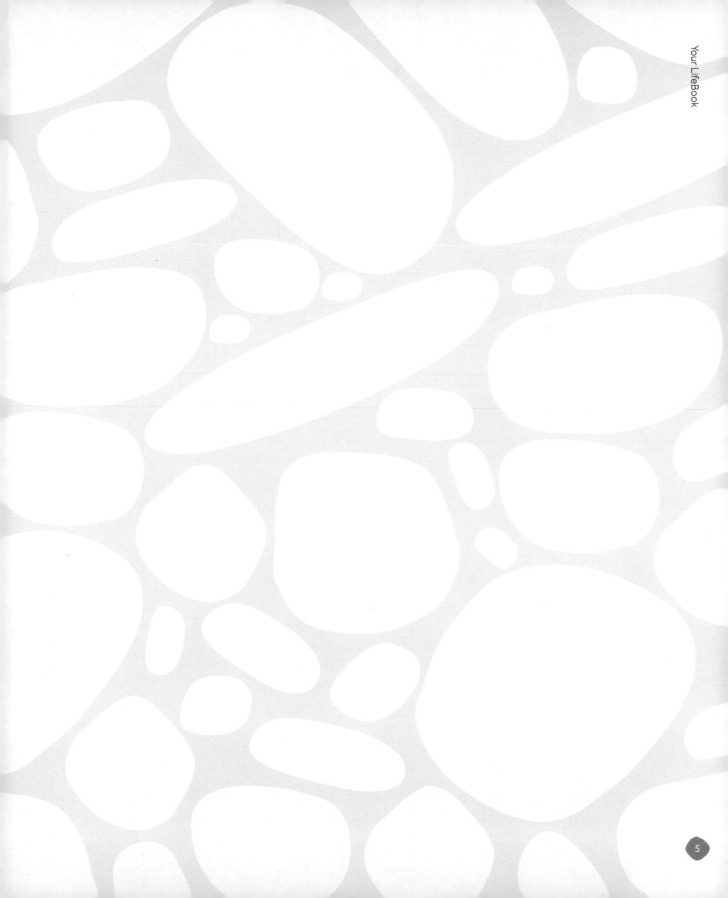

One of the biggest and most powerful realizations we can ever have is to know that our life path is not fixed. The way you think, the way you act, the people you spend time with, and even the world you live in can all be changed.

All things are possible. You have the capability over time, with specific focus, guidance, and practice, to become the dominant force in your life.

From where you sit today, you might rightly think that what I am saying isn't possible. You might ask exactly how I can have a clue about your life? In fact, you're probably thinking I'm a bit full of myself.

Well, I know we've only just started this book together but I need to tell you that you're wrong.

Years ago, things were different. I was certainly different. But that was a long time ago. Today, I am full of confidence and certainty in my approach and understanding, which is based on the firsthand experience of thousands of people, from every walk of life, who have transformed their lives.

These people are not strangers. They are my family, my friends, and a community of clients and coaches who all made a decision to take control of their health and lives. What they share is a willingness to reach out for help and embrace a different way of approaching their lives.

Their approach has gone from focusing on what's wrong in their lives to a mindset of asking, "How can I change, what do I need to learn, and how can I include others in my journey?"

These individuals have rewritten their stories so they are the central characters in amazing journeys of transformation. I'll share some of their stories as part of the Habits of Health experience.

Today, reading this, you now have the opportunity to write the next chapter of your health and your life. Believe me. I understand that the idea may seem scary. Based on your past experiences, you might not even think it's something you can do. In this chaotic and unstable world, in times of accelerated change, everything seems to be beyond your control.

Your life does not have to be one of those things.

THE HABITS OF HEALTH TRANSFORMATIONAL SYSTEM

The Habits of Health Transformational System is your pathway out of a reality that doesn't appear to be within your control. The system will give you the opportunity to take a different path and equip you with what you need to write a different story from today onward.

This system will give you a new sense of direction and put you in the driver's seat, so you can take control and travel along a new path toward better health and improved wellbeing.

This is your companion guide to accompany you on an exciting journey to optimal health and wellbeing. In the original version, this guide was structured as a workbook used to help people learn the components of the Habits of Health System.

I've made Habits of Health 2.0 into a much more valuable tool that helps you as you learn and practice the Habits of Health as part of the Habits of Health Transformational System.

Rather than simply gathering information and filling in the blanks as we did before, this new companion becomes an interactive documentary of your advancement toward a healthier and more thriving life.

In short, it is *Your LifeBook*, expressing your story as you move forward. It is here to guide you and lay down the foundations—at your pace —to help you build a new future. *Your LifeBook* will also give you the opportunity to make notes on what is working (and what isn't) so you can measure your daily progress on your journey.

Like a science experiment, I want to uncover what works for you specifically so I can guide you to your new future. *Your LifeBook* will help track your progress and provide powerful feedback as you grow and advance on the path to better health and wellbeing.

Remember, this is your story. So, because it is absolutely unique, I want to support you in the ways that work best for you. *Your LifeBook* is designed to do just that. You will be able to customize and adjust the Elements to fit your talents, your genetics, and your priorities.

HOW THE PARTS OF THE SYSTEM WORK TOGETHER

There are three parts to the Habits of Health Transformational System. There is the Habits of Health book in a new and updated version. You're holding *Your LifeBook* in your hand. And then there is the Habits of Health App. Let's briefly explain why they all matter and how they interact with each other.

Dr. A's Habits of Heath

This is the main textbook; its contains much more detail about the different aspects of the Habits of Health. It reflects on the latest science of wellbeing and outlines a huge amount of important information about nutrition, sleep, exercise, and more. Think of this as the part of the system that lives on your bookshelf and you will reference it often.

Your LifeBook

This is a day-to-day journal packed with really useful tips, hints, and advice on your journey to optimal health. Each progressive Element represents a central core component which will forge a rock-solid foundation for your progress to optimal health and wellbeing. As a completely joined-up summary of the main book, it's designed to be easy to carry around and perfect for jotting down your thoughts, your progress, and your challenges—so you can reflect on your achievements and know your weaknesses! Think of this as something you can keep with you throughout the day and on your bedside at night, and over the next 12 months you will use it to create and write your new healthy story.

Habits of Health App

Using the latest technology, I've created an app that will help you manage crucial aspects of your journey to optimal health. Using the App, you can set alerts for mealtimes, store and refer to dietary information as well as recipes, and keep a dynamic record of your daily levels of activity. It will also allow you to better manage your emotions.

The three critical parts can work independently of each other but because they're all based on the same principles and with the same aim—of getting you to optimal health—they're far more effective when used together.

There's one important thing you should know: Your journey will not go perfectly. It will be full of challenges and setbacks but they are all part of the life-building process.

But if you stay the course, use the life lessons as learning opportunities, and are willing to be open and curious then this story will be a happy beginning to a thriving life. When you are doing what you want to do, becoming good at it, and sharing it with those you love and care about, you will have written a great story.

ROCKS, PEBBLES, AND SAND

Before you start writing your own story,
I would like to set the stage by retelling a story
I have heard (and told) many times. It's a story
about rocks, pebbles, sand, and a mason jar.

A teacher places a mason jar filled with rocks in front of his class and asks if the jar is full? "Yes" the kids say. He takes a pail with smaller pebbles and pours them into the jar, shaking it until they fill the spaces between the rocks. "Is the jar full?" he asks. "Yes", they say again. The teacher then adds a scoop of sand to the jar. The grains fall between the larger and smaller rocks. "Is the mason jar full?" he asks. The class inspects the jar; there is no more room for anything else. The teacher smiles, grabs a pitcher with water and proceeds to fill the jar to the brim.

The teacher explains that the demonstration is an analogy. He tells them that the jar is your life. The rocks are the big things in your life such as family, your partner, your health, and your hopes and dreams.

The pebbles are other things that give life meaning, like friendships, a job, or hobbies. And the sand and water are the small things that fill in the rest of our time.

The point of the demonstration is that if you fill your life with the small stuff, how will you ever be able to put in the big important stuff? Everything fits in the jar just like the components of your life but you need to consider how the small stuff fits around the bigger things, not vice-versa.

I love this story for several reasons. Its principle lesson is the very building block of the Habits of Health Transformational System. Life is a series of choices and some of them are more important than others. As you will soon learn, it is the prioritization of those choices that creates the motivation which drives everything you can accomplish.

Since the origin of the story is unknown, I am going to adopt the visual analogy it offers and make it a way of explaining and describing our system. It is the perfect structure to visualize and empower your new story and your journey.

The reality is that we live in an obesigenic world, surrounded by so many things that can have damaging effects on our weight and our health. As I describe in Part 1.1 of *Dr. A's Habits of Health*, *It's Not Your Fault That You're Struggling*, with your weight, your health, and your wellbeing. And this chaotic, unhealthy, fast-food-filled, stressful world is not going to change in the near future.

The Habits of Health Transformational System is like the mason jar, as it creates a microenvironment of health to protect you from your unhealthy surroundings. The MacroHabits of Health are the foundations of optimal health and wellbeing. These six key foundational categories are like the rocks. We will place them in the jar first to create lifelong transformation and to protect you from the modern world's negative side effects.

MICROENVIRONMENT OF HEALTH

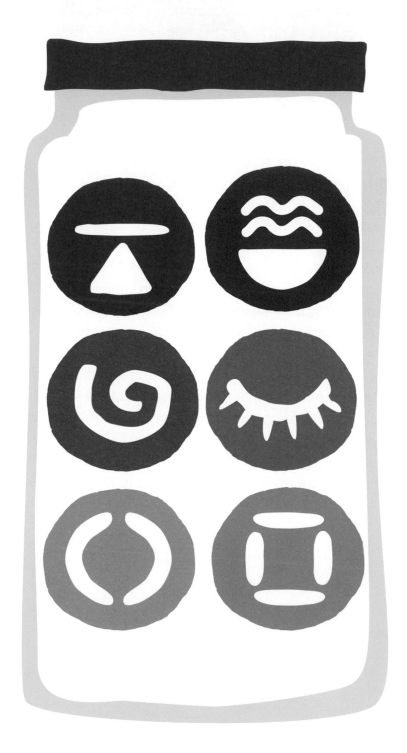

MACROHABITS OF HEALTH

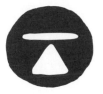

**Healthy Weight
Management**

**Healthy Eating
& Hydration**

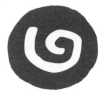

**Healthy
Motion**

**Healthy
Sleep**

**Healthy
Mind**

**Healthy
Surroundings**

Addressing all six of these MacroHabits of Health is critical. Taking time to focus and place these rocks in our jar is the first step in building the foundation necessary for our long-term success. If we fail to tackle each of these keystones of our microenvironment of health, the structure will be weakened and decrease our chances to withstand the effects of our modern world. Next, we have to introduce the primary and secondary habits that are derived from the six MacroHabits. These are the pebbles. These actions surround, reinforce, and actually arise from the foundational rocks. These Habits of Health can be further broken down into the microHabits of Health which are extremely small positive actions— they're so small that we can always do them.

MicroHabits are the thousands of small choices that are a part of our daily life. For example, we make over two hundred decisions about food each day, and each micro-action either adds to our health and life or detracts from it.[1] The sand, therefore, represents what appears to be insignificant choices on their own but, when placed in the jar and mixed with water, they become the concrete that makes the jar rock-solid and a formidable force against any external challenges to your health and wellbeing.

1 *Exploring Comfort Food Preferences across Age and Gender, Physiology and Behavior* – Wansink, B 79 (4–5,2003):739–47

How to use Your LifeBook

Think of this guide as a combination of a guidebook and a personal journal. I would encourage you to make it as personal as possible. You can attach photos of your progress, write about your successes and your challenges, or sketch a favorite meal. The key thing is that the LifeBook is special to you.

Each Element will have a central theme and a goal and will end with a review of that principle and how you have applied it to your life. Each principle builds on the previous one to lay a foundation for your daily life. Once learned and installed, we can step up on your path to give you a firm footing for your ascent to optimal health and wellbeing.

If you have a coach or professional helping you, they will help make sure you have mastered each Element before you move on to the next. They have been trained to help you get the most from *Your LifeBook* and the process.

Your LifeBook is designed to accompany you throughout your day so you can take notes in it and refer back to key takeaways later. This will be important to remember breakthroughs and insights and to identify triggers from which future days can be built.

Your LifeBook will also allow you to track your progress; so, fill it with notes on experiences and maybe even setbacks. It will help you remember the key things that you are working on.

It cannot be said enough that reviewing your notes, events that lead to "aha" moments, and just coordinated repetition will allow you to go over where you are in your Element and your journey. This can lead to amazing breakthroughs.

'This knowledge is most valuable when you decide to "become" through the act of doing, which will lead to the results you are really after.

Not only should you review your current and completed Elements often, but you should also share your insights and thoughts with your coach or mentor.

What I really hope is that *Your LifeBook* ends up on your nightstand so that you will transcribe your key thoughts from the day into it as one of your habits. Whether it is expressing your gratitude, a list of key takeaways, notes, or reminders of how you will start your day tomorrow, it should become a part of your life as you journey to your transformation.

Your LifeBook has much in common with a traditional journal but our approach gives it structure.

Each Element is a permanent step toward a better understanding. It will equip you with increasing skills and act as a reference so you can proceed safely on your climb to optimal health and wellbeing.

Each Element will have enough structure and information for you to master it. And, if you are not used to writing things down and journaling (it took me a while to get used to this when I first started), it will give you default boxes to check off when you make progress and provide questions to assist you on your journey. Using *Your LifeBook* is a key Habit of Health that you can successfully install. It will become an automated part of your day, like all of the other Habits of Health.

Your LifeBook is designed to chronicle your first year of building your new healthier life. It will also document your increasing mastery of the key Elements as you become a higher version of yourself. There are 26 progressive Elements for the next 52 weeks which gives you, on average, two weeks to progress through an Element. Some of the lessons you will be able to complete sooner, and some may take a little longer. There is no set schedule because we want you to proceed at your own pace. I will provide an average time I think is reasonable to complete each Element simply for your reference.

A quick look inside Your LifeBook

Your LifeBook has been designed to be as interactive as possible. That's about you writing in it, carrying it around with you, and turning to it when you need inspiration, advice, or a reminder about how far you've come.

Let's take a quick look at how each Element works.

1. Each Element starts by setting goals and being clear on why it matters

2. We'll also ask you to write about your experiences so far

3. And we'll tell you what you'll learn

4. We include lots of helpful tips and advice

5. You'll see references to the main Habits of Health book

6. Your coach will help assist you to master each Element

If you are ready to start, proceed to the first Element.

For those of you who have already started the journey and are losing weight and getting healthier, congratulations. We can pick up from here because the journey to optimal health and wellbeing isn't just about a restricted period of time when you are losing weight.

It is about fundamentally changing your habits one at a time until you have created sustainable transformation. Those new habits will provide a microenvironment of health to armor and protect you against whatever this crazy world throws at you for the rest of your life.

In Health,
Dr. Wayne Scott Andersen

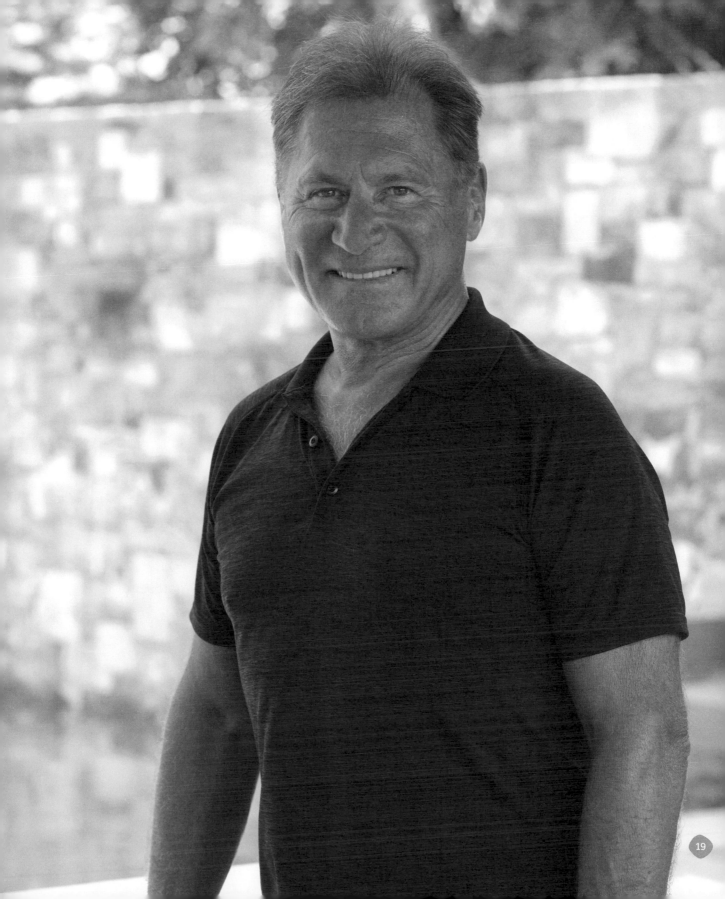

YOUR CURRENT STORY:
HOW IS YOUR LIFE?

"Knowing your current reality
is the first step in creating
your new life."

Dr. Wayne Scott Andersen

The idea behind *Your LifeBook* is that it will help you keep a dynamic record of the transformation that will take place over the next year— from your current reality to a life of optimal health and wellbeing. Along with the Habits of Health, it will help you learn and master a series of fundamental Elements that will be at the heart of the story you write of your new life.

Let's begin by documenting your starting point.

Note: Although this may not be an exercise that excites you, it is important because it will give you a reference point. It's like taking the "before" snapshot that you'll compare with the "after". Everything is going to change as you improve in your health and your life. This snapshot will provide a reference point to your old story.

Why does writing in this journal matter?

Before you start, I want you to realize that this is a safe space in which you can tell your current story. This is *Your LifeBook*, which means it is your private interactive journal and guide. It is unique to you. You will have time for self-reflection, plenty of space to take notes, and more than enough of the insights I have gathered over the last 20 years or so to help you write your new story at your own pace. In this digital age where everything is electronic, I believe that there is real power in using a pen and writing our past and current thoughts and observations in our own hand.

Much like writing down our goals, the written word has magic in it.

The structure of this section and the future Elements have been designed to increase your self-awareness so you become more aware of who you are and where you are starting. This will allow you to methodically build and master the Elements, thereby creating lifelong transformation. The idea is that you will develop a deep desire to continue to learn, grow, and develop.

Our focus will be on your lifestyle habits because you have full control over them and, as you strengthen them, they will provide a solid foundation for creating overall wellbeing. In the coming Elements, we'll explore the core building blocks of health and wellbeing. Before we gather some of your information and ask you a few questions to see where you are now, I would love you to write a brief introductory piece about who you are.

LET ME TELL YOU A LITTLE BIT ABOUT ME

First though, let me introduce myself properly.

I am Wayne Michael Scott Andersen. I am 66 years old and I have an amazing life. I get up every morning in a state of great health and approach the day with the enthusiasm of someone a good deal younger. I am active, fully engaged in my life, and I have a ton of energy. I have two beautiful daughters and a love of nature and the outdoors. I would characterize myself as a highly spiritual person. I love my vocation (it's really my avocation) because it fills my day with rewards. I feel I am bringing value to the world.

The story of my past was not so optimal and there were many areas of my life where I was far from thriving. That's why I hope you are confident I can help you to help yourself. It is the application of the principles in the Habits of Health Transformational System that have allowed me to grow and transform to the thriving state I now find myself in.

Recently, completely and unexpectedly, I lost my soul mate and wife Lori. Although it is a tremendous loss, having the foundations and Elements have allowed me to continue to live fully and with purpose. The support and guidance during this adjustment has enabled me to be fully present for my daughters.

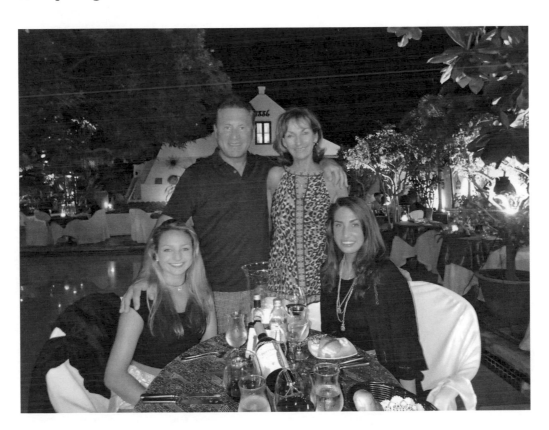

Dr. A, Lori, Savannah, and Erica in Aruba, Christmas 2017

Let's find out about you

Okay, now it's your turn. Tell me a bit about yourself and create a powerful snapshot:

Your current story is only your current story based on the habits of your past and current life. We're here together to help you improve and become a higher version of yourself.

We need to start by gathering the current state of your body, mind, life, and work.

Making a note of your current numbers

Current chronological age:

Height in inches:

Weight in pounds:

BMI (see chart on page 155):

Current waist circumference (at belly button) in inches:

Allergies:

Current medications:

Current illnesses:

Assessing your overall wellbeing and how you are managing your days will start to give you an insight into your world.

We know that eating right will improve our health yet, in the moment, we can't help grabbing a cheeseburger or a sugary doughnut because one burger or one doughnut can't really lead to obesity or diabetes, can it? We know we should be more physically active but our favorite TV show is on. My kid has a baseball game tonight but I am buried at work and he won't mind. My friend has asked me out to dinner three times but I blow them off because I am just too busy. I find myself going shopping every time I really get stressed and yet, when I get my credit card bill, I am under even more pressure.

Let's see how you currently stack up in the parameters that determine the quality of your life.

The design of *Your LifeBook* allows you regular opportunities to check boxes which will give you some measurable parameters. But the areas where I ask you to write your thoughts in your own words are equally important. I do that because I am asking you to take ownership of your situation and write— in your own words—your observations, thoughts, and "Aha!" moments.

Let's do a wellbeing evaluation.

Go online to HabitsofHealth.com to complete the comprehensive Habits of Health Assessment but use the shortened version here to get started.

HOW IS YOUR PHYSICAL HEALTH?

Physical health includes many key areas, like reaching and maintaining a healthy weight, developing healthy eating habits, engaging in robust physical activity, slipping into high quality sleep time for relaxation, and being within a healthy, safe, hazard free work, home, and play environment.

In these key areas of physical health, give your best estimate as to where you think you are on a scale of 1 to 10, with 10 being optimum.

Here are some ideas to help you rate your current position on the scale:
- How competent are you at managing your weight?
- How much energy do you have throughout the day?
- What kind of food are you putting into your body?
- What is your level of activity each day and do you exercise?
- Do you get a good restful night's sleep?
- How good are you at handling stress? And do you make sure you have evaluated the potential hazards in your world?
- Have you removed unhealthy food from your workplace and house?
- Do you get medical checkups and maintain yourself?

How safe is it where you work and live in terms of exposure to health risks such as steep stairs, poor water quality, crime and so on?

If you are not exactly sure where you are, don't worry. Take your best guess and we will gather more detail later. For now, complete the answers and then put your total score at the bottom.

	Bad		Poor		Fair		Good		Optimum	
Weight Status	1	2	3	4	5	6	7	8	9	10
Eating Habits	1	2	3	4	5	6	7	8	9	10
Physical Activity	1	2	3	4	5	6	7	8	9	10
Sleeping	1	2	3	4	5	6	7	8	9	10
Relaxation	1	2	3	4	5	6	7	8	9	10
Safe & Healthy Surroundings (Work/Home/Play)	1	2	3	4	5	6	7	8	9	10

Score_____ /60

Your current score in physical health is only a snapshot of what your score can become as you apply the principles and adopt the Habits of Health in your life.

Your physical health is primarily determined by your current habits and, to a lesser extent, your genetics (they account for roughly 30% of your physical health).[1]

In the space below, it will be useful to describe, in your own words, your current physical health. Use the questions I presented on the previous page to help guide your writing.

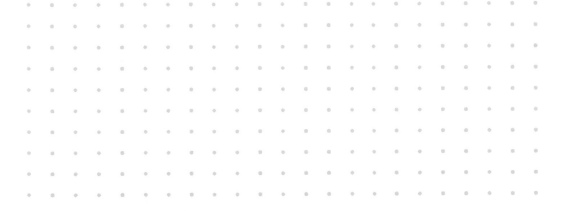

HOW IS YOUR MENTAL HEALTH?

Mental health includes many key areas, including strong relationships, a sense of community, making time to follow spirituality, and finding engagement and motivation at your job, hobbies, and so on.

In these key areas of mental health, give your best estimate as to where you think you are on a scale of 1 to 10, with 10 being optimum. If you are not exactly sure where you are, take your best guess and then put your total score at the bottom.

Here are some ideas to help you rate your current position on the scale:
- Do you have deep meaningful relationships with friends and family?
- Do you have passion for your job, enjoy what you're doing, and feel fully attentive and focused throughout your days?
- Do you believe that you can accomplish whatever you put your mind and body to?
- Are you hopeful and optimistic about the future and act thoughtfully on your emotions when they arise?
- Are you resilient and learn from the past?
- Do you have meaning and purpose and savor the small pleasures of life?
- Do you feel that life is happening through you and that you're connected to your faith and spirituality?
- Are you connected to your community in service?
- Are you having fun, relaxing, and connecting to nature with hobbies and free time for yourself?

	Bad		Poor		Fair		Good		Optimum	
Most Relationships	1	2	3	4	5	6	7	8	9	10
Attitude at Work	1	2	3	4	5	6	7	8	9	10
Meaning & Purpose	1	2	3	4	5	6	7	8	9	10
Spirituality Time	1	2	3	4	5	6	7	8	9	10
Community Service	1	2	3	4	5	6	7	8	9	10
Hobbies/Fun	1	2	3	4	5	6	7	8	9	10

Score_____ /60

Your current score in mental health is only a snapshot of what your score can become as you apply the principles and adopt the Habits of Health in your life.

Your mental health is primarily determined by how you take responsibility for your thoughts and actions. As we work together, you will learn to be able to place your thoughts and mind where you want, for as long as you want, to become the dominant force in your life. It will require you to go to a place called the mental gymnasium and install some powerful Habits of a Healthy Mind.

Your mental health is also heavily influenced by your physical health, brain health, the quality of your relationships, and the individuals you associate with.

Take a few moments to describe your current mental health in your own words. Use the descriptions I presented as a reference point for writing about your own experience in terms of how much abundance you have or desire.

HOW IS YOUR FINANCIAL HEALTH?

Financial health encompasses many key areas, which includes abundance (the feeling that your life is full in terms of resources). It is important to feel like you have the means to create experiences and memories with family and friends. It also includes the confidence that comes from knowing you can pay your bills and care for your family.

In these key areas of financial health, give your best estimate as to where you think you are on a scale of 1 to 10, with 10 being optimum. As before, if you are not exactly sure where you are, make a guesstimate because we'll add more detail later. Put your total score at the bottom.

Here are some ideas to help you rate your current position on the scale:
- You sense you have what it takes and know that with gratitude, hard work, and direction you can bring what you want into your life.
- You do good deeds for others that are unexpected.
- You have resources so you don't have to spend your days worrying how you will pay your bills.
- You plan and control your finances so they don't control you.
- You have discretionary income and the time to be spontaneous as well as focus on creating health and wellbeing.
- You have developed the resources to create special experiences of travel and events with your loved ones and friends.
- You have the resources to give back to your community and favorite charities.

	Bad		Poor		Fair		Good		Optimum	
Abundance	1	2	3	4	5	6	7	8	9	10
Resources to Minimize Stress	1	2	3	4	5	6	7	8	9	10
Money Management	1	2	3	4	5	6	7	8	9	10
Money to Do What You Want	1	2	3	4	5	6	7	8	9	10
Resources to Create Memories/ Experiences	1	2	3	4	5	6	7	8	9	10
Community Contribution	1	2	3	4	5	6	7	8	9	10

Score_____ /60

Your current score in financial health is only a snapshot of what your score can become as you apply the principles and adopt the Habits of Health in your life.

Your financial health is primarily determined by how you take responsibility for your thoughts and actions. As we work together, you will learn to be able to place your thoughts and your mind where you want, for as long as you want, to become the dominant force in your life. It will mean a visit to the mental gym, but it will be worth it.

Your financial health is also heavily influenced by your physical health, brain health, and the quality of your relationships and individuals you associate with.

Although the Habits of Health is not a course on financial planning, these habits will prepare you to become a higher version of yourself in all your daily actions!

Take a moment to describe your current financial health. Use the descriptions I presented as a reference point for writing about your own experience in terms of how much abundance you have or desire.

We have just taken a really important step. We have evaluated your current reality in terms of your health and wellbeing.

I'd now like you to go back and get your scores in the key areas of wellbeing.

Fill in the scores for the three key areas in the table below. Take note of the areas you are the strongest in and the areas in which you could use some help. Remember, there is a more in depth health assessment available on the website, if you would like to dive deeper than we did here.

	Bad	Poor	Fair	Good	Great	Optimum
Physical Health	10	20	30	40	50	60
Mental Health	10	20	30	40	50	60
Financial Health	10	20	30	40	50	60

What stands out to you?

Were your scores as you expected? In what areas were you higher or lower?

What have you learned about yourself by going through this exercise?

Okay. I'd like you now to take your three cumulative scores, add them up, and create a combined score.

What was your cumulative score?

	Failing	Poor	Surviving	Above Average	Thriving	Optimum
Overall Wellbeing	30	60	90	120	150	180

Your cumulative score emphasizes a couple of very powerful points. First, it's possible to be doing well in some areas of your life but they seem independent and unrelated. I can tell you that they are not. In fact, they are interdependent to such an extent that ignoring one area will almost always have an effect on the others.

That is why the Habits of Health are more than a way to improve your mind and body. Your score gives you a good idea of how you are currently running your life, and wellbeing is a great measure of how you are doing in terms of the quality of your life. If it needs improvement and you want to do something about it, you have come to the right place. If you have been operating mindlessly and have allowed your short-term desires to dictate your daily lifestyle, I can help you choose a different path. Together, we will build a life that matters and allows you to thrive in what is most important to you.

The idea of optimal health is to organize your life around the key areas that we have identified, which empowers you to create wellbeing and makes sure your daily choices support those long-term objectives! In the next Element, we will start building the process that will construct a new pathway to guide you on your journey to optimal health and wellbeing.

And it starts with knowing why. In the next few Elements, we will explore why you want to change, what needs to change, and what we need to tweak in your life!

1 In October 2010 Science magazine(ii) published an important paper that reviewed the notion of the "exposome"— the idea that the environment in which your genes live is more important than your genes themselves. What this suggests is that applying genomics to treat disease is misguided because 70–90% of your disease risk is related to your environment exposures and the resultant alterations in molecules that wash over your genes.

ELEMENT 01:
BEING CLEAR WHY YOU ARE HERE

Average time to complete: **1 week**

In Element 01, we will:

• Identify why you are here.

• Share the importance of intrinsic motivation in your life.

• Explore, in your words, why you are ready to begin now.

WHY ARE YOU HERE?

I am not sure why our paths are crossing at this moment in your life, but I imagine it is because you are ready to make a change.

I'm glad you're here.

I admire your courage in stepping out from the masses and making the crucial decision to improve yourself.

Let me say before we go on that helping people transform their lives is a mission that I care about very deeply. I know that if you are ready to make changes in your life to improve your health and wellbeing then this system can help you.

For many, it may start with losing weight, becoming more active, sleeping better, and reducing stress. These are great starting points in improving health. They are what I describe as the MacroHabits of Health.

We will take one small step at a time to help you achieve what you want.

In conjunction with *Dr. A's Habits of Health* book, in each Element of *Your LifeBook* we will discover, explore, and install a specific Element that will allow you to sustain a lifelong transformation. We'll fill your life with the rocks, the pebbles, the sand and, finally, the water.

Element *def.*
a fundamental and essential
piece of the whole

So, let's get started with the first basic Element: Why are you here?

LET'S UNDERSTAND YOUR "WHY?"

Understanding your "why?" or your motivation for change is a key Element. It's essential to making lasting change in our behavior and habits.

As you read this, you may be feeling pressure from your significant other, your healthcare provider, your boss, or your friends. Or it could just be a voice in your head saying "I should" or "I ought to" make a change.

It's very important to take note of those reasons, but in this Element we are going to start by taking a closer look at what is really important to you rather than any emotional conflict that may have brought you to this point (motivation that's driven by loved ones and interpersonal conversation will not last long. If you want to find out why, take a look at Part 1.3 of *Dr. A's Habits of Health, Are You Really Ready to Change?*).

If we are motivated by those types of emotions and feelings, we are likely to look for quick fixes and to find help from someone else rather than look to ourselves. When we look outside of ourselves, we give away any power we have to make real change in our life. We are going to tap into something much more powerful: the core Element of all real change.

Your "why?" is your intrinsic motivation and your highest stimulus for change. It drives you into action because it's what you want to do. It inspires you to grow and be better. And when you're doing something that inspires, you want to share your desire with others and increase your level of engagement. It creates a "whatever it takes" mindset and becomes a powerful ally in your path to success.

That level of engagement and passion might have eluded you for quite some time; perhaps even since childhood. The default program for adult life is one of distrust, caution, and an inner voice that says "no you can't." Our biology likes to stay the same, and our mind likes to stay the same too.

THE SAME OLD STORY

I would like to close that old book and open this first chapter of your new story by asking you a few questions. I want you to answer them from your heart or your gut. Don't overthink or rationalize whether you think you can or cannot.

Ready? Okay.

Do you really care about getting healthy?

Do you want to improve your life?

I thought so.

It tells me that you do value your health and your life.

Put what you think you can do to one side for the rest of this Element, and explore why you want to change and what is possible. For the moment, let me worry about how we are going to make your transformation a reality. This is a journey that we will be on for the rest of our lives, so we've got plenty of time.

Let me give you some examples of our vision as you step forward into this journey.

We will be exploring what is important to you and how you can create a better life through awakening possibilities. We will then set you into a specific process and do the work. The path I am going to lay out for you in the Elements of *Your LifeBook* will allow you to stay focused on what comes next. Step by simple step, we will lay the foundation for amazing things but only if you are willing to do the work and stay the course.

I am talking about filling your days with vibrancy in your physical health. Achieving a state of calm, joy, spiritual strength, and having great relationships with family and friends. Getting up every morning and loving what we fill our days with. And we'll create security in our resources and hugely supportive surroundings with time to enjoy it all.

These types of transformations can be possible if you are willing to grow and do the work. I will share stories of transformation throughout our time together.

Before we get into the questions, let me say that it's fine if you just want to lose some weight, but filling out your "Why?" in terms of your health and wellbeing is a powerful way of tapping into your deepest aspirations and unlocking your potential for more in your life. It is worth the time it will take. Remember, we are starting to write the next chapter in your story and we want to awaken the inspirational thoughts and things that are important to you, which will give you lasting satisfaction.

" I would define optimal health as a state characterized by anatomic, physiologic, and psychological integrity and optimization which supports optimal wellbeing. It's the ability to perform at a highly effective and satisfying level. You will be able to/are able to fulfill valued family, work, faith, and community roles by developing the ability to deal with physical, biological, psychological, and social stress while maintaining internal equilibrium and external stability. "

Dr. Wayne Scott Andersen

WHY ARE YOU READY?

Please find a quiet time to complete this exercise.

Include a description of why you want to change. Make sure these are things that motivate you to create health and bring what you want into your life. Avoid writing negative reasons for stopping or phrases built around problem solving such as "I hate the way I look", or "I am so unhealthy."

To get you started, here are some common reasons for change given by other people I've worked with who've made the same decision as you.

Check the ones that apply to you:

Quick Fixes: I am done with quick fixes and want to create sustainable changes

My Health is Important: I am ready to put my health and wellbeing first

Decision: I am ready to get off the fence and go for it

More than Weight Loss: I want to create health and wellbeing

In Charge: I am ready to be in charge of my health

Integrated: I want to focus on my overall health for my future and family

Results: I know what to do now, and I want to actually do it

Best Version of Myself: I am ready to become more

Need Blueprint: I need a plan to make it reality

Mind in Charge: I need to build my mindset

I Want More: I want to move from where I am now and become healthier

Now that you are thinking about some concrete reasons for your change, it is important for you to add some of your own words, emphasizing what we are for instead of what we are against. There is power in wording your why around what you want. For example : I want more energy, I want to be more active, I want to feel great, I want to travel, I want to live longer in a healthy state, I want to be here for my grandkids, and so on.

How does it feel to express this in your own words? It doesn't matter if it's a small tangible change for now. Why you are here right now may be as simple as wanting to lose a few pounds. Based on your current story, the ability to accomplish more than that may feel like a dream to you today.

The good news is that is okay. We can work with that. These concrete small "Why's" are a powerful way to get you started. When you see the immediate benefits of making a change, it becomes a strong motivator to start now and do the daily actions. As you start feeling moments of success and move past the small baby steps, you will start to think bigger.

In the next Element, we will define and explore the areas you want to work on in more detail. I just want you to know that a different future is possible, even as you start writing your new story.

So, with that in mind, why don't we have some fun?

Describe, in as much detail as possible, something you would love to do in the future that gets you really excited but which you cannot do in your current reality.

"Dreaming about a healthy future was not something I'd even considered when I started this program. Frankly, at nearly 400 lbs, I started the program with little hope.

I thought perhaps I could lose 25 or maybe 50 lbs in an attempt to avoid a premature death. Fortunately, two weeks was all it took for me to see how effective this program was in improving my health. It was then that I started to dream BIG, as I hope many of you will choose to do!

What did I dream for? Some of them were simple things, like wanting to be able to go to the grocery store without being exhausted when I got home or to go to a theater and be able to comfortably fit in the seat. I looked forward to being able to buy cute clothes at the store and to be able to wear heels without pain. I was excited about the prospects of being able to fly in an airplane without a seat belt extender, to be able to take trips with lots of walking, and to have the energy and stamina to enjoy it. Roller coasters were a big draw for me too, as well as swing dancing with our son at his wedding. I wasn't opposed to being a "trophy wife" for my dear husband— something that would have never occurred to me before! Setting a good example for others who wanted better health inspired me too. I also looked forward to the day when our grandbabies would arrive. I wanted to be the vibrant grammy who could sit on the floor to play with them and have the energy to enjoy going down the slide at the playground with them, instead of watching from a park bench.

What's really wonderful is that all those dreams and many more have come true. I've lost 215 lbs*, and because I've incorporated the Habits of Health into my life and have the ongoing support of my coach, I'm not afraid the weight is ever coming back![1] "

Shirley Mast

*Average weight loss on the Optimal Weight 5&1 Plan® is 12lbs. Average fat loss is 10lbs.

We have now explored and documented the first Element: Knowing your Why and why it is important to you. We'll come back to this many times as a fuel source and we will expand on it as you experience success.

In Review:

Your "Why?" is your intrinsic motivation and your highest stimulus for change. It drives you into action because it's what you want to do. It inspires you to grow and get better. When awakened, you will want to share your desire with others, increase your engagement, and create a "whatever it takes" mindset. It's a powerful ally in your success.

At this point, write your "Why?" on a note card or sticky note. Put it on the mirror in your bathroom, carry a copy with you in your bag, or put it on your screensaver on your phone, computer, or Habits of Health App.

Here is an example of a client's note card:

My Why:
I am changing and focused on improving
my health and wellbeing because:

- I want to like the way I look in the mirror

- I would like to feel healthier

- I want my husband to be proud of how I look

- I would like to have more energy and stamina

- I want to be a great example of health for my grandkids

- I want to travel on a Safari in Africa

My Why: I am changing and focused on improving my health and wellbeing because I

I want to congratulate you for being open to doing the exercises. Hopefully, your juices are flowing. Once you have awakened to the possibilities and have a desire to create a better future for yourself and those around you, you will have an energy source to build the necessary habits to ensure you flourish in this fast-paced world.

I know now that you want to be healthy and thrive in your life.

I also know that you might have come to this book because you may have had limited success in the past. Your current conditions may not be ideal, and you have some life challenges. Let me ease your apprehension: we have you covered.

The Habits of Health Transformational System is a dependable blueprint that allows you to build a series of small changes and habits. If you follow the process, are patient and consistent you have a great shot of being successful. Your current conditions are no match for your powerful transformation.

Knowing your "Why?" was the first step in your self-discovery process.

In Element 02, *Knowing What You Want To Accomplish*, we will explore what you are going to work on and in Element 03, *How Do You Create What You Want?*, we'll look at how it all works.

These Elements will clarify how all of this will sink in and help you to make permanent changes.

Notes to yourself:

Note: We will end each Element with three questions that will set the stage for you to reflect on what you have learned. I highly recommend that you write down everything you are experiencing in this section and share it with your coach or mentor. Also review these notes often during your journey to increase your learning and reflect on your better understanding and your growth as you become a higher version of yourself.

Please write down your thoughts guided by the following questions:
What does this Element mean to you right now?

What does this Element give you the opportunity to reflect on?

What actions are you going to take as a result of this Element?

1 Average weight loss on the Optimal Weight 5&1 Plan® is 12 lbs. Average fat loss is 10 lbs.

ELEMENT 02:
KNOWING WHAT YOU WANT TO ACCOMPLISH

Average time to complete: **1 week**

In Element 02, we will:

• Identify what you want.

• Develop a strategy to help you start creating your desired change.

• Explore how ready, confident, and willing you are to engage
  in each of the six MacroHabits of Health.

In Element 01, *Being Clear Why You Are Here,* we explored why you want to make a change.

The idea was to awaken you to what is really important to you. Once you're awakened and focused on your personal desire and the reasons that will drive your change, you are ready for the second Element.

WHAT DO YOU WANT?

Although I am not sure what is most important to you personally, I'm a fellow human being, so I can guess. You probably thought about better health, great relationships with family and friends, being part of your community, having stress-free joyful days, and feeling like you have the resources and time for your spiritual and recreational fulfillment.

Our goal is to help you create immense success and satisfaction in your personal and professional life.

And yet, the things that will enhance our health and our lives seem difficult to obtain in this chaotic world. Our days move along at a frenzied pace, and there never seems to be enough time or energy. Our to-do list never ends. We barely have time to sleep, let alone proper time to work on our health and wellbeing.

It's probably true that we spend more time planning our vacations than we do planning our day-to-day lives. In the meantime, our health and our life are getting away from us.

Letting another week, month, or year slip by without making the decision to intervene and take control of your life is too easy.

In this Element, we are going to begin executing a strategy and start the process that will help you make the desired changes to create the life you choose to live.

There are many different ways you can live your life. You are reading this book because you have discovered that your current way is not delivering the results that you want for your future.

I also know that the intervention you are making may be occurring at an inconvenient time. The truth is there is never a good time to change your familiar routines and habits, but if they're currently leading you to poorer health and wellbeing, there will never be a better time than right now!

Let me take a moment and provide some insight—based on my perspective as a physician—into the *inconvenience* of disease.

If your daily choices are robbing you of energy and vibrancy and you are gaining weight and becoming less fit, it will not get any better unless you take time for yourself right now. The inconvenience of being tied to six or more medicines and having to take them multiple times a day will be a constant reminder that your health is on the decline. Remembering when to take them, and coping with their debilitating side effects will drain both your time and resources.

TV commercials are selling sickness in a way that is almost irresponsible, as their adverts glorify the importance of medicines by showing people using pharmaceuticals and thriving in their lives. Let me tell you there is very little radiant health or wellbeing that comes from the long-term use of medications. If you picture a future full of the inconvenience of multiple healthcare providers appointments, constant pain and suffering, and the time you will need to allocate to dealing with sickness and disease later in life, I hope you can see how this is the perfect time to take control of your health and life.

In an upcoming Element, we will contrast your present and future self and how different your story will be as a result of making this decision and creating a new life. *Your LifeBook* is going to be central to guide and record your new story that starts by exploring strategies, tools, and areas that will be integral in your journey.

Hopefully, you'll see that the work we did in Element 01, *Being Clear Why You Are Here*, will serve you well as we identify what we are going to work on.

Let's start with a review of how ready you are to begin this journey. As you gather your thoughts, let me clarify a few things.

First, I am not going to ask if you think you can create optimal health and wellbeing. You can't possibly know the answer to that question because you have not done it. That is my job.

I know you can create optimal health because the system we're going to use, and which I established, creates predictable transformation. As you write your new story, you will be learning, growing and getting better. I will deliver you a realistic plan, complete with strategies, tools, skill development, support, and other cool ways to proceed at a pace that works for you.

What we are doing right now is making sure you are ready.

On a scale from 1–10, where are you right now with your desire to improve your health and wellbeing?

This is a readiness ruler—a tool to help you evaluate where you are right now and how much "juice" your "Why?" has to put you into action.

Readiness Ruler

0	1	2	3	4	5	6	7	8	9	10

I am **not** ready to change
I am **almost** ready to change
I am **very** ready to change

What is your score?

If your score is less than seven, then your current level of motivation is probably not high enough to support the focus and energy needed to make a meaningful change to your health and wellbeing. I would suggest you go back to the first Element, read the early sections in Dr. A's Habits of Health, or consider asking for help from a coach or mentor.

For those who have scored more than seven, congratulations.

You are ready to start your journey.

It's time to design your personal strategic approach and begin the real work of developing your new story. Our goal, step by step, is to help you create lifelong transformation that will provide immense satisfaction in both your personal and professional life. It's a system designed to create long-term change. Let me take a moment to frame what I mean by this.

When we talk about what we want, it is usually tied to a pleasure principle rather than lasting satisfaction. We confuse the things that bring us immediate pleasure with the things that lead to lasting fulfillment. Most of the things that create pleasure are only present while we are doing them.

When we eat, we feel pleasure, and when we stop the pleasure does too.

As an example, when you are eating ice cream out of a carton, it is really hard to stop. It has been said that 75% of the time we're eating we're not hungry—the only reason we continue is so the pleasure doesn't stop. We'll address how you can take control of mindless eating later.

Satisfaction—rather than pleasure—occurs when you create, do, or bring things into your life that have a lasting effect or value. Today, you may come home from work tired and stressed, and want to sit on the couch, watch the TV, and eat something salty or sweet.

Instead, you put on your running shoes and go out for a walk and get some exercise with your partner, your dog, or both. When you are done, you will be glad you did it and that sense of satisfaction will last beyond the action. The things that bring you satisfaction will last beyond the effort needed to complete them.

Contrast this with something we want more and more of and yet brings us less and less satisfaction—an addiction. My role is to anchor you in things that will give you an enduring sense of satisfaction and make it easier for you to adapt to a constantly changing world.

In the Introduction, we talked about the big rocks: the ones that are essential for optimal health and wellbeing. These MacroHabits are the foundational stones that we want to put into your very own mason jar to give you the highest chance of transformation in your health and life.

The Habits of Health are the things we will bring into our lives that will live on and their benefits will far outweigh the work and time it takes to learn and install them.

What we need to do is to review what habits are represented by those big rocks and examine each one in more detail. You are in charge of your transformation, and it's important for you to decide what you are the most excited about working on. We have included the readiness ruler for each major category to help you decide which area you are most interested in changing.

Since almost two thirds of us are overweight or obese, the MacroHabit of Healthy Weight Management will be where most of us will start, and that is generally where most people are ready to make a change.[1]

You may not be at the same stage of readiness in other Macrohabits or realize how your choices in these other areas are contributing to weight gain and your overall health and wellbeing. The purpose of this exercise is to explore your readiness and how you assess your current ability to change in the areas that will determine your future health.

In each of the MacroHabits sections, you need to write down the three things you would like to change.

Check which areas you want to work on now, and then circle how ready you are to change (it's a simple scale, from a state of "not at all ready" to "very ready indeed").

Then write down at least three things you want to change in that category.

MACROHABITS OF HEALTH

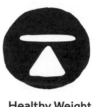

Healthy Weight Management

Healthy Eating & Hydration

Healthy Motion

Healthy Sleep

Healthy Mind

Healthy Surroundings

Healthy Weight Management

Most of my clients, patients, and readers start their journey here, so you are not alone in making this an area of focus.

Around 70% of people struggle to reach and maintain a healthy weight.[2] Apart from stopping smoking, there is no more important area to address than learning how to reach and maintain a healthy weight. We will give you some great ways to make it simple so you can create early successes. As you lose weight, your confidence and motivation will increase and set the path for many other microHabits.

As you feel better, have more energy, and are losing weight safely, you will be motivated to discover more ways you can improve your health. As you reach a healthy weight, we will continue to add more new habits that will help you maintain your ideal weight. It's an eating plan specifically designed to move you through a fat-burning stage to a recalibration stage and then to an optimizing stage in which your metabolism is working at its most efficient.

Answer the following questions to work out how important this is to you and how confident and ready you are to address the issue and place this rock in your mason jar.

How *important* is it to make a change in your weight right now?

Willingness Ruler

0   1   2   3   4   5   6   7   8   9   10

I am *not* ready
to change

I am *almost* ready
to change

I am *very* ready
to change

What led you to pick this number?

1.

2.

3.

If possible, what would help you pick a higher number?

1.

2.

3.

How *confident* are you that you can reach a healthy weight right now?

Confidence Ruler

0   1   2   3   4   5   6   7   8   9   10

I do *not* think I
will reach my goal

I have a *50%* chance of
reaching my goal

I will *definitely*
achieve my goal

What led you to pick this number?

1. . . . .

2. . . . .

3. . . . .

If possible, what would help you pick a higher number?

1. . . . .

2. . . . .

3. . . . .

How *ready* are you to make a change in your weight management
right now?

Readiness Ruler

0   1   2   3   4   5   6   7   8   9   10

I am *not* ready
to change

I am *almost* ready
to change

I am *very* ready
to change

What led you to pick this number?

1.

2.

3.

If possible, what would help you pick a higher number?

1.

2.

3.

Eating Healthier and Better Hydration

The new habits that you started installing while reaching a healthy weight will continue to encompass a number of healthy eating and hydration behaviors. I will talk about portion control, meal frequency, and eating a balanced diet. Together, we will continue to improve your fuel sources so your body is receiving the right vita-nutrients. I will help you discover the foods that add flavor and texture (and that you will actually like), which will support optimal health for the rest of your life. I will also address the importance of water and proper hydration and help you optimize the efficiency of your body, even if you are struggling to drink enough water at the moment.

How *important* is it to make a change in your eating habits and hydration now?

Willingness Ruler

| 0 | 1 | 2 | 3 | 4 | 5 | 6 | 7 | 8 | 9 | 10 |

Not important
at all

About as important as
everything else

Most important
thing in my life

How *confident* are you that you can make a change in your eating habits and hydration now?

Confidence Ruler

| 0 | 1 | 2 | 3 | 4 | 5 | 6 | 7 | 8 | 9 | 10 |

I do *not* think I will
reach my goal

I have a *50%* chance of
reaching my goal

I will *definitely*
achieve my goal

How *ready* are you to make a change in your eating habits and hydration now?

Readiness Ruler

| 0 | 1 | 2 | 3 | 4 | 5 | 6 | 7 | 8 | 9 | 10 |

I am *not* ready
to change

I am *almost* ready
to change

I am *very* ready
to change

Write three things that you can start doing that will help you install the Habits of Healthy Eating and Hydration right now.

1.

2.

3.

Write three things that you can stop doing to help you eat healthier and hydrate better right now.

1. · · · · · · · · · · · · · · · · · ·

2. · · · · · · · · · · · · · · · · · ·

3. · · · · · · · · · · · · · · · · · ·

Moving More

I'll ease you into the right amount of physical activity at the right moment in your development. While your movement plan may include formal exercise, it's more often made up of fun activities and clever strategies that make moving your body easy and fun—including some you've probably never even considered. We pioneered a way to increase your ability to create activity throughout the day with our NEAT leisure and work and emphasized its importance. NEAT or Non Exercise Activities Thermogenesis represents all the ways, outside of exercise, that we move during our waking hours. By focusing on moving constantly we can increase our calorie expenditure but also off set the negative affects of sitting all day. We will spend lots of time helping you become a perpetual motion machine to offset our sedentary modern lifestyle. Recent studies support the need for daylong movement to counter the disease producing effects of a progressively sedentary society.[3] Even among those that exercise for more than 7 hours a week, people who spent the most time sitting had a 50% greater risk of death from any cause.[4] Put simply, all-day motion is a necessity.

How *important* is it to make a change in your activity level now?

Willingness Ruler

0   1   2   3   4   5   6   7   8   9   10

Not important
at all

About as important as
everything else

Most important
thing in my life

How *confident* are you that you can change your activity level now?

Confidence Ruler

| 0 | 1 | 2 | 3 | 4 | 5 | 6 | 7 | 8 | 9 | 10 |

I do *not* think I
will reach my goal

I have a *50%* chance of
reaching my goal

I will *definitely*
achieve my goal

How *ready* are you to change your activity level now?

Readiness Ruler

| 0 | 1 | 2 | 3 | 4 | 5 | 6 | 7 | 8 | 9 | 10 |

I am *not* ready
to change

I am *almost* ready
to change

I am *very* ready
to change

Write three things that you can start doing to help you install the Habits of Healthy Motion right now.

1.

2.

3.

Write three things that you can stop doing to help you move more right now.

1.

2.

3.

Sleeping Better

The effect of regular sleep patterns on health is often underestimated, but sleep is one of the most critical factors in creating overall health and wellbeing. It also has a direct impact on losing weight and keeping it off. Skipping that necessary extra hour of sleep decreases your wellbeing, productivity, health, and your ability to think.

How *important* is it to make a change in your sleep habits now?

Willingness Ruler

0	1	2	3	4	5	6	7	8	9	10

Not important
at all

About as important as
everything else

Most important
thing in my life

How *confident* are you that you can change your sleep habits now?

Confidence Ruler

0	1	2	3	4	5	6	7	8	9	10

I do *not* think I
will reach my goal

I have a *50%* chance of
reaching my goal

I will *definitely*
achieve my goal

How *ready* are you to make a change in your sleep habits right now?

Readiness Ruler

0	1	2	3	4	5	6	7	8	9	10

I am *not* ready
to change

I am *almost* ready
to change

I am *very* ready
to change

Write three things that you can start doing to help you sleep better right now.

1. . . . .

2. . . . .

3. . . . .

Write three things that you can stop doing to help you sleep better right now.

1. . . . .

2. . . . .

3. . . . .

A Healthier Mind

Your long-term success depends on choosing the best strategic actions to support your health. These include taking time to examine how you make choices, understanding your patterns and triggers, and helping you maintain a sense of calm and resilience regardless of what life throws at you. With greater self-awareness, we will increase your capacity to thrive in a rapidly changing world. I will also encourage you to adopt new behaviors by helping you master the art of habit installation so that you will no longer have to rely on willpower to carry on with positive actions and, more importantly, avoid unhealthy behaviors. I will help you create real focus so that you can put your mind where you want, anytime you want, in any situation. We will build self-efficacy by creating generative motivation, supporting what is most important to you, and working within your current ability to change and improve key life skills.

How *important* is it to make a change in your thoughts, feelings, and actions now?

Willingness Ruler

| 0 | 1 | 2 | 3 | 4 | 5 | 6 | 7 | 8 | 9 | 10 |

Not important
at all

About as important as
everything else

Most important
thing in my life

How *confident* are you that you can make a change in your thoughts, feelings, and actions right now?

Confidence Ruler

| 0 | 1 | 2 | 3 | 4 | 5 | 6 | 7 | 8 | 9 | 10 |

I do *not* think I
will reach my goal

I have a *50%* chance of
reaching my goal

I will *definitely*
achieve my goal

How *ready* are you to make a change in your thoughts, feelings, and actions right now?

Readiness Ruler

| 0 | 1 | 2 | 3 | 4 | 5 | 6 | 7 | 8 | 9 | 10 |

I am *not* ready
to change

I am *almost* ready
to change

I am *very* ready
to change

Write three things that you can start doing to help you have healthier thoughts, feelings, and actions right now.

1.

2.

3.

Write three things that you can stop doing to help you have healthier thoughts, feelings, and actions right now.

1.

2.

3.

Better Surroundings

The *people*, *places*, and *things* you surround yourself with can enhance or diminish the success of your other Habits of Health. I'll show you how to build a "health bubble" that will help you take control of your personal environment and create conditions that support long-term health. This will be particularly important in helping you establish support systems. As with any good strategy, the first steps make the next steps easier to do. I'll help you build the support system that works best for you, whether that's me, a friend, a group of friends, a coach, or a whole network of people. This will help you build lasting relationships and a stronger sense of connection.

How *important* is it to make a change in your surroundings now?

Willingness Ruler

0	1	2	3	4	5	6	7	8	9	10

Not important at all   **About as important as everything else**   **Most** important thing in my life

How *confident* are you that you can make a change in your surroundings right now?

Confidence Ruler

0	1	2	3	4	5	6	7	8	9	10

I do **not** think I will reach my goal   I have a **50%** chance of reaching my goal   I will **definitely** achieve my goal

How *ready* are you to make a change in your surroundings right now?

Readiness Ruler

0   1   2   3   4   5   6   7   8   9   10

I am *not* ready   I am *almost* ready   I am *very* ready
to change   to change   to change

Write three things that you can start doing to help you have healthier surroundings right now.

1.

2.

3.

Write three things that you can stop doing to help you have healthier surroundings right now.

1.

2.

3.

Other Areas

Any other important areas that we have not addressed in the above questions should be written down as we begin your new journey. They may be factors that will alter your focus, decision-making, and time, and we will need to build a pre-emptive plan so these new factors do not derail you. It's important that you realize obstacles in our lives can be turned into areas of growth, and we will look at them to help you adjust on your journey.

Our goal will not be to solve but to create the desired outcome you want to bring into being.

Take a moment to list any concerns and issues we have not addressed in these six MacroHabits.

How *important* is it you make a change in this area right now?

Willingness Ruler

0	1	2	3	4	5	6	7	8	9	10

Not important at all   About as important as *everything else*   *Most* important thing in my life

How *confident* are you can make a change in this area right now?

Confidence Ruler

0	1	2	3	4	5	6	7	8	9	10

I do *not* think I will reach my goal   I have a *50%* chance of reaching my goal   I will *definitely* achieve my goal

How *ready* are you to make a change in this area right now?

Readiness Ruler

0   1   2   3   4   5   6   7   8   9   10

I am *not* ready   I am *almost* ready   I am *very* ready
to change   to change   to change

Write three things that you can start doing to help you create the desired outcome right now.

1.

2.

3.

Write three things that you can stop doing to help you have the desired outcome right now.

1.

2.

3.

We have now outlined the six major components of MacroHabits that we'll address in the days, weeks, and months to come. We have also addressed other concerns or areas that are important to you as you write your new story.

We have now explored and documented Element 02, *Knowing What You Want To Accomplish.*

Let's take a moment to review

We have touched on the key Elements that we will focus on during your journey to optimal health and wellbeing. These are the largest rocks in your mason jar.

It may seem like a lot, but the great news is we are going to proceed at a pace that makes sense, supports your ambition, and will actually help you gain momentum.

It's worth remembering, as you set out on what seems like a massive task, that the best way to eat an elephant is one bite at time (and although we want to decrease your consumption of red meat, this is the perfect metaphor for your journey).

We reviewed these key areas because we need to use an integrated approach to your health and wellbeing. So, if you want to create lifelong transformation, we needed to do a complete 360 on the big rocks in the mason jar.

At this point, we're picking the low-hanging fruit. Now that you have defined what you think is most important, you think you can do it, and you are ready to change that area, we have everything working for us.

Looking back on your recent answers, write down the three areas that are most important for you to change right now (the three highest ruler scores).

1.

2.

3.

Write down the three areas that you are the most confident you can change right now (the three highest ruler scores).

1.

2.

3.

Write down the three areas that you are the most ready to change right now (the three highest ruler scores).

1.

2.

3.

The most important area I want to work on is:

The area I'm most confident I can change is:

The area I'm most ready to change is:

As we finish up this second Element of your new story, I hope you can see that we have uncovered some very powerful information. Once you know why you want to change and what you want to change, you already have the building blocks of proper motivation and a clear sense of what is really is important to you.

Make sure you review all your notes and this Element often.

Also, share it with your coach and spend time discussing how these possibilities will become a reality.

We will install habit formation for the things that you desire to change now. It's helpful if you have a high-degree of confidence that you can change. When it comes to the things you are less confident about but are ready to tackle, we'll break them down into smaller steps so they also will become yours to master.

In the next Element, we will show you how to make these new habits a reality.

Notes to yourself:

Now that you have completed Element 02, *Knowing What You Want To Accomplish*, write down your thoughts guided by the following questions:
What does this Element mean to you right now?

What does this Element give you the opportunity to reflect on?

What actions are you going to take as a result of this Element?

I encourage you to connect with your coach, so you can share your thoughts and actions as soon as possible. Sharing your thoughts with your coach will help them become a reality. Make sure you review all your notes and this Element often.

1 According to data from the National Health and Nutrition Examination Survey (NHANES), 2013–2014 2, 3, 4, 5 more than 2/3 of us are overweight or obese.

2 *Americans Struggle with Long-Term Weight Loss* – Penn State, Science Daily, 5 September 2010, www.sciencedaily.com/releases/2010/09/100903104830.htm more than 2/3 of us are overweight or obese.

3 *Too Much Sitting : A Novel and Important Predictor of Chronic Disease Risk* – British Journal of Sports Medicine 43(2) 81–83.

4 *Is Sitting a Lethal Activity?* newyorktimes.com /2011/04/17/magazine/mag-17sitting-t.html.

ELEMENT 03:
HOW DO YOU CREATE WHAT YOU WANT?

Average time to complete: **1–2 weeks**

In Element 03, we will:

- Discuss the strategies, tools, and methods we are going equip you with to create optimal health and wellbeing.
- Explore the steps you can take to create what you want.
- Discover the tools that will help you move forward, creating sustainable and long-term change.
- Empower you to evaluate your progress and adjust as necessary along the way.

"We first make our habits,
then our habits make us."

John Dryden

In Element 01, *Being Clear Why You Are Here*, we explored why you want to make a change.

In Element 02, *Knowing What You Want To Accomplish*, we figured out what you want to create in terms of your health and wellbeing. We started to outline what is most important to you and where you want to start this journey.

The goal in the first two Elements was to awaken what is really important to you and explore the areas you are willing and able to work on right now.

This is the point where we move from the discovery phase to the creative and work phase. It's where the rubber meets the road. We'll discuss the strategies, tools, and methods we are going to equip you with to create optimal health and wellbeing. This is where we start making your new story a reality.

HOW DO YOU CREATE WHAT YOU WANT?

At the core of this Element is giving you the means of building new healthy habits to support your new behaviors and to then create the desired outcomes you want for your health and for your life. In *Dr. A's Habits of Health* Part 1.5, *The Bedrock of Transformation: Successful Habit Installation,* there is plenty of information covering the details and science of habit formation. It is essential to remember that the most important Element in actually creating the sustainable transformation of your weight, health, and wellbeing is the development of your own ability to take ownership of your choices.

This capability comes from your mastering the ability to create a series of small sustainable changes in your daily choices that will—over time— create long-term change. These are the small daily habits that are going to be the backbone of your new story as we build your new behaviors.

The Habits of Health Transformational System is set up to organize your new habit installation in a way that is easy. It will deliver a process that will provide a reliable, consistent way to transform your current and past behaviors to new sustainable habits that will serve you for the rest of your life.

This process allows you to organize your goals in a way that will help you focus on your primary habits. Through its four steps you will build in the pieces that make it easy to get it right the first time.

Step One: Use structural tension to organize your MacroHabits
Step Two: Set up a habit loop for a specific Habit of Health
Step Three: Identify the microHabits to install
Step Four: Connect present action to immediate and long-term rewards

It starts by addressing the MacroHabit (MHoH) category. I have found that it is easier to work on one MacroHabit category at a time. That way you can focus your energy and time making sure you consistently and effectively install a habit before you go on to another category. You may add microHabits from another category. This is good because they all affect each other to help you reach the big goal of long-term health and wellbeing. Once you have decided which MacroHabit category will be your starting point (for most it will be Healthy Weight Management), then you will pick the specific habits that you are going to work on.

STEP ONE:
USE STRUCTURAL TENSION TO ORGANIZE
YOUR MACROHABITS

Step one begins by picking which primary choice you are focusing on and what secondary choices support the transformation in that category (these are the pebbles that are derived from each MacroHabit). Each of the six MacroHabit categories has a series of primary choices that are essential for mastering that area of transformation. The secondary choices are the Habits of Health actions that support you to reach the desired outcome. See Part 1.3 and 1.4 in *Dr. A's Habits of Health* for a much more detailed explanation of structural dynamics and primary/secondary choices.

We're going to start by building your first structural tension chart to help organize both your desired outcome and the secondary action steps that structure the Habit of Health installation.

For most of us, our struggle is with our weight, so I will use the category of **Healthy Weight Management** as an example.

You can use the same content from the example to get you going or you can start customizing it immediately. Remember, it's *Your LifeBook* and you are starting to write the next chapter in your health and life. This is your opportunity to document the first year of your new healthy life. Having made a decision to change everything, it provides a chance to chronicle this amazing time in your life.

In this example, we are setting up my desired outcome in the weight management MacroHabit category. My desired healthy weight is 175 lbs and a waist circumference (at belly button level) of 33 inches.

Structural Tension

CURRENT REALITY	SECONDARY CHOICES	DESIRED RESULT
Overweight 195 lbs Muffin Top 35 inches	Portion control 6 meals / day Eating breakfast everyday Low-glycemic carbs only Lean and Green / 1 daily 8 glasses of water / daily	Healthy Weight 175 lbs Waist 33 inches

My current reality is that I weigh 195 lbs and have a waist circumference of 35 inches. The secondary choices I have listed are some individual habits that I can develop to reach my primary goal of a healthy weight. Once they are installed, it will be much easier to maintain my healthy weight. I know that once I have decided that reaching a healthy weight is important on my journey to optimal health, I will have contrasted how I feel at my current reality and why I want to be at a healthy weight.

When I visualize my desired weight goal and how I feel now in relationship to how I will feel when I reach my healthy weight, it creates a powerful tension that needs to be resolved. It also awakens a desire to install the secondary choices that will allow the generative improvement in my health and weight.

Now it is your turn to build your first structural tension chart. If you are going to work on your weight management, then feel free to follow my basic example and fill in your desired and current weight and waist circumference next to mine. If you want to start from scratch, I have provided a blank structural tension chart for you to use.

Structural tension is a very powerful force in helping you create better health and wellbeing. It's a process you will use in each category as you establish what you are going to be working on.

Structural Tension

CURRENT REALITY	SECONDARY CHOICES	DESIRED RESULT

I suggest you read Part 1.3 and 1.4 in the Habits of Health to increase your understanding of structural dynamics—we'll be using these principles and ST charts as key tools of the creative process on your journey to optimal health and wellbeing.

Now that you have created your structural tension, we'll move on to Step Two—which is setting up your habit loop for your secondary choices.

STEP TWO:
SET UP A HABIT LOOP FOR A SPECIFIC HABIT OF HEALTH

Habit loops are described in much more detail in *Dr. A's Habits of Health* but, for now, it's most important to know that they activate an important area in your brain that helps when learning your new healthy habits. They work beautifully as a means of installing the secondary choices you have decided will help you reach your desired outcomes.

What I'd like you to do now is to review the visual of each of the three pieces of a habit loop. First, there is the **cue**—the stimulus that activates the new habit. It can be any kind of reminder that will signal the brain to begin an action or habit. We can create a new **cue** or anchor it to an already functioning behavior.

We then outline the action, secondary choice, or ***routine*** we want to install.

And the third part of the habit loop is to provide an immediate ***reward*** or benefit to reinforce the installation of the behavior.

The Habit Loop

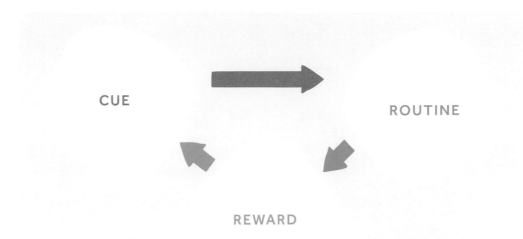

CUE

ROUTINE

REWARD

If we look at the example l used in my structural tension chart (to reach a healthy weight), one of the secondary choices I listed was eating six times a day. If I want to make sure I start installing that new habit, I need to eat every three hours. So I will create a habit loop labeled "fueling" every three hours.

That starts with picking a *cue* to initiate the new habit I want to create. I will set my phone to remind me every three hours as my *cue*, and the Habits of Health App will do this automatically for me. The point is that I need this *cue* as a stimulus to start my routine. The *routine* is to eat a small portion-controlled meal or fueling. It is important I have the ability (and the means) to do this when the *cue* comes. This is easily accomplished by either having a prepackaged fueling or having a healthy meal pre-prepared—we will discuss this in the coming Elements. The *reward* is immediate taste satisfaction, the feeling of fullness, and noting how great I feel in the hours that follow because I ate something healthy.

The Habit Loop—Fueling Every Three Hours

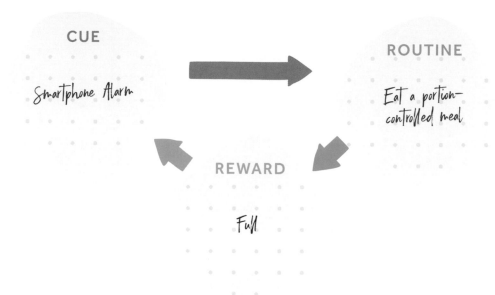

Now it is your turn.

Pick one of the actions from your secondary choice list, and set up a habit loop. You can pick a new **cue** to activate your **routine**, or a new habit, you can connect it to something you are already doing. Actually, I find that most of my new habits are connected to an existing healthy habit. For example, I put a dish of dental sticks or a roll of dental floss next to my toothbrush to remind me to floss once I have brushed my teeth.

It's important to remember to create a closely linked benefit or **reward** to enjoy once you complete your new habit. It can be as simple as just saying "Good job!" to yourself as you complete your new **routine.** I accept it may sound silly, but installing these new habits over time will give you almost unlimited power to improve your life.

My Habit Loop

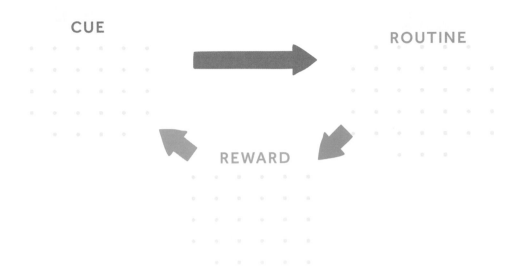

You now have two very important skills, and a process to install all of your Habits of Health. You have the ability to organize your daily choices specifically around what is going to create the new healthy habits, and you have the basic habit loop with which to install the actual new habits. These powerful tools will allow you transform your overall health and wellbeing.

Remember that even with a system **consistency** is key.

We need to make sure that you can repeat your **routine** every single day so the new behavior will become automated.

We do that by making sure nothing gets in the way of you being able to practice your new **routines** and to make them easy enough so that you can do them every day.

This leads us to a powerful tool in our arsenal:
our **microHabits of Health (mHoH)**.

STEP THREE:
IDENTIFY THE MICROHABITS TO INSTALL

Sometimes the habits you are working on will be easy enough, so that you will only need steps one and two to organize and build a new habit.

Other times we will have to do some more preparatory work to make sure we effectively install the new habit. In Part 1.5 of *Dr. A's Habits of Health, The Bedrock of Transformation: Successful Habit Installation,* I explain in detail how critical it is to make sure you automate these new behaviors.

There are three questions you need to ask as you prepare to install a new habit:
1. Is it appealing? Do I want to do it?
2. Is it achievable? Can I actually do it?
3. Is it easily activated? Is there a prompt that reminds me to do it?

Is it so appealing that I can do it every day because this **routine** brings me such joy I look forward to it? If that is the case then great—just do it. But if it is something that will take effort or it is not something you love to do then we need to proceed to the second question.

In order for it to be achievable, you have to be able to do it every day. That means that even on the days when your motivation and willpower are low you can still do it and on the days when you are overwhelmed you can still do it. It also means knowing you have the time and the ability to do this activity.

This is the vital role of *microHabits.* They allow you to install behaviors that will automatically sustain your health in an effective way.

A *microHabit of Health (mHoH)* is, by definition, easy to do and always within your ability in terms of ease or effort. They take into account other limiting factors such as time constraints.

I know that today life can be extremely complex. *MicroHabits* will help ensure that even when life gets in the way you will always be able to carry out the habit.

Imagine that your secondary Habits of Health have been made so small in terms of effort that you can do them even on your worst days. When your willpower, discipline, and motivation are almost zero, you will be unstoppable. And on the days when your motivation is higher, you can do more. The base level of effort is so easy and simple that the daily repetition necessary for installation is never in question.

You can always do it.

It is this consistency and predictability that creates the new behavior. By definition, a *microHabit* is a small doable behavior that can always be completed.

And on the days when you do more than is required we call that *mHoH Plus,* which is defined as the ability to add more reps on the days when your motivation or conditions are favorable. The vital role of daily consistency is visually represented by the daily checks on the calendar that create a chain or streak.

As we discussed in *Dr. A's Habits of Health*, it takes an average of 66 days to install a new habit. It could be as low as 18 days for easy habits or several months for more complex new behaviors.

The way you'll know that it has been installed is it will start getting a whole lot easier.

mHoH Routine

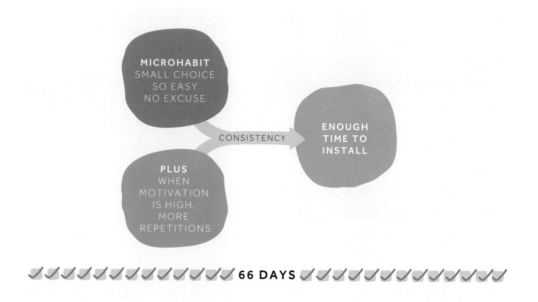

✓✓✓✓✓✓✓✓✓✓✓ **66 DAYS** ✓✓✓✓✓✓✓✓✓✓✓

What follows is an example of a small microHabit I was working on to overcome a long-term tendency:

I would often describe the environment I trained in as a critical care physician as a war zone. It was in the era of Miami's cocaine cowboys. We seldom had more than a few minutes to eat between taking care of patients who were in critical condition and had a good chance of dying if they didn't receive nonstop attention. I developed a very poor habit of wolfing my food down. I fed as voraciously as my Labrador retrievers.

Unfortunately, it became an ingrained habit. The effect on my health was significant (and obvious). I decided to use my mHoH system to retrain my habit.

I committed to the microHabit of chewing my food at least five times before swallowing. Today, on days when I am more aware and not in a rush, I actually chew as much as 15 times. Initially, it took two months to retrain, but my pace of eating has slowed down and I enjoy my food more. As a result, I very seldom eat more than I have put on my plate.

This is now a microHabit in my MacroHabit of Weight Management category!

My mHoH Routine—Increasing awareness of time to slow down during fueling

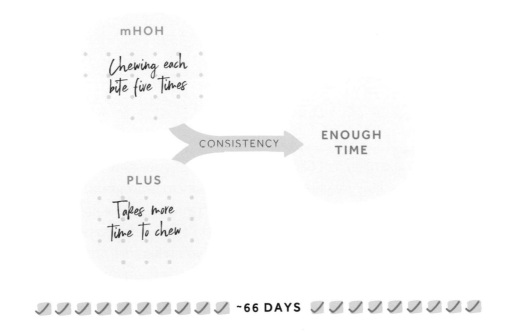

Now that I've shared my own challenge and the way I resolved it, it's your turn to pick a microHabit from the structural tension chart (the one above) or one of your secondary choices.

Make sure you spend the time to make it small enough so that you are positive you can do every day.

The great news is you can start this new habit immediately.

Your mHoH Routine

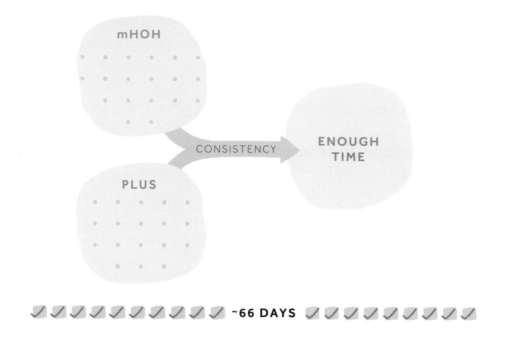

Now you have the means of decreasing the size of your new habits you can be sure of its daily installation. That's the key to reprogramming the brain and mind to automate a new behavior. If you do miss a day, make sure you make it your number one priority the next day. If you miss two days, it becomes critical not to miss a third. If you do, you will most probably need to go back and start all over again. Why? Because the brain disregards patterns that are not consistent.

Note: Use my Habits of Health App to make sure you never break a streak!

There are a couple more powerful ways you can make your habit installations easier and more successful. Let's explore them next.

For those who are thinking, "How can one push-up or sit-up or writing twenty-five words in *Your LifeBook* make a difference?" Let me give you an example. I was working with a grandmother who had lost considerable weight and who was starting to increase her activity in the Habits of Healthy Motion. I asked her what she wanted to work on, and she said that she would like to have more strength in her upper body so she could carry her grandchild in her arms.

She said she wanted to start doing push-ups. She suggested doing five a day to start. I asked her how many she was capable of doing currently. She actually had difficulty in doing one. We modified her technique, and she could do five against the wall standing straight up. We ended up settling on her doing one a day against the wall. Over the first month, she never missed a day. By the third month, she was able to do a traditional push-up and switched to this being her mHoH. In the last month, she averaged five a day and, more importantly, sent me a picture of her holding her grandson. All things are possible if we are willing to use the process of microHabit installation.

STEP FOUR:
CONNECT PRESENT ACTION TO IMMEDIATE AND LONG-TERM REWARDS

As you are writing in *Your LifeBook* and you are beginning your journey, it is very helpful to envision your optimal healthy future.

As you stand in the future and envision how your health and wellbeing will be improved, it provides valuable guidance to help inform your daily activities. In Part 1.6 of *Dr. A's Habits of Health, You in Charge of Yourself: Setting Up for Success*, we discuss our inability as individuals to consistently connect our present actions to our future health benefits. In fact, the next illustration shows that when it comes to our choices we are more likely to make decisions based on what we want right now than for any long-term benefit.

How many times have you gone to bed and said you are going to get up in the morning and exercise and yet when morning comes you are once again hitting the snooze alarm and saying I will start tomorrow? Or how often have you spent time on vacation saying how you are going to eat healthier when you get home and yet the next day you find yourself at the local doughnut shop getting a jelly doughnut and coffee?

Building Your Future Health and Wellbeing

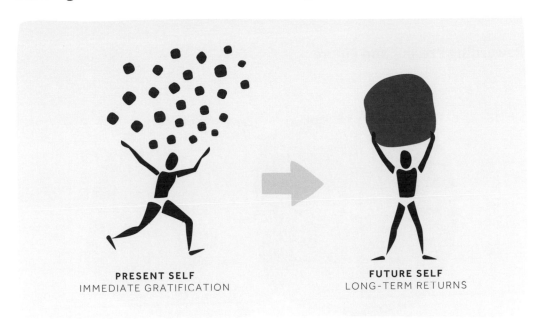

PRESENT SELF
IMMEDIATE GRATIFICATION

FUTURE SELF
LONG-TERM RETURNS

How can we connect our future self back to our present self so we make decisions that are in our mutual best interest? We need to bring immediate feedback to actions that create future benefits.

If we can connect our current routines to future benefits by creating present consequences, we can create mutual benefits.

In essence, we need to connect our present and future self so that the daily choices we make benefit both of our selves. See the diagram below.

Rewarding Present and Future

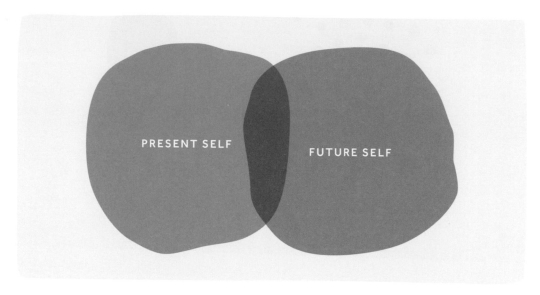

In my own example of reaching a healthy weight, I know that all of the habits I installed would help my future health and as a result I would become healthier, look better, and be more likely to live longer free of disease. Those are great long-term benefits. But if we examine this more closely, I can now see immediate benefits to installing each of those secondary choices.

If I eat smaller fuelings every three hours (or six meals a day), I will have more energy throughout the day. If I eat breakfast, I know I will be less hungry and more likely to eat healthy today. If I eat low-glycemic carbs, I will have more even blood sugar and less mental fog at work. If I drink eight glasses of water, I will be less hungry and more alert throughout the day.

Hopefully, you can see that tying in immediate benefits of new choices will make it more likely that you do them. In essence, we're building in immediate rewards to celebrate our present choices and, at the same time, we're supporting our long-term Habits of Health benefits.

Weight Management

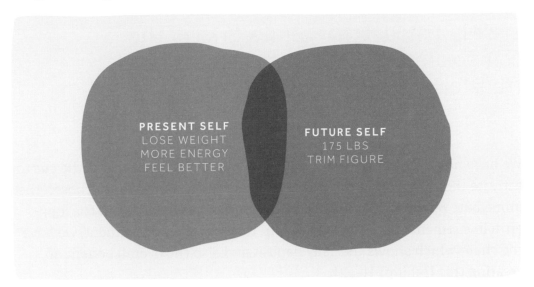

You will always want to connect the daily action to immediate positive feedback to tie in your present self as well as the long-term compounding effect of installation. At all levels, using the habit loops, which consist of **cue, routine**, and **reward,** is important for the sustainable transformation necessary for creating optimal health and wellbeing.

You can also create negative immediate consequences for things you have decided but are having trouble initiating. Say you have decided that you want to get up and run in the morning, then why not call a friend who lives nearby and ask them to run with you in the morning?

That way in the morning when the alarm goes off you will decide to get up rather than push the snooze alarm because the immediate consequence of letting a friend down forces you into action.

As it gets easier and the loop of a jog with a friend becomes desirable (the reward of companionship and a flow of endorphins), you will start seeing this amazing transformation beginning and your story will get even better.

We will finish this last step by creating a mechanism to journal this transformational process.

CREATE A TRANSFORMATIONAL CYCLE

Here is a model that connects all of the components of habit installation in one transformational cycle.

We have now picked the habit we are installing. We have decided the **cue** to activate the actual habit or action being ingrained, and we have chosen the immediate **reward** to reinforce and give immediate feedback to the long-term investment that is being made. In the long-term investment, we have the chain which shows the daily deposit and also the overall benefit of creating this Habit of Health.

We now have created the transformational cycle that connects the immediate and long-term benefit within a long-term feedback accountability tool.

Habits of Health—Transformation Cycle

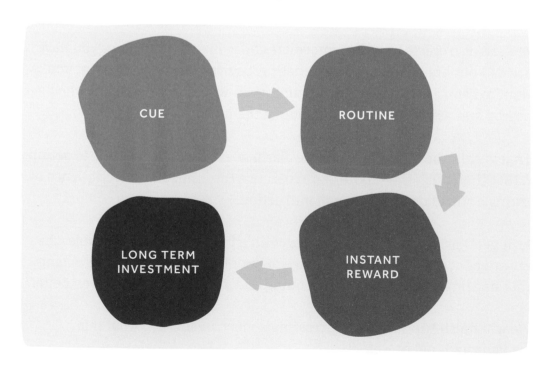

If we use my example of fueling the body every three hours (and the related *cues*, *routines*, and *rewards*), I can track the daily long-term investment in my health. In so doing, we are connecting all of the necessary ingredients to create a transformational habit.

Habits of Health—Healthy Weight Transformation Cycle

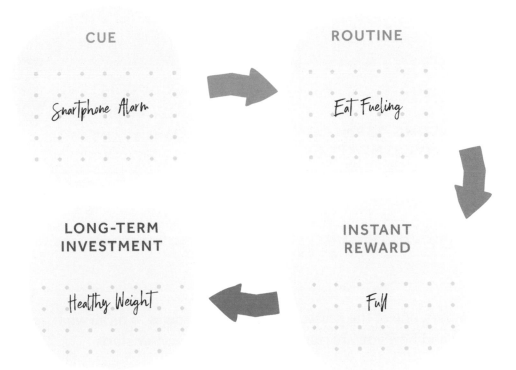

Now it's your turn to take the habit loop you have selected and put it into this transformational cycle. This will give you all the variables to install your new habit, so it supports both your immediate and long-term health and wellbeing.

Habits of Health—Transformation Cycle

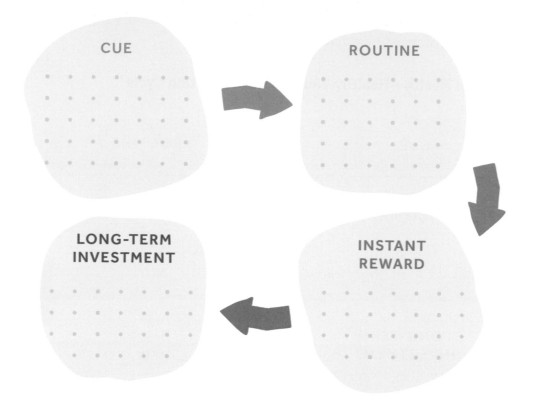

In summary, one of the key ways to learn and grow is to recall what you are learning and how you are going to apply it to your new story.

Please take some time and write down the new ways you are going to install your habits.

How do you see these *microHabits* empowering you to be successful in the creation of new healthy behaviors?

What are you most excited about so far? Make sure you often review all your notes and this Element. Also, share it with your coach, and spend time discussing how these possibilities will become a reality.

In the next Element, we will focus on how the people, places, and things in your surroundings can be modified to serve you in creating your new story.

Notes to yourself:

Now that you have completed Element 03, *How Do You Create What You Want?*, write down your thoughts guided by the following questions:

What does this Element mean to you right now?

What does this Element give you the opportunity to reflect on?

What actions are you going to take as a result of this Element?

I encourage you to connect with your coach, so that you can discuss your thoughts and actions as soon as possible.

Sharing your thoughts with your coach will help them become a reality.

Make sure you review all your notes and this Element often.

ELEMENT 04:
BUILDING A
HEALTHY MINDSET

Average time to complete: **1–2 weeks**

In Element 04, we will:

- Understand how the people, places, and things in your surroundings can be modified to serve you in creating your new story.
- Realize the power and importance of self-awareness.
- Give you tools for building a healthy mindset.

You have now acquired some powerful tools contained within the Habits of Health Transformational System. They're designed to help you learn and install your new behaviors. Hopefully you now understand that real change isn't just possible, it's inevitable. That is, if you're willing to become a student of the creative process and put the time in to make the necessary changes to install the Habits of Health. In order to overcome and move past your current behaviors and tendencies and make your weight, health, and wellbeing sustainable, we need to add Element 04, *Building a Healthy Mindset.*

MY GOAL IS FOR YOU TO BECOME
THE DOMINANT FORCE IN YOUR LIFE

When I say my goal is for you to become the dominant force in your life, I am being very serious. When you have internal stability and external equilibrium each day of your life will become all-out magical. You will possess a habit that most have never even thought about.

So, what am I talking about?

It's the ability to respond to whatever life throws at you, to respond in a way that will always help you in your life-building process.

And believe me, life is going to get in the way.

We will eventually talk about how you can modify your surroundings to help the people, places, and things in your life support you in your quest to improve your health and life.

But right now, we are going to focus on you.

So let's get started.

Who is responsible for your current health and wellbeing?

- Your parents
- Your environment
- Your spouse
- Your genetics
- Your friends
- You

The correct answer is YOU.

If you disagree, I consider it important to understand why. In fact, I would encourage you to write why you think so. Most people have a natural tendency to look outside of themselves to explain why life is happening to them. In fact, our ancestors survived because of their ability to detect and respond to threats. Like a neural tripwire, we would immediately go into a defensive position, shut down, and release a series of chemicals that would allow us to either fight, flee, freeze, or faint without thinking about it. There was no time to evaluate because you would be eaten, stung, bitten, or otherwise badly hurt.

Let's talk about who's in charge of your life.

Let's explore a little more about how your mind works.

Today, most of the things that could have killed you (sabre tooth tigers for example) are in the past. Today, your alarm system has been hijacked and survival is about protecting ego, identity, and beliefs.

The focus has shifted to a need to be right, the need to not look bad, the need for social approval, and the fear that we don't have enough stuff. For many, this becomes a feeling where we think life is *happening* to us.

Part 1.6 of *Dr. A's Habits of Health, You in Charge of Yourself: Setting Up for Success*, explains how we evolved since ancient times. There will be a much more detailed discussion of how our brain, mind, and our emotions are designed when we unpack the Habits of a Healthy Mind later.

For now, it is important for you to understand who is leading you on this journey to optimal health and wellbeing.

Most people are sleepwalking through their days, unaware and not conscious of what's happening around them. They are not sensitive to the reactive state they live in and how they are responding on a daily basis to the people, places and things in their lives. They do not know how to treat themselves.

Life is happening to them. So how about you?

Let me ask you to answer the questions below so that we can assess how you are responding currently to your world.

Choose only one answer for each.

Your intelligence is:

- Something very basic about you and cannot change

- You can learn new things but you can't really change how intelligent you are

- Fixed by the age of five and cannot change beyond then

- No matter how much intelligence you have, you can always significantly change it

Your character as a person is:

- Set and there is not much you can do to change that

- Flexible so you can do things differently but the important parts can't really be changed

- Determined by your family and cannot really be altered

- Is changeable and you can always modify basic things about the kind of person you are

When presented with a challenge I...

- Find myself getting upset most of the time

- Usually shy away from it and hoping someone else will take care of it

- Find myself making excuses

- Look to see what I can learn

When I am in an argument I...

- Find it important to be right above everything else

- Find myself quick to point the blame

- Feel sorry for myself

- Seek to understand what the other person is saying

When something bad happens in the world I...

- Find myself focusing on whose fault it was

- Find myself wondering why the world is not different

- Find myself blaming people who hold other beliefs

- Seek to understand what can be learned from it

When I find myself overeating I...

- Blame it on someone else

- Blame it on something else

- Blame it on myself

- Look to understand why

When I find myself getting upset because someone makes me look stupid I...

- Find myself unable to think straight

- Look to blame it on someone else

- Feel very angry

- Realize only I can upset myself

In the diagram below, where do you place yourself (most of the time) as you go through your day? Are you above or below the line?

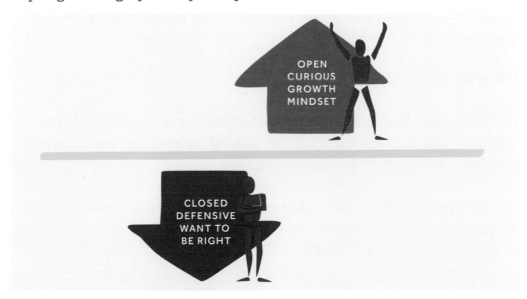

If you find yourself mostly below the line and answered anything other than number four in the questions above, you are not taking as much responsibility as you could.

I've said this before, and I'll say it again: it's not your fault. You are most likely still allowing your ancient brain to run the show. You're not alone, and it does not make you a better or a worse person. It simply means that you are operating your life at a mostly unconscious level.

Welcome to the human race.

Most people think the world should be a certain way, and that in itself is a recipe for anxiety, upset, frustration, or letting our thoughts become entrenched. We blame our surroundings, others, or ourselves for our current state. We become closed, defensive, and consumed with being right.

Why is it important to move above the line and to take responsibility for how we respond to the world and the people that live in it? Well, besides being a sure way to make this world a better place to live, moving above the line is essential if you want to reach your healthiest self and live in a state of optimal wellbeing.

In fact, this is the keystone in installing the Habits of a Healthy Mind. At this early stage in your journey it plays a vital role in helping you take charge of your health and life.

It starts with self-awareness.

It's really important to understand that if you're unaware that you are operating at a subconscious level and making choices that are not in your own best interest, then you cannot improve.

Secondly, you absolutely need to decide that you are going to take responsibility for your behavior and your results. This is very different from placing blame or responsibility on something or someone outside of your control.

In psychology, how an individual responds to their world is referred to as the locus of control. In other words, do I make life happen or is it happening to me? Who is in charge?

When we place blame on others, we give away our power and surrender control, and we place the cause and reason outside of ourselves. When we decide we are the dominant force in our lives, we are taking back our power and responsibility, and the cause now lies inside ourselves.

Most people play the victim and wonder why life is happening to them.

Others play the villain and blame what is happening on someone else or on themselves. The third group—the heroes—hate conflict and pain. They avoid dealing with them by overcompensating and arriving to save the day. When you take responsibility, you are refusing to get caught up in the Drama Triangle that's illustrated below:

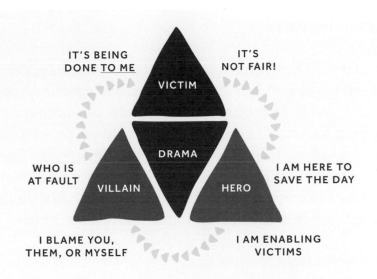

People get caught up in this triangle because something happens or goes wrong, and they are fearful that they will look bad, get in trouble, and have their ego damaged. And so the drama continues. Many times the players shift roles (as indicated by the arrows). The effect of blaming, feeling shame, and fear that things will not go their way happens because the locus of control is outside those who are caught in the triangle. This leads to a state of internal unrest, anxiety, and a highly stressed state, all of which are unhealthy for your body, mind, and overall wellbeing.

It also leads to bad habits, like emotional eating, increased alcohol intake, drug dependency, internet and smartphone addiction, gambling, stress, and depression. Rather than succumbing to the Drama Triangle (which we now know exists and can prepare for), we're going to create a new triangle that will help empower you and others.

This new triangle—of empowerment—is the basis of the creative process that forms the building blocks of the Habits of Health.

Here's how this new triangle can help. First, when you find yourself drifting below the line, don't fall back into your previous tendency to feel like a victim. Instead, take responsibility as the creator of your new story. Equipped with structural tension as your new form of generative motivation, you are going to focus on your desired outcome rather than reacting to what happens.

Second, you will challenge yourself when something happens and be curious enough to use these challenges to learn, grow, and improve rather than finding someone to blame (which is easier, and ultimately offers you no long-term reward). The obstacles in your life will now become the way that you get better—the means by which you change your life—rather than being any reflection on you. And when you are responding to others, you can take the crucial decision to not drift down into their drama. Instead, you will help to empower rather than enable others.

This new model looks like this:

The Empowerment Triangle

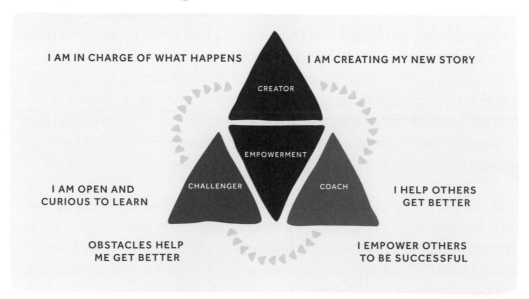

How do we make this work for you on a practical basis and give you the means of installing this new way of responding to your world? You need to be your own chief advocate on your journey and have the ability to minimize anything or anybody throwing you off track.

If you're feeling overwhelmed by these new concepts, and the idea that you can be in control of your destiny, remember that I am right here with you on this journey. We'll take this process like we do all the Habits of Health you acquire: in baby steps, one *microHabit* at a time.

Think of this as taking regular trips to the mental gymnasium. We will start with some really useful and interesting tools to help you but, first, we need to take a look at how the world works and why many fail when they try to change.

When you escape your hectic schedule and are on vacation, spending some time alone, or on a quiet walk, then your health and wellbeing intentions will make sense. You know that it is important to lose some weight, start to move more, and make sure you get more sleep.

Without the constant stream of what seems like negative information, it would be easier to install your new habits and stay on the plan. But sadly, your great intentions seem to wilt when life gets in the way and, unfortunately, we can find ourselves reacting in a way that may not be in our best interest.

That's why we can be in charge one minute, then find ourselves acting like a spoiled kid the next, doing something that we know does not serve our best interests.

The rational brain (our thinking brain that knows what is best in times of calm) is barely, if at all, aware when your lower brain senses something is wrong. Most don't stand a chance as they sleepwalk through life in an unconscious state.

The stimulus creates an immediate response from our emotional brain without a gap or time for thinking.

It looks something like this:

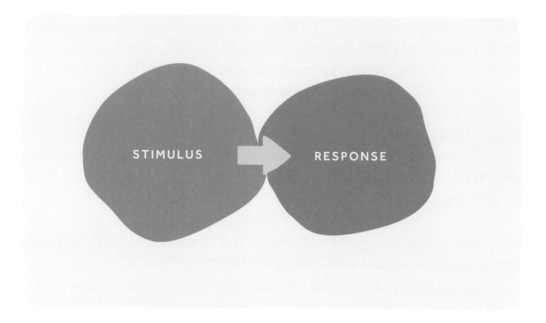

I explained this earlier and in Part 1.6 of *Dr. A's Habits of Health*, You're in Charge of Yourself: Setting Up for Success, we will further discuss how our emotional (or Labrador) brain reacts at a subconscious level. When something happens to us, we respond at a reactive level. It activates us, and we drift below the line into the Drama Triangle. We eat, act, and respond in ways that do not serve our new desire to create optimal health and wellbeing—the things you have created in your thinking brain.

Can you recall a situation where your reactive brain dominated your response rather than your rational brain?

Without conscious awareness, all the above-the-line attributes, which are so important in developing your new story, will never get online and so have no chance of taking charge.

In the visual below, you can see that the stimulus does not have time to reach the thinking brain before you've already eaten the doughnut, yelled at your kids, or shown a single finger to a passing motorist (burning very few calories in the process).

Our Lower Brains

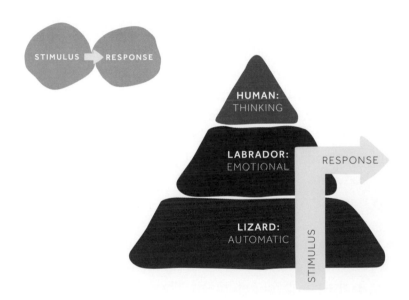

The key to regaining control starts with self-awareness. We need to create a pause in our lives—even a momentary one—so that we create time for areas of higher thought to be present. The conscious thoughts can take over and put you back in charge.

How do we break the stimulus response that triggers reactive behavior and gains control over our automated brain and subconscious mind?

STOP. CHALLENGE. CHOOSE.™

This is all about becoming fully aware at the moment when the stimulus or event happens so that you can choose to delay the immediate response from being triggered. To do this, we engage our thinking brain.

Self-awareness is the first step in changing your previous programming. It will be one of the most important Habits of Health that you will learn. It will develop throughout your journey, and you'll use it on a daily basis. There are many ways to work on becoming more aware, which we will develop together, including a focus on your breathing and the important use of meditation as a Habit of Health. For now, I am going to give you some cues your body serves up when it's about to go "prehistoric" on you. These will give you ways to start breaking the stimulus-response behavior instantly. It begins by becoming more aware of your body and detecting the signals coming up from your unconsciousness as they rise to the surface.

Anytime you feel that something isn't quite right, you will sense your breathing change, your heart rate increase, a lump forming in your throat, a queasiness sitting in the pit of your stomach. These are all signals that should make you *stop* before saying or doing anything.

These sensations are a sign of your awareness that an emotion is rushing through your body. It is usually connected to an action.

Let's run through the Stop. Challenge. Choose.™ response.

Stop: Your mind and body are tightly linked. The physical sensations, like that feeling in your gut, are cues that signal you to immediately take control of your current condition.

Challenge: By becoming good at stopping, you are putting yourself in a position to know how to control your response to a negative feeling or emotion.

In the chapters that follow of the healthy mind, we will go into this in much more detail. For the moment, once you have stopped the immediate response, there are some things you can do to cool off.

Usually, negative feelings are generated when our ego and identity are somehow threatened. It takes about two minutes for the emotion to pass (once you recognize it), and it will take its natural course. I find if I drink a glass of water before talking or take a deep breath before acting then I can fully engage my rational brain and decide what action will move me forward in my health, my relationships, and my overall wellbeing. Triggers, such as your immediate urge for sugar, chocolate, a salty snack, or another habit of disease, will cause your body to send out similar signals that you can now detect to prevent mindless eating.

Choose: This book is making you aware, teaching you the principled Habits of Health so that you will have a growing repertoire of better choices to make in every circumstance. Like all other habit installations, using Stop. Challenge. Choose.™ will take time and practice to learn and install but over time they will become automated.

If you think about it, we're right back to the trio of *cue, routine,* and *reward.*

Your detected feeling is the *cue* which signals **Stop**, the **routine** is your thinking **Challenge** of sorting out what is going on, and **reward** is making the right choice by **Choosing** an action that turns a potential negative action into a positive choice. This will give you a sense of accomplishment.

Below, we show the ability of Stop. Challenge. Choose.™ to delay the stimulus response and activate the thinking brain to choose a healthy habit rather than a habit of disease.

Engage Our Thinking

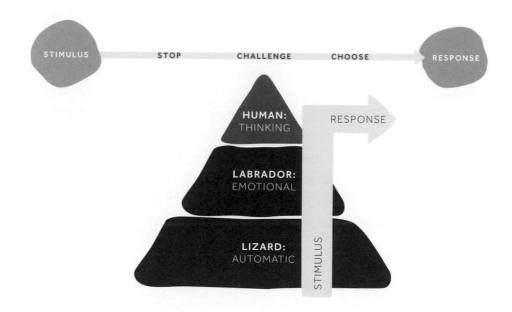

I think you will find Stop. Challenge. Choose.™ to be a powerful tool that helps you start to gain more control over your world. You will find that you are no longer competing with the people around you. Instead, you are looking within to get better at being in control of your inner world.

What are some of the immediate ways you can start using Stop. Challenge. Choose.™?

1.

2.

3.

Name three things you want to stop doing immediately.

1.

2.

3.

Write down ways that you are currently using Stop. Challenge. Choose.™ to increase your

Awareness:

Self-control:

CONSCIOUS BREATHING SKILL

When we are buying a car they give us two different fuel consumption ratings: City and Highway.

Fuel consumption is erratic in the city, with all the frequent stops and gos but once you get out on the superhighway the engine settles into a coherent rhythm that allows fuel efficiency to increase. We want our breathing to have the same coherent, efficient rhythm.

When we are emotionally upset, stressed, or overthinking, our breathing becomes shallow and chaotic, originates from the upper chest and neck, and over time it creates considerable wear and tear on our body. We are usually not conscious of this daily condition until we make a decision to pay attention and become aware of when we are in this erratic state. It is your normal conditioning, which served you 10,000 years ago as part of the physiologic state, stimulated once again by your emotional brain.

The great news is you can rapidly take control of this physiological chaos with your breathing. The simple awareness of your breathing can actually create physiological coherence which allows you to rapidly regain the human (thinking) brain control so that you can now **Challenge** it and **Choose** a rational desirable outcome.

Changing the state of breathing can help bring all your physiology back in line, much like the conductor turns the potential chaos of an orchestra into beautiful harmony.

The conscious control of your breathing is not unique to the Habits of Health Transformational System but plays a central role in helping you become the dominant force in your life.

Our approach is not to address every aspect of breathing but to focus on a few key Elements which will have the biggest and most rapid effect of helping you gain control.

The key is for it to feel natural and not contrived.

First: Constant Rhythm
Establish a constant rhythm so you have the same cadence on inhalation and exhalation.

Four-second count in / six-second count out or use a five in five out. Pick the ratio that is the most natural to you.

Decide what ratio relaxes you most:

Inhalation: . . . . count

Exhalation: . . . . count

Make sure you use that first breath to take full command of your breathing and become fully present.

Second: Even Flow
Create an even flow of air so that the *speed* of inhale and exhale are the same. This insures a consistent flow rate that helps establish a smoothness to go along with a constant rhythm.

Third: Create A Positive Emotional Experience
Focus on your heart or the center of your chest as you take these rhythmatic even flow breaths and feel the positive emotional experience as the chaos starts to pass, which will give you a sense of calm and control.

Note: Not to confuse you, but I am talking about sensing your heart region as the center of your emotions, which will help you regain coherence with your breathing. From a mechanical standpoint, proper breathing will come from successfully engaging your diaphragm rather than your upper neck and chest. You can check this by placing your hand over your belly and feeling the expansion of your abdomen with each breath.

I would like you to practice taking over your breathing several times a day. This will prepare you to be able to respond quickly and effectively as soon as you sense it's time to *stop* when any situation, event, or person starts to scramble your thinking!

As soon as you sense negative feelings, shift your physiology by initiating that first breath of control. This will help you build the habit of emotional freedom.

How many times a day are you creating conscious breathing?

Describe how it is working:

Before we complete this Element, let's go back to the visual of playing above the line to demonstrate how powerful your ability is to look at the world from your new perspective.

Now that your thinking brain is in charge, you can look at everything from the perspective of a new question: how can I learn and grow from this experience? There is no longer a need to be closed and defensive or to always be right.

Carol Dweck has labeled this state a growth versus a fixed mindset. Her studies have shown that people with this growth mindset are much more successful and experience a far higher level of wellbeing.[1] She is correct, but mine and Robert Fritz's work* shows that it is really more about focusing on your desired outcome than what we think about ourselves.

*Identity, Robert Fritz and Dr. Wayne Andersen. Newfane Press 2016

Those that have a fixed mindset think they have finite ability, and everything they do reflects on them personally, so they spend most of their time in the Drama Triangle. They have a need to defend their position and as a result they struggle. You, on the other hand, have a creative mindset which keeps you focused on the desired outcome. You are open and curious and have both the tools and knowledge to make the necessary adjustments to continue to improve slowly but steadily. And when something new is needed, you have the built-in inventiveness to move forward, despite the obstacles that will challenge you. This will be very important as you start to write the new story of you and focus on creating optimal health and wellbeing for yourself.

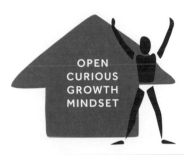

**OPEN
CURIOUS
GROWTH
MINDSET**

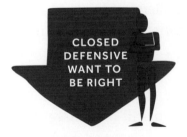

**CLOSED
DEFENSIVE
WANT TO
BE RIGHT**

So now when you sense something is happening, you can apply Stop. Challenge. Choose.™ to immediately shift back above the line and move into the growth mindset. The following diagram shows how you can catch yourself and shift above the line, using challenges as a time to learn and improve. By catching yourself as you begin to drift, you prevent descent into the Drama Triangle, where it is more difficult to recover.

Healthy Mind Shift

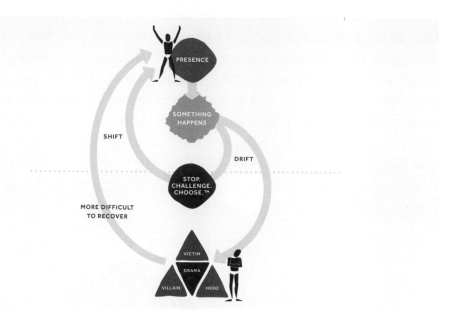

Remember: we all go below the line on occasion. It is the ability to catch yourself when you are drifting down into the reactive mode and to shift into a growth or creative mindset that marks you as different to the majority. What this means is you have a series of daily opportunities to develop the *microHabit* of Stop. Challenge. Choose.™ and it's this that makes every situation an opportunity to get better. Your Habits of Health App allows you to do this daily.

When these moments arise, describe (in your journal) some examples over the next week where you start to drift but you've stopped yourself, challenged why you were thinking that way, and made a conscious effort to shift and choose an outcome or behavior that is part of your new story. Make sure you review all your notes and this Element often.

Also, share it with your coach and spend time discussing how these possibilities will become a reality in helping you be the dominant force in your life. In the next Element, we will move from the powerful forces and strength you have within you to take a look at your surroundings and see how we can recruit the people, modify the places, and change the things that touch your world.

Notes to yourself:

Now that you have completed Element 04, *Building A Healthy Mindset*, write down your thoughts guided by the following questions:

What does this Element mean to you right now?

What does this Element give you the opportunity to reflect on?

What actions are you going to take as a result of this Element?

I encourage you to connect with your coach, so you can share your thoughts and actions as soon as possible.

Sharing your thoughts with your coach will help them become a reality.

Make sure you review all your notes and this Element often.

1 *Mindset* – Carol Dweck PH.D. Random House 2006.

ELEMENT 05:
OPTIMIZING YOUR SURROUNDINGS

Average time to complete: **1–2 weeks**

In Element 05, we will:

- Look at your surroundings and see how we can recruit the people, modify the places, and change the things that touch your world.
- Discover how to create a microenvironment of healthy relationships.
- Provide you with tools, resources, and tips that will help you improve your relationships.
- Examine the value of community and surrounding yourself with like-minded people.

" *Your goal is to create a microenvironment of health: a protective bubble to shield you against obesigenic forces and nurture your growth and transformation.* "

Dr. Wayne Scott Andersen

Now that you have taken responsibility, determined that you will play above the line, and decided to take total accountability for your health and life, everything will change. In situations that present themselves you will get progressively better at being able to recognize when you are drifting below the line.

This new way of being has a side effect. You will start interacting with your world in a different way, and it's worth considering that those around you may not be making similar choices. This may present challenges, and that's what we will now discuss in Element 05, *Optimizing Your Surroundings*.

In the last Element, we worked on your relationship with yourself and equipped you with a very simple structure—Stop. Challenge. Choose.™

As you get better, making your daily choices in line with your goals will get easier. You will see your ability to control your behavior and maintain calm in contrast to others who are quick to react and lose their composure over trivial things.

In order to minimize the effect on your progress by those around you who are not quite there or simply don't support you, we need to talk about the dynamics of relationships, interactions, and connections with others.

This section will help you gain the support of others, which will be an incredibly important part of your daily life this year as you design and create new chapters in your life.

OPTIMIZING YOUR RELATIONSHIPS

Relationships are critical to everything we do in life. We are hardwired to be social, and our sense of connection, belonging, and attachment to other people is one of the most fundamental of all human needs. This connection not only serves us on our journey to health and wellbeing but is essential in living a longer healthier life. People that lack these fundamental human relationships of companionship and connection are at a forty-five percent greater risk of dying earlier.[1]

If these positive connections support and enhance our journey, how do we create more of them and deepen our existing relationships?

Let's first address how you can enhance your current relationships and build strong allies who might even join you on your mission.

Let's do a quick review using our above the line visual as a guide. Remember, you have decided to take full responsibility for whatever happens during your day. You also know that sometimes you will drift below the line. The keystone habit you are building is to be able to shift back above-the-line using Stop. Challenge. Choose.™ to help you keep your thinking brain as your guide versus the reactive, emotional, Labrador brain.

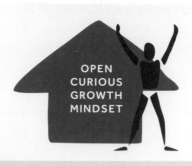

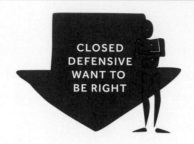

There is a very practical way of thinking about how to manage the two states we find ourselves in daily.

The emotional, or Labrador brain, has been referred to as a *Hot or Go System*. In ancient times, it helped us survive. When we were threatened the amygdala, a concentrated group of nerves that control the emotional brain, would hijack our thinking and shut off cognitive, high-level activities and instead begin pouring out emotional energy to put the body into action. The body prepared itself to run with increased blood flow to muscles. No thinking or pondering, just high-energy reactions and below-the-line thinking! It's how little kids (and quite a few teenagers) tend to think.

The *Cool or Know System* is the second operating system. It is run by our thinking brain and allows you to have meaningful conscious conversations that are mutually beneficial. The body is in a very relaxed state with a slow heart rate, normal blood pressure, and a sense of alertness. It allows us to thrive. It is the Habits of Health default state and our goal as you design your authorship of your life.

These two systems play very different roles.

10,000 years ago, the *Go System's* hair trigger helped protect you and your tribe.

Unfortunately the perceived threats we feel today are mostly to our ego, and they trigger the *Go System* when, in almost every case, we would be better served by our *Know System*.

Let's say you're in a meeting and you perceive someone is mocking an idea you have just shared. Your *Go System* is activated, and you want to tear his head off. You release a litany of aggressive language, your face goes beet red, and you adopt an equally threatening body position. After work, you throw down two drinks without thinking to calm you down, only to find out later that his comments had nothing to do with your proposal.

The sum total is Full *Go System* activation: Increased blood pressure, too much alcohol, damaged relationships, potential loss of job advancement, and poorer health.

Next time: Stop. Challenge. Choose.™ Have a glass of water, and achieve understanding by using the *Know System*, so that you progress toward better health and wellbeing, and maybe even a promotion.

As you become more aware of your current behavior and you work on developing your healthy mindset, this simple analogy offers you the opportunity to improve your interactions with those around you.

It's a *Know Go* that can help!

Let's break down how we can help influence your world to serve your needs and support your journey.

Your self-awareness really means knowing yourself, your emotions and what triggers them, and how you normally react to specific people and places. This will help your *Know System* dominate.

It is really as simply stopping and asking yourself: "What is happening here?"

If we can help you make sense of your emotions and recognize when they are starting to reveal themselves, we can intervene and prevent them from hijacking the thinking brain. In turn, this will mean we can respond in a way that best serves us and keeps the *Go System* switched off. Building this powerful *microHabit* of responding rather than reacting changes everything.

This gives us great power over our emotions.

In the last Element, we talked about the importance of sensing the types of changes in your body that herald the rise of an emotion and the beginning of the activation of the *Go System*. Early detection helps us to create a gap and gives us time to prevent *Go System* activation. We can then use our *Know System* to challenge our response and choose an outcome that moves us forward on our journey.

If you can recognize and become fully aware of the emotion, then you can understand what is causing it.

The beauty is that it usually represents a symptom of something we need to address in ourselves or our relationships. It can help you understand something important about yourself as you shift back above the line and learn from it. You can ask yourself what triggered it, if you need to respond, and if you can avoid feeling that way by reframing what you heard to serve you in a more constructive way?

Many times, you will find that your ego is at play. If you resist the temptation to interpret these interactions as a real threat, you can immediately defuse those disturbing feelings. If it is a genuine threat to you, then you will be able to respond in a more reflective way that builds your case rather than destroying it.

Ask yourself, does it matter what I think about myself in this situation? Most of the time, unless it is a tangible threat to your job or runs the risk of you being physically hurt, it is more likely to be an imagined threat to our ego and self worth. It is a default state response, which is left over from our self-generated story. It does not serve the new you. We will unpack this more in *Dr. A's Habits of Health*.

In the space below, think of a moment you identified an emotion. Do not judge, but just observe. Make a note of whether you were successful at using Stop. Challenge. Choose.™ and your *Know System* to respond in a way that's different from before.

Regulating your Emotions (Example)

Emotion:

When my daughter leaves the kitchen in a mess, I feel angry

Past response:

I would yell, and create stress and bad feelings. Why would I respond with anger? I want her to be successful and make great choices.

Current response:

I see the mess, and turn to yell, but I immediately stop, let the feeling pass (that lasts about 90 seconds on average) and ask my daughter to clean up. Once she has finished, I hug her and tell her I love her.

PS
After a few false starts I now have a clean kitchen and a great relationship with my daughter.

As an exercise, pick different emotions you experience during the day, observe and identify the real reason you are feeling those emotions (if known), then observe how those emotions are affecting others, and how you are using Stop. Challenge. Choose.™ to change the outcome. You can decide to watch the emotion run its course, engage in a constructive way, or leave the situation if you feel that this is necessary.

Emotion

Know or Go?

Emotion:

Know or Go?

Emotion:

Know or Go?

Our emotions are a powerful source of energy for action. If we fail to harness it, Go energy can easily see us slip into unhealthy behaviors in both our choices and our interaction with others. Being able to feel our emotions fully and determining our own choice of how to constructively express them is our goal.

The first step is being aware and the previous exercise allows you to reappraise and move from *Go* activation to a smarter choice.

There will be people in your life that can activate your neural tripwire more easily than others. Try to avoid confrontational people and situations until your Stop. Challenge. Choose.™ habit is fully installed and they no longer have the ability to trigger negativity in you.

It's going to be helpful to record the following: for the next week track who and what type of situations push your buttons and activate your *Go System*.

We'll discuss how to manage behavior very shortly. What I'd like you to do next is write down some avoidance strategies to help you manage the kind of situations you've experienced above.

If this person or situation presents itself, then you will:

"Check Yourself Before You Wreck Yourself"
I saw this on a sign at the entrance to a ski park. I thought it was a perfect reminder that if we want to improve our conscious control of our behavior, then it is important to figure out what we can change in our relationships to help them be more supportive on our journey.

MANAGING OUR EXPERIENCES

Regulating your behavior will be easier as you become more aware of your emotions and that will allow us to start managing responses better.

If these positive connections support and enhance our journey, how do we create more of them and deepen the existing relationships we have?

Let's first address how you can enhance your existing relationships and build strong allies who might even join you on your mission.

Besides using Stop. Challenge. Choose.™ there are other things you can do to improve your response to bad situations. These ideas will allow you to start building the habit of control and take responsibility for healthier outcomes.

Using this reflective assessment will give you tremendous power over your emotions. You will build self-efficacy so that it becomes easier to interact with everyone in your world. Remember the *Know System* is at the heart of the Habits of Health experience.

It is going to take some work but inch by inch everything's a cinch.

Tips to help you stay above the line

Here are some ways to help you stay above the line when the situation feels like it's getting out of control.

Stop. Challenge. Choose.™

- Immediately sense your breathing
- Feel the hot energy cool down before you speak or act
- Open your water bottle slowly and take a drink before speaking
- Think of how your response can improve your health before choosing
- Count to ten before responding
- Sleep on it before responding
- Get a better night's sleep
- Smile and be appreciative
- Be open, curious, and desire growth when challenged

Check the ones you're going to implement into your interactions with the people around you.

Write the other things you're learning or using to help you regulate your emotions and your behavior below. What else can you do to make increasing your awareness and self-regulating your response easier?

Question:
Who Can Upset You?

Answer:
Only You

Here are four questions that can help you take a bad situation and diffuse the drama. It uses above the line thinking (being open, curious, and wanting to learn and grow) as you write your new story.

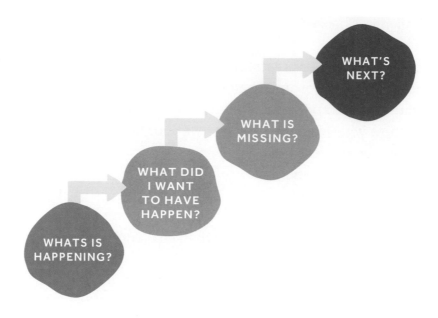

These four questions can keep you out of the Drama Triangle and allow you to pull others out as well.

With these new strategies on how to improve how you act, model, and respond to others, let's shift the focus to how you can help people around you become allies in your new healthy story.

YOUR SOCIAL CONSCIOUSNESS

Now that you have started to self-regulate and to consider how you will respond when you are angry, sad, or joyful, you are in a position to learn how to be aware of other people's emotions and what's going on inside them.

It's an incredibly important shift. Our connection to others can be strong, supportive, and build powerful bonds that have a dramatic effect on both our relationships and our health and wellbeing. When you truly reach out and seek to understand others, you will find that even those not yet ready to change will be more inclined to support you if they feel that their perspective is validated.

The key Habit of Health here is to listen with the desire to understand people from their vantage point.

Listening is not something we learn or do naturally. We are much better at being transmitters of information. We talk about our point of view, our views, our world, and our story. So, when we seek to understand things from someone else's world and their path, everything opens up in our relationships.

How do we do a better job?

When someone is talking to us, how much do you think is communicated through:

Actual words	%	(7)
Tone of voice	%	(38)
Body language	%	(55)

Body posture and tone can give us a powerful insight into what others are thinking and they go a long way to avoid potential confrontation, stress, and otherwise unhealthy outcomes. This is why it's better to discuss something important in person rather than use text or emails. How many times have we either upset someone or been unintentionally rattled by relying on the trivial seven percent of words available by text or email?

You can also listen to understand, avoid looking at your phone or screen while people are talking, step into someone else's shoes, and seek to understand the whole picture.

Assignment

Make a decision to listen to what someone else is communicating until they are completely done talking (and by that I mean when they have finished their last syllable) before even formulating your response. Strive to listen to understand so that you get the person you're talking to and you can appreciate them as a fellow human. Then, replay what you heard them actually say.

Write down examples of how that changed the conversation or has improved your relationships:

Try this with people you are close to as well as those with whom you have some friction!

IMPROVING RELATIONSHIPS

One of the critical roles to optimize our relationships is to become better at managing the difficult ones. These conversations are usually filled with drama and excessive stress. They sabotage us most frequently and are often the ones we have with family members, bosses, coworkers, or anyone that frequents the Drama Triangle. If we can improve these interactions, it will go a long way to keep life from getting in the way of your day-to-day interactions.

Since most of us do not handle stress well, your decision to improve your own emotional behavior and become more aware of the emotional state of others can go a long way to improve difficult conversations. It will also help keep the others *Go Systems* from being activated.

Your decision to stay above-the-line and respond in a rational way to someone else's below the line behavior is a huge step in improving your daily interactions because these connections are a key part of thriving in our work and in our play.

In addition, as you spend more time building stronger relationships beyond infrequent interactions, you will build trust and rapport.

Being open, curious, and wanting to understand and learn from another person's perspective is a powerful demonstration to them that you respect and honor the differences you have.

Take a moment and pick five people who are important in your life and who you would like to improve your connection with.

1.

2.

3.

4.

5.

How will improving these relationships affect your health and wellbeing?

Our connections with the people that come into our daily life have a profound effect on our mood, our productivity, and our health and wellbeing.

I know you probably didn't expect to spend so much time discussing this area of your life in this book, but our emotional and relational soundness is a powerful Habit of Health that we will be talking and writing about daily as you build your new story. By taking responsibility for these critical relationships, you are building a platform to make life happen through you, with less chance of derailment.

Since you are most influenced by the people you hang out with at home, work, and play, the more you can be a positive influence on them, the greater chance there is of a ripple effect on all of your lives. You can exercise with a friend, walk your dog with a neighbor, join a healthy living organization, or even partner with a group on the Habits of Health, and practice installing the Habits of Health together.

Take a few moments to consider some of the ways you can recruit your friends to help improve your health and wellbeing. Jot them down.

If you want to understand the power of relationships and the effect they have on your life take a look at Part 1.7 in *Dr. A's Habits of Health, Optimizing Your Surroundings: Creating Your Microenvironment of Health.*

As you create your new healthy life, you should draw your friends close and move away from your accomplices. A friend is someone who will help you on your journey. An accomplice is someone who actively helps you to get in trouble.

List five friends   List five accomplices

Having like-minded people around you is a powerful motivator.

That's why it's a good idea to preemptively stack the deck with people that can assist you on your journey to a healthier you. When managing your accomplices, make sure that when you are socializing with them you avoid environments where they can influence your behaviors. It may be better to take a break from them until your habits are installed and you are stronger.

Your decision to change your health and improve your wellbeing is life-changing but only if you are willing to take responsibility and make some secondary choices that may seem hard right now; however, I promise it will pay dividends down the line. It is important to understand that your authorship of the story of your health and wellbeing will occur in a series of small steps or chapters. They will unfold with feedback, practice, and coaching and—like a seed planted today—will grow over time.

Avoiding Traps

One of the key areas you are going to have to work on is family members, friends, and others creating scenarios that are well-intended but put you in a position that would create behavior that is not supportive of your new path and story.

We all have a well-meaning grandmother that makes our favorite pie and expects us to eat everything we're served. It is important to use your new skills here to address a potential relationship issue if you say no. Remember, the offering is the other person's expression of love or gift to you and they may not have the same mindset as you.

The best thing you can do is politely explain why you are choosing to not eat the pie. I recommend a big hug, an "I appreciate the thought," and an "I love you", if it is appropriate. You can also ask them to respect your request to support you because it is very important to you. Also, to give you strength, you can even share with them your why from Element 01, *Being Clear Why You Are Here*, which explains all the important reasons you are making these changes. If they truly love you, they will get it, and if they don't, they should be considered an accomplice!

Places

The environment around us shapes our daily behavior. This section has two main categories. We will first look at a place of support to assist you on your journey. Then, we'll explore the underlying structure of your environment.

Support can come from many different places: I am here to help coach and assist you. Beyond the help I can provide, the idea of being coached, or part of a group may be appealing to you, or you may be more comfortable as a self-help individual. Remember, this is your new adventure and you need to proceed at your pace and your comfort level.[2] That said, there is a lot of evidence that having a variety of sources of influence and assistance in this type of journey can enhance our chances of success.

My experience has shown that we all learn in different ways but that there are some important catalysts to enhance your ability to master your new habits. Learning and practicing are important, and you have probably heard about the 10,000 hours that are required to achieve mastery of a particular action. The part that is often overlooked is that it is deliberate practice that makes the difference. This is best accomplished by using accurate mindfulness, feedback, coaching, and deliberate practice.

In the following diagram you can see the progression:

Four Stages of Learning the Habits of Health

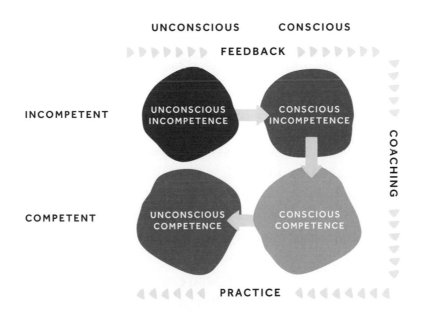

Stage One: Unconscious Incompetent

This is our starting point. We may have some ideas about how to transform a particular Habit of Health, but it is usually incomplete. We've also not shown any ability to consistently perform a certain skill or behavior.

Stage Two: Conscious Incompetent

By reading *Dr. A's Habits of Health* and through feedback from others, you are now aware of what you need to do to accomplish the skill or habit.

Stage Three: Conscious Competent

Through applying the installation tools, using *Your LifeBook*, and having the support of a coach or some other form of assistance you are learning and repeating the new skill or habit which is transforming your behavior in an effective way.

Stage Four: Unconscious Competent

This is the point when the skill, ability, or habit is fully installed and you do it without thinking. You are transforming your behaviors to create and support optimal health and wellbeing so you reach your goal and it lasts a lifetime.

This is the goal of the Habits of Health Transformational System:

To allow you to take full authorship of your health and life and for you to become the dominant force in your life.

The Habits of Health Transformational System is designed to move you through the four stages in a logical fashion. Its design will go a long way to help provide information and skills which will, in turn, provide feedback, coaching, and some great tools. In addition, I highly recommend you seek additional support to help you practice and achieve the goal of mastering your habits and behavior.

Support could come from role models who exemplify optimal health or wellbeing, or you can start by recruiting a friend to join you in this new path to health. It can be as simple as a buddy, your spouse, or even neighbors. Essentially, you need someone who can provide an easy, convenient opportunity to be together. Earlier, you listed some of the ways and people you associate with that can encourage you or give you a helping hand.

Having like-minded people around you is a powerful motivator. Whether you are best served by a drill sergeant, a cheerleader, or getting the occasional encouraging word from a friend, it is nice to be around people who desire to improve their health and their lives alongside you.

Beyond the Habits of Health Transformational System and your close friends or family, there are many powerful influencers you can use to help you become a strong unconscious competent in your health and life.

Throughout the book, I will refer to the robust community that I have helped design and build to provide an amazing support network of people who have developed a culture of optimal health and wellbeing. This dynamic social structure has already affected the lives of over a million people.

In this structure, OPTAVIA®, of which I am the Co-Founder (and which you may already be part of) offers the guidance of a coach who uses the Habits of Health Transformational System to assist people in the journey to optimal health. Think of coaches as fellow travelers who have decided to help others as well as themselves to become a higher version of themselves. If you are part of our community, I hope you are taking full advantage of your coach as a caring partner that can play a vital role in your transformation. Also, our community is a rich environment of support, role models, knowledge, and common goals. It also values many other intangibles that connect and enhance the experience.

I have found that the clients who are plugged into our community have a much higher rate of success.[3] If you are alone then you fail alone and, potentially, might give up. If you are plugged into our community and you fail, you are encouraged, inspired, and reminded that this is simply a temporary setback and by continuing you will build the ability to succeed. It also leads to many people to also decide to become coaches and help themselves as they assist people they work, play, and socialize with to develop better health and share a higher state of wellbeing.

Help can come from formal settings like behavioral groups, medical facilities, wellness programs, commercial programs that involve group meetings, and from online communities. It can also come from trainers, wellness coaches, health professionals, and others who specialize in helping others create health in their lives.

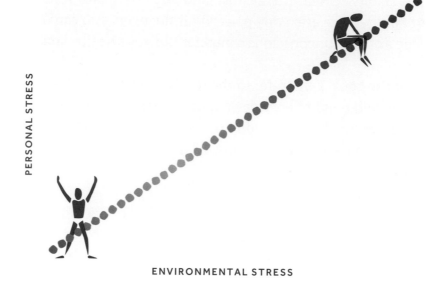

PERSONAL STRESS

ENVIRONMENTAL STRESS

In addition, you will start noticing that there are other things which increase your tendency to make unhealthy or healthy choices.

It will be very important as you progress in *Your LifeBook* to start making note of things that throw you off. It is equally important to note when certain things or conditions make it easier to make healthy choices.

Lastly, it is always good to ask yourself the following:

What is your Kryptonite?

What things, places, or persons have the tendency to throw you off your game?

The Electronic Leash

One of the distractions that has crept into modern life and has created an almost insatiable craving is our relationship with our digital devices. And yes they provide the incredible benefit of continuous connection to our family and friends but it is not without a cost to our health and wellbeing. Our attention span has dropped over the last decade from 12 to 8 seconds, which is shorter than that of a goldfish. It's a source of stress and causes a decrease in productivity and physical ills such as neck pain, elevated blood pressure, and all out exhaustion.[4]

Check the boxes as you adopt these basic techniques which are *microHabits* that can improve your relationship with your electronic devices:

- Turn off push notifications to reduce the constant stimulus response and check your device at convenient times instead. This will break the stimulus response that can be so addictive and exhausting.
- Perform a phone stack at lunches and dinners or actually put the phones out of sight. Recent studies have shown that just the presence of your phone has a negative and exhausting effect on your relationships and health.
- Change your screen to black and white which will decrease the appeal and vibrancy that continually grabs our attention.
- Pick periods during the day that are digital free times. A good way of doing this is to leave your phone at your desk when you get up every hour to move. This way you are incorporating two Habits of Health into one time period.
- Make your bedroom a digital free room and invest in a good old-fashioned alarm clock.
- Stop multitasking and focus on one screen at a time because when you switch back and forth it is disruptive to our thinking and creates anxiety.
- Read a book on paper rather than digitally as your mind processes abstract information more effectively when it is printed.
- Hold your phone and place your digital devices at eye level to decrease neck strain.
- Use the 20-20-20 rule. Look up from your device every 20 minutes and look 20 feet away for 20 seconds.

In Conclusion:

What is the main keystone behavior that seems to make everything fall into place?

The beauty of *Your LifeBook* is that you now are able to start identifying the patterns and things that get in your way. You can now address those areas and add in a pre-emptive plan.

When you find something that typically throws you off, you can now say:

If   happens, I will now choose to

Providing this contingency allows you to have an automatic response so that it is easy to avoid activating the *Go System* and allows you to make Stop. Challenge. Choose.™ almost automatic.

In the next Element, you will start using many of the things you have been learning in the previous Elements to start improving your health.

Notes to yourself:

Now that you have completed Element 05, *Optimizing Your Surroundings*, write down your thoughts guided by the following questions:

What does this Element mean to you right now?

What does this Element give you the opportunity to reflect on?

What actions are you going to take as a result of this Element?

What does healthy community mean to you? Do you currently have one?

I encourage you to connect with your coach, so you can share your thoughts and actions as soon as possible. Sharing your thoughts with your coach will help them become a reality. Make sure you review all your notes and this Element often.

1 *Loneliness in Older Persons: A Predictor of Functional Decline and Death* – Carla M. Perissinotto, MD, MHS; Irena Stijacic Cenzer, MA; Kenneth E. Covinsky, MD, MPH. July 23, 2012. Arch Intern Med. 2012;172(14):1078 – 1084. doi:10.1001/archinternmed.2012.1993.

2 *The role of social support in weight loss maintenance: results from the MedWeight study* – J Behav Med. 2016 Jun;39(3):511-8. doi: 10.1007/s10865-016-9717-y. Epub 2016 Jan 22. Karfopoulou E(1), Anastasiou CA(1), Avgeraki E(1), Kosmidis MH(2), Yannakoulia M(3).

3 Greater weight loss associated with more coaching contacts
  • Individuals who talked with their OPTAVIA® coach more often lost twice as much weight
  • Emphasis on Habits of Health, not just weight loss
    OPTAVIA® Clinical Study 2018 with Chicago Research Group.

4 *Computers in Human Behavior* – 31 (2014) 373 – 383 The dark side of smartphone usage: psychological traits, compulsive behavior and technostress.

ELEMENT 06:
YOUR PATH TO A HEALTHY WEIGHT

Average time to complete: **1 week**

In Element 06, we will:

- Set a goal to help you reach a healthy weight as part of a lifelong transformation.
- Explore the Phases of Weight Management.
- Determine where you are, and learn new habits to begin creating your healthy weight.

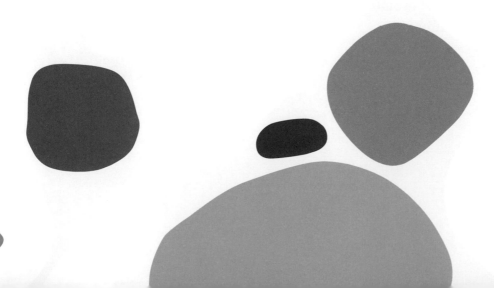

HOW DO YOU CREATE A HEALTHY WEIGHT?

The answer is really embedded in the question. You **create** a healthy weight. And that is what we are going to start doing for you in this Element.

In fact, the creative process will be at the center of all the key aspects of your transformation.

This next twelve months are going to be exciting as we work together to install the key Habits of Health.

The last five Elements have set you up with the proper motivation, and a clear understanding of where you are currently in terms of your health and wellbeing (The Wellbeing Evaluation). You have decided which areas you are ready to work on and the outcomes you desire. In addition, you now understand the creative process and how we take those desired outcomes and place them in a structural tension chart to focus on what we want to create.

We then determined the secondary choices that will take us to our desired outcome. We use the habit loop daily to install our new choices and build the new behaviors that result in our improving health and wellbeing.

And to leave nothing out in the big wide world that can catch you off guard, we have prepared you for real life getting in the way and have given you some skills and tools to work on to help you manage your emotions and environment in a progressively skillful way. And hopefully you have one of our coaches who has been trained to help you successfully use *Your LifeBook* to progress towards a healthier and more fulfilled life.

KNOWING WHERE YOU ARE GOING FROM THE START

Over 45 million individuals in the U.S. go on a diet to lose weight each year,[1] desperately seeking to shed the extra fat they have accumulated. For the vast majority, the decision is emotionally driven, triggered usually by a negative consequence of the way we look, the way our clothes fit, external pressure from those around us, or a potential looming medical issue. Feeling bloated, tired, and unhappy, most run to the latest weight-loss fad and start what has become a series of attempts to get rid of their belly fat.

These diets, typically, are a period of time where you restrict what you eat to force your body into a starvation mode which is neither fun nor necessarily healthy.

Approximately 85% of people who go on a diet gain all their weight, and then some, back within two years. The only habit they ever create is the habit of dieting over and over again. It is insanity.

Of course, if you restrict your calories and put very little in your body by dieting for a period of time, you will usually (not always) lose weight, but as soon as you stop and go back to the way you have always been, your body will seek to go back to its original size.

Your improving weight management will be a byproduct of a simple, baby step approach to creating overall optimal health and wellbeing.

As outlined above, we have left nothing to chance and our goal is to help you reach a healthy weight as part of a lifelong transformation.

So, let's get this story started.

In the beginning of Part 2.1 in *Dr. A's Habits of Health, The Habits of Healthy Weight Management*, I outlined the different phases of weight management.

Your Weight Management Phase

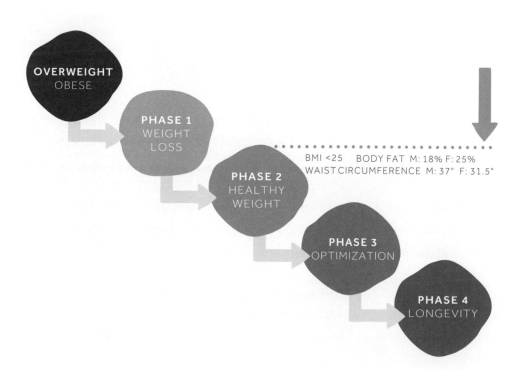

We will use three different measurements to assess your current phase in your weight management. You can do this on your own or have your coach help you figure out where you are starting in terms of your weight management.

Body Mass Index:

This is the gold standard because of its simplicity. When combined with your waist circumference, it provides an accurate assessment of whether we are at a healthy weight. The chart below can help you quickly calculate your current BMI. You can also use one of our online calculators.

Body Mass Index Chart

WEIGHT (LBS)

HEIGHT	100	110	120	130	140	150	160	170	180	190	200	210	220	230	240	250	260	270	280	290	300	310	320
4'5"	25	28	30	33	35	38	40	43	45	48	50	53	55	58	60	63	65	68	70	73	75	78	80
4'6"	24	27	29	31	34	35	39	41	43	46	48	51	53	55	58	60	53	65	68	70	72	78	80
4'7"	23	26	28	30	33	35	37	40	42	44	46	49	51	53	56	58	60	53	65	67	70	72	74
4'8"	22	25	27	29	31	34	36	38	40	43	45	47	49	52	54	56	58	61	63	65	67	69	72
4'9"	22	24	26	28	30	32	35	37	39	41	43	45	48	50	52	54	56	58	61	63	65	67	69
4'10"	21	23	25	27	29	31	33	36	38	40	42	44	46	48	50	52	54	56	59	61	63	65	67
4'11"	20	22	24	26	28	30	32	34	36	38	40	42	44	46	48	50	53	55	57	59	61	63	65
5'0"	20	21	23	25	27	29	31	33	35	37	39	41	45	45	47	49	51	53	55	57	59	61	62
5'1"	19	21	23	25	26	28	30	32	34	36	38	40	42	43	45	47	49	51	53	55	57	59	60
5'2"	18	20	22	24	26	27	29	31	33	35	37	38	40	42	44	46	48	49	51	53	55	57	59
5'3"	18	19	21	23	25	27	28	30	32	34	35	37	39	41	43	44	46	48	50	51	51	55	57
5'4"	17	19	21	22	24	26	27	29	31	33	34	36	38	39	41	43	45	46	48	50	51	53	55
5'5"	17	18	20	22	23	25	27	28	30	32	33	35	37	38	40	42	43	45	47	48	50	52	53
5'6"	16	18	19	21	23	24	26	27	29	31	32	34	36	37	39	40	42	44	45	47	48	50	52
5'7"	16	17	19	20	22	23	25	27	28	30	31	33	34	36	38	39	41	42	44	45	47	49	50
5'8"	15	17	18	20	21	23	24	26	27	29	30	32	33	35	36	38	40	41	43	44	46	47	49
5'9"	15	16	18	19	21	22	24	25	27	28	30	31	32	34	35	37	38	40	41	43	44	46	47
5'10"	14	16	17	19	20	22	23	24	26	27	29	30	32	33	34	36	37	39	40	42	43	44	46
5'11"	14	15	17	18	20	21	22	24	25	26	28	29	31	32	33	35	36	38	39	40	42	43	45
6'0"	14	15	16	18	19	20	22	23	24	26	27	28	30	31	33	34	35	37	38	39	341	42	43
6'1"	13	15	16	17	18	20	21	22	24	25	26	28	29	30	32	33	34	36	37	38	40	41	42
6'2"	13	14	15	17	18	19	21	22	23	24	26	27	28	30	31	32	33	35	36	37	39	40	41
6'3"	12	14	15	16	17	19	20	21	22	24	25	26	27	29	30	31	32	34	35	36	37	39	40
6'4"	12	13	15	16	17	18	19	21	22	23	24	26	27	28	29	30	32	33	34	35	37	38	39
6'5"	12	13	14	15	17	18	19	20	21	23	24	25	26	27	28	30	31	32	33	34	36	37	37
6'6"	12	13	14	15	16	17	18	20	21	22	23	24	25	26	27	28	29	30	31	32	34	35	37

■ UNDERWEIGHT ■ HEALTHY ■ OVERWEIGHT ■ OBESE

Waist Circumference:

This allows us to evaluate the visceral or organ fat accumulation and it is a very good indicator if your extra fat poses a health challenge.

To correctly measure waist circumference:
· Stand and place a tape measure around your middle, just above your hip bones
· Make sure the tape is horizontal around the waist
· Keep the tape snug around the waist, but not compressing the skin
· Measure your waist just after you breathe out

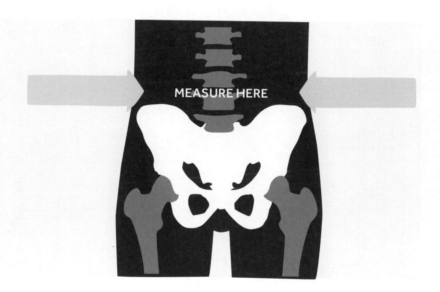

Your health is at risk if your waist is

Men	Over 94cm (about 37 inches)[2]
Women	Over 80cm (about 31.5 inches)[2]

Body Fat (Optional):

Tracking body fat (if you have an accurate source available) can offer a third source of measurement to assess your current weight management. It also helps you to see that you are losing fat and not muscle. Our Habits of Health programs are designed to minimize muscle loss. In Phases 2, 3, and 4, body composition becomes important to make sure you are building muscle and not just adding fat! For now, if you have access to a Bod Pod, DEXA, or someone who can help you use a set of skin calipers then you can also use this number to determine your current phase.

Note: Most electrical impedance devices are not very accurate but may give you a trending option.

SEX	FATNESS	BODY FAT% AGE 20 – 39	BODY FAT% AGE 40 – 59	BODY FAT% AGE 60 – 79
MALE	UNDERFAT	<8%	<11%	<13%
	NORMAL	8 – 20%	11 – 20%	13 – 25%
	OVERFAT	20 – 25%	22 – 25%	25 – 28%
	OBESE	>25%	>28%	>30%
FEMALE	UNDERFAT	<21%	<23%	<24%
	NORMAL	21 – 33%	23 – 34%	24 – 36%
	OVERFAT	33 – 39%	34 – 40%	36 – 42%
	OBESE	>39%	>40%	>42%

As recommended by The American Council on Exercise.

WHICH PHASE ARE YOU IN CURRENTLY?

Current Reality: Overweight or Obese
This is the current state most people find themselves in. If you are like two thirds of Americans, this is the current starting point for your journey.[3]

BMI >24.9

| Waist Circumference: | Male >40 | Female >35 |
| Body Fat (optional) | Male >18% | Female >25% |

We will start with a quick review of why you are here and then dive right into our weight-loss phase.

Phase I Weight Loss
Until BMI <25

| Until Waist Circumference: | Male <37 | Female <31.5 |
| Until Body Fat (optional) | Male <18% | Female <25% |

We will provide a couple of options to choose from to guide your weight loss journey.

Phase II Healthy Weight[4]
BMI <25

| Waist Circumference: | Male <37 | Female <31.5 |
| Body Fat (optional) | Male <18% | Female <25% |

The general guidelines for healthy weight is a body mass index (BMI) of 24.9 and a waist circumference of 32.5 inches for a woman and <37 inches for a man. Having a healthy fat composition is also important. It is age dependent, but as a general guideline we will want to lower your body fat to less than 25% for women and 18% for men.

We will move you into eating healthy for life. This will lead you into the second MacroHabit: Healthy Eating and Hydration.

Phase III Optimization

BMI <25

| Waist Circumference: | Male <31 | Female <31 |
| Body Fat (optional) | Male <18% | Female <25% |

This is an exciting phase when we will modify your food intake and energy expenditure to optimize your health and wellbeing for your age and lifestyle.

Phase IV Longevity[5]

BMI 21–24.9

| Waist Circumference: | Male <32 | Female <29 |
| Body Fat (optional) | Male <12% | Female <17–22% |

In the third part of the book, once you have optimized your health, we'll explore the things you can do to create Ultrahealth™ and potentially live a longer healthier life.

Your Current Reality (Starting Point)

Your current phase · · · · · · · · · · · · · · · · · ·
My BMI is · · · · · · · · · · · · · · · · · ·
My waist circumference is · · · · · · · · · · · · · · · · ·
My body fat is · · · · · · · · · · · · · · · (Optional)

The phase you are currently in is just that: a phase which you will move through as you get better at managing your weight. Do not get caught up on the absolute numbers of exactly what weight gives you a BMI of under 25. It is a target which, for most, will seem far off as you start but over time will seem much more doable.

In fact, for now, write down how much weight you would like to lose.

Write down a time in your life when you were healthier.

· ·

What has changed between now and then?

· ·

Write down what it would be like to be back to that healthy weight and wellbeing again? In terms of:

How you feel.

· ·

What you can do.

· ·

How you connect with friends and family.

· ·

Is there anything else you want to write down now that you know where you are going and why?

· ·

CREATING YOUR FIRST STRUCTURAL TENSION CHART FOR WEIGHT MANAGEMENT

We laid out how to create a structural tension chart in Element 03, *How Do You Create What You Want?*, and Part 1.3 and 1.4 in *Dr. A's Habits of Health* went into much greater detail about the power of this advancing structure in terms of creating a sustainable transformation in your weight and health.

In the desired result space on the following page, write down your healthy weight goal and, in the current reality space, write down your current weight. You should also put a date when you would like to be at your goal weight. Although, at this time, it is really just an estimate.

You will have many actions and steps that you will add to your secondary choices as we design the series of habits that will support you to reach and optimize your weight management.

For now, you can see the secondary choices or action steps I put down in my example as key tactics to create long-term weight management. We will explore these essential habits in the coming Elements. You can fill in these secondary choices now or work with your coach. You can continue to add to the list as we build your new story.

Structural Tension

CURRENT REALITY	SECONDARY CHOICES	DESIRED RESULT

Overweight 195lbs
Muffin Top
35 inches

Portion control 6 meals / day
Eating breakfast everyday
Low-glycemic carbs only
Lean and green / 1 daily
8 glasses of water/daily

Healthy
Weight 175lbs
Waist 33 inches

My example:

CURRENT REALITY	SECONDARY CHOICES	DESIRED RESULT

Summary

As we conclude this Element, it should be much clearer to you now how you can create a healthy weight without going on a diet. In fact, in the space provided below, write down the key differences in how we are structuring your path to a healthy weight and share your reflections below with your coach. Remember to review this often.

Three Key Points in Creating a Healthy Weight

Please spend some time and reflect on what each of these key points means to you at this stage of your journey, and make some notes to yourself. Also, share and review with your coach.

1. Your focus will be on building health, which is something you really want to create. This will motivate you each day. Remember, when you feel a little better a problem caused by emotional conflict will lose its energy and you will be much more likely to quit!

Notes:

2. You will use structural tension to help you to move from your current weight to your healthy weight. This will set up the actions to make this a reality.

Notes:

3. Your healthy weight will be built on learning a series of new habits which will create new behaviors that will make managing your weight much easier. Unlike willpower, which cannot be counted on during tough days, habits actually transform your previous actions into an automated state of new choices that require little thought and yet support long-term health.

Notes:

Starting in Element 07, *Creating A New Leptogenic World*, we shall develop our secondary choices or Habits of Health that will be integral in developing your mastery of the MacroHabit of Healthy Weight Management.

1 *The Big Number: 45 Million Americans Go On a Diet Each Year* – www.washingtonpost.com/national/health-science/the-big-number-45-million-americans-go-on-a-diet-each-year/2017/12/29/04089aec-ebdd-11e7-b698-91d4e359.

2 These guidelines are based on World Health Organization and National Health and Medical Research Council recommendations.

3 *Selected health conditions and risk factors, by age: United States, selected years 1988–1994 through 2015–2016* – www.cdc.gov/nchs/hus/contents2017.htm Table 53.

4 These guidelines are based on World Health Organization and National Health and Medical Research Council recommendations.

5 *A pooled analysis of waist circumference and mortality in 650,000 adults* – Cerhan JR, Mayo Clinic Proceedings. 2014;89:335./ Healthy weight: Assessing your weight. Centers for Disease Control and Prevention. www.cdc.gov/healthyweight/assessing/Index.html. Accessed May 10, 2017./Despres JP. Waist circumference as a vital sign in cardiology 20 years after its initial publication in the American Journal of Cardiology. American Journal of Cardiology. 2014;114:320.

ELEMENT 07:
CREATING A NEW LEPTOGENIC WORLD

Average time to complete: **1 week**

In Element 07, we will:

- Focus on making simple, powerful changes in your surroundings to make it easier to make healthy choices.
- Connect time and place with your food choices to optimize health.
- Explore and implement strategies to adjust your surroundings to create your leptogenic world.
- Feel amazing while making these changes!

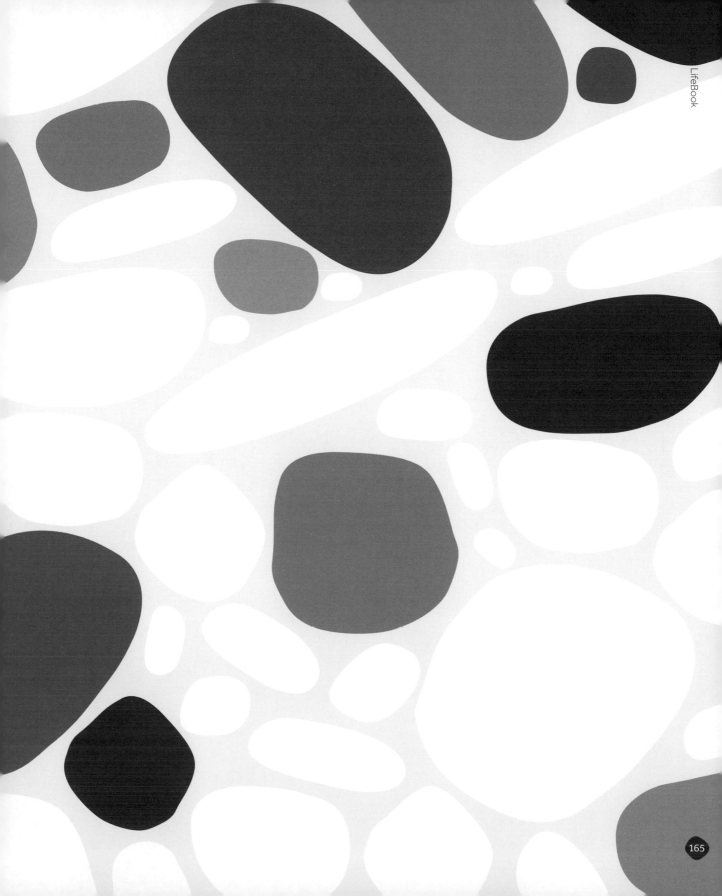

We live in an obesigenic world. This is a major reason why so many of us struggle with our weight. What if we could create a leptogenic world? Surroundings that help you become thin!

In this Element we will focus on making simple yet powerful changes in your surroundings to make healthy choices easier.

YOU BUY YOUR WILLPOWER AT THE GROCERY STORE

Most people think they make poor choices and gain weight because they lack willpower. They feel low and run to food for comfort.

But if you only bought healthy food at the grocery store and it's not close at hand you can instead *Stop*, *Challenge* and without any temptation *Choose* something healthy to eat or an activity on your health path.

Over the last several years we've discovered that willpower is not something you have or don't have but a resource that becomes depleted and, like a battery, can be recharged.

Remember your days in school during finals week when you were using your willpower to study and everything else suffered. My girls deteriorated from being perfectly turned out young women who made healthy food choices, to wearing sweatpants with no makeup and living on pizzas, cheeseburgers, and fries during exam week. When your willpower is depleted you are more likely to make your decisions based on your surroundings. After those tough days at the office, you are much less likely to make the effort to prepare a healthy meal or exercise, so it is important to eliminate potential unhealthy temptations when you're more vulnerable to poor choices.

In this Element we are going to introduce the habit of connecting time and place to coordinate where you are throughout the day and make small but critical changes in your surroundings. In the next Element this will evolve into your own personal habit clock. This will make it easier to do the Habits of Health and harder to fall into the Habits of Disease. We are, in essence, going to reduce the need to use willpower by creating a new healthy leptogenic world for you.

Review choice architecture in *Dr. A's Habits of Health* Part 1.7, *Optimizing Your Surroundings: Creating Your Microenvironment of Health*.

Let's spend some time and go through your day. We need to consider what we can do in your current day to put obstacles in place and to increase the steps needed to make bad choices. At the same time, we need to eliminate some steps to make it easier to make good choices.

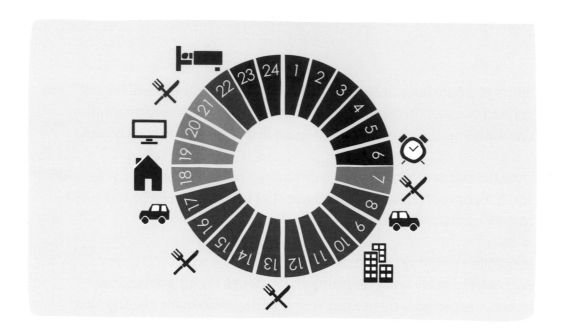

As you can see there are multiple times during the day and night when we can make interventions. We are going to concentrate on your bedroom, car, work space, meal times, and home (specifically the kitchen, pantry, and living spaces).

Food Environment Design in Your House

Let's start with the center of food storage, preparation, and serving in your kitchen and pantry. You will want to read Part 2.2 in *Dr. A's Habits of Health, Your Blueprint: Safe Weight Loss and Health Gain,* which will give you specific foods to toss as well as ones to replenish your shelves. I will discuss some basic principles and I want you to log what you have changed and whether it is helping you make better choices in your surroundings.

Pantry

The pantry is the place where most processed foods are stored. You will want to eliminate all ultra processed foods that have sugar or refined flour as the first few ingredients.

Why? In Part 1.1 in *Dr. A's Habits of Health, It's Not Your Fault That You're Struggling,* we talk about how the food industry encourages you to consume large amounts of ultra processed food by manipulating taste, salt, and texture. They are also responsible for creating sugar and refined flour addiction.

Important note here. Our fuelings* are designed to do the opposite. Because they are low-glycemic, portion-controlled, provide balanced protein and carbohydrates, have lower calorie, and work with the body to turn off the metabolic switches, they turn us into a fat-burning healthy state. These fuelings are healthy food designed to help you manage your weight and health.

Get rid of tempting foods that could sabotage your healthy eating choices and don't use this time to finish off that bag of cookies you find! If you have children or teenagers, this is a great chance to help them eat healthier too. But if you must keep foods for them in the house that don't fit your plan, put them in a low, out-of-the-way cupboard and don't go near them!

Start by getting rid of:
• white rice, white flour, white bread, crackers, rice cakes, croutons, and breadcrumbs
• hydrogenated vegetable oils, including hard or semi-soft margarine and shortenings such as Crisco, and partially hydrogenated oils
• white potato, potato mix, cornmeal, and corn grits
• refined cereals (whole grain is okay) and flavored oatmeal
• cookies, candy, cakes, and muffins
• chips, crackers, pretzels, and popcorn

* Fueling is used generically to mean giving the body energy through healthy food and also to describe our prepackaged meals.

Write down all of the things you are throwing out:

· ·

· ·

The key reason for writing down all of these unhelpful unhealthy foods can be summed up in one sentence: I don't eat these foods because I have chosen to create optimal health and wellbeing in my life.

This is a very different approach from when you may have told yourself that you couldn't eat these foods because they were not on your diet. Previously you may have said "can't" which creates a feedback loop that points out the restrictions and limitations of what you can and can not do. It sets you up for failure because you are, in essence, saying: I am being forced to do something I do not want to do.

If we go back to our hierarchy of choices then we are making secondary decisions because they support what is most important to us: Optimal health and wellbeing. You are giving your body a gift of health rather than a restriction of instant pleasure.

"Out of sight out of mind" plays out big time as we redesign your surroundings so you are no longer even having to make a decision. By the way, the same thing applies to going out to restaurants. Do not enter unhealthy eating establishments because even if they have healthy options you are putting your willpower to the test and that is a gamble we do not want to make in the Habits of Health Transformational System.

In this Element, we want to explore how we make everything healthy and supportive of wellbeing easier. We also want to eliminate or make it harder to make poor choices.

So let's start populating your pantry with healthy food such as olive oil. whole grains, high fiber breads and pitas, whole-wheat flour, walnuts, almonds, and pistachios, a variety of beans, and different spices and herbs. These are all healthy choices once you have reached your healthy weight.

(If you are in the weight loss phase your choices will be more limited than these healthy examples).

In fact, put below some of the things you can have in your pantry during weight loss Phase I (see Part 2.3 in *Dr. A's Habits of Health, The Catalyst to Reaching a Healthy Weight*):

E.g. Almonds, walnuts, pistachios

. . . .

. . . .

It is a good idea to run this list by your coach before you purchase the above items. Also, check the guide that comes with your fuelings.

List the fuelings you have in your pantry and start making notes of which ones you love, like, or want to pass on in future. I find that I settle into about a half dozen favorites that I will use for most of my fuelings and over time add or delete ones I get tired of (see Part 2.3 in *Dr. A's Habits of Health, The Catalyst to Reaching a Healthy Weight*).

. . . .

. . . .

One last note on choice architecture in your pantry, place the healthiest items at eye level and if you have other family members that are not yet eating healthy request that they place their processed foods either out of sight or in areas which require more work to reach.

Refrigerator

Here's what needs to go from the fridge:

- Whole-fat dairy products such as milk, cheese, yogurt, butter, cottage cheese, and mayonnaise
- Processed deli meats, bacon, hot dogs
- Sugary sodas and juices
- Beer and wine

- Foods high in calories, fat, or sugar, including peanut butter, jellies, and salad dressings (except low fat and low calorie)
- Sweet pickles, relish, ketchup
- Puddings, applesauce

Write down here all of the things you are tossing:

Describe how that feels:

Now fill your fridge back up with:

- Low-fat protein sources such as lean chicken and meats, tofu, hummus, and eggs
- Fresh vegetables (and vegetables for the freezer)
- Condiments such as mustards, pickles, and vinegars
- Mineral water, sparkling water, unsweetened ice tea
- Olives, capers
- Herbs and spices

In fact, list below some of the things you can have in your refrigerator during weight loss Phase I (see Part 2.3 in *Dr. A's Habits of Health, The Catalyst to Reaching a Healthy Weight*):

It is a good idea to run this list by your coach before you purchase the above items. Also, check the guide that comes with your fuelings.

Freezer

Here's what needs to go from the freezer:

- Frozen fruit with added sugar
- Frozen vegetables with seasoning that contains sugar
- Orange juice, lemonade, other fruit concentrates
- Bread, rolls, etc.
- Frozen entrees containing rice and pasta,
- Frozen pizza
- Frozen desserts, ice cream, sorbets, cakes, cookies

Write down all of the things you are tossing:

Describe how that feels:

Now fill your freezer back up with:

- Frozen vegetables like broccoli, spinach, cauliflower, green beans
- Unsweetened fruits like blueberries, peaches, raspberries, strawberries
- Frozen shrimp, fish, seafood without sauces/sugar
- Lean beef, poultry
- Veggie burgers from soy, beans, no grain potato, or sugar

In fact, list below some of the things you can have in your freezer during weight loss Phase I:

Preparation and Storage

In terms of preparation there are many ways we can use design to help us eat healthier.

One of the keys to eating less is to serve less and this can be accomplished in four very practical ways:

Smaller plates: Move from 12 inch to nine inch plates. We will discuss why this is so important in my healthy eating system for life.

Make a note of where and when you will change your plate size:

Check here when it is done. See Element 15, *How To Eat Healthy For Life,* which explains Dr. A's Healthy Eating System before making purchases.

Colored plates: When your plate color contrasts with your food the size of the portions sticks out and we sense we are eating more. When they blend in the amount does not register and we eat more. Buying green plates makes sense as its okay to eat bigger portions of green vegetables. During the weight loss phase filling half your plate with vegetables can help create fullness.

Serve from kitchen only: Put your portion on your plate and do not bring serving bowls for seconds to the dining table.

Use plates that are green and have a high color contrast with foods that need to be eaten in moderation only. For example, do not put rice or potatoes on a white plate.

Make a note of where and when I will change to this new behavior:

Make sure it is a consistent change

. . . .

. . . .

Large glasses of water with a pitcher of water for refill on the dining table: As we will discuss in a future Element always have a large glass of water with you including at the dining table. Our hunger can always be diminished by drinking more water.

Other design thoughts in your kitchen surroundings.
When storing leftovers, wrap any unhealthy food that family members have eaten in aluminum foil so it is not visible. And wrap your healthy leftovers in plastic wrap so they are visible. Also, store healthy food in bigger containers so they are more visible when going into refrigerator and unhealthy ones in smaller ones or I actually toss them. Once you have reached a healthy weight display a large bowl of fruit in a high trafficked area to encourage consumption. It cannot be said enough, do not bring anything into your house that is not healthy and good for you. To accomplish that make sure you are not hungry or stressed when you go to the grocery store. And only shop around the perimeter of the store.

One more word on emotions and stress: they stimulate areas of your brain that make you crave sugar, fat, and salt. When you start feeling that uneasy uncomfortable feeling I like to call the "icky sauce" coming on make sure you stop, drink some water, and remove yourself from any surrounding environment that has even the hint of unhealthy food.

When eating out keep the following in mind: *Keep portions in check by design.*

Car
In the morning on your way to work please avoid the Starbucks or Dunkin' Donuts drive through with the 500 calorie mocha or other fancy coffees and tempting muffins. Also avoid driving into or even by fast food joints, places like gas stations that sell snacks, and anywhere else that can tempt you such as Dairy Queens, juice bars, and so on.

Let's address eating out in general:

Restaurants

Restaurant servings have become out of control. An occasional treat is fine, but if you eat out often, you need to develop an overall strategy for portion control. Here are a few tips:

- Visualize the divisions on the nine-inch plate.
- Order two appetizers instead of an entrée, such as soup and a dinner salad, or shrimp cocktail.
- Split a meal with your dining companion.
- Don't rely on the chef or waiter to serve you the proper amount of food. Surveys show that people generally eat everything that's put in front of them, whether they wanted it or not.[1]
- Ask for a leftovers container right when you place your order. When your meal comes, eyeball your proper portion right away and put the rest into the box to take home.

More later but also: Stay away from cream sauces and soups, butter, oil, au gratin, breaded, Alfredo sauce, gravy, and anything battered or fried. Blackened entrees are usually dipped in butter or oil, covered with spices, and then pan fried with a higher probability of toxic effects on our health.

Don't be afraid to take charge of your meal. Choose only lean cuts of red meat such as loin and flank. If you're having chicken, remember that white meat contains less fat. Ask for your meat, fish, or poultry to be prepared with minimal oil and butter or prepared "light". Have the chef trim all excess fat before cooking and be sure to remove the skin from poultry before you eat.

Request that vegetables be steamed with no added sugar or butter. Optimal cooking methods are baked, broiled, grilled, poached, or steamed. And of course, fresh is best!

Let's now go to your bedroom:

Healthy Surroundings: Ready Your Bedroom

Creating an environment that optimizes sleep quality is critical to good health. In fact, several studies confirm that poor sleep directly contributes to poor eating habits.[2] We'll spend considerable time in Phase II on this MacroHabit both in *Dr. A's Habits of Health* and in a future Elements giving you some tips to improve your sleep, but right now here are a few simple steps to make your bedroom more conducive to healthy sleeping:

1. Organize your bedroom and put away clutter.

Done:

Describe how that feels:

2. If you have a TV in your bedroom, remove or unplug it.

Done:

Describe how that affects your sleep:

3. Choose a bedtime that means you get eight hours of sleep and stick with it.

Done:

Describe how that feels:

4. Keep your room cool while you sleep.

Done:

Describe how that feels:

5. Never eat in bed.

Decided:

Describe how that has changed your sleeping:

Now you understand the importance of making changes in your surroundings so you are no longer reliant on willpower to make good choices and stay away from bad ones.

List the three adjustments you have made to your surroundings that are making an immediate difference to your health and life:

1.

2.

3.

Make sure you review all your notes and this Element often. Also share it with your coach and spend time discussing how these possibilities will become a reality.

In Element 08, *Learning To Eat Every Three Hours,* we will explore eating every three hours as integral in you developing the mastery of the MacroHabit of Healthy Weight Management.

Notes to yourself:

Now that you have completed Element 07, Creating a New Leptogenic World write down your thoughts guided by the following questions:

What does this Element mean to you right now?

What does this Element give you the opportunity to reflect on?

What actions are you going to take as a result of this Element?

I encourage you to connect with your coach, so you can share your thoughts and actions as soon as possible.

Sharing your thoughts with your coach will help them become a reality.

Make sure you review all your notes and this Element often.

1 www.foodpsychology.cornell.edu/discoveries/92-clean-plate-club.

2 Matthew Walker, a UC Berkeley professor of psychology and neuroscience and senior author of the study published Tuesday, Aug 6 in the journal Nature Communications. University of Arizona Health Sciences researchers found that nighttime snacking and junk food cravings because of sleep difficulties are factors in medical problems. Their findings were presented at the 32nd Annual Meeting of the Associated Professional Sleep Societies LLC in Baltimore.

ELEMENT 08:
LEARNING TO EAT
EVERY THREE HOURS

Average time to complete: **1 week**

In Element 08, we will:

- Learn the value and benefits of eating every three hours.
- Identify the key to reaching a healthy weight.
- Use the Habits of Health Clock to create a fueling
  plan that works!
- Explore the ways that you can install the habit of eating
  every three hours.

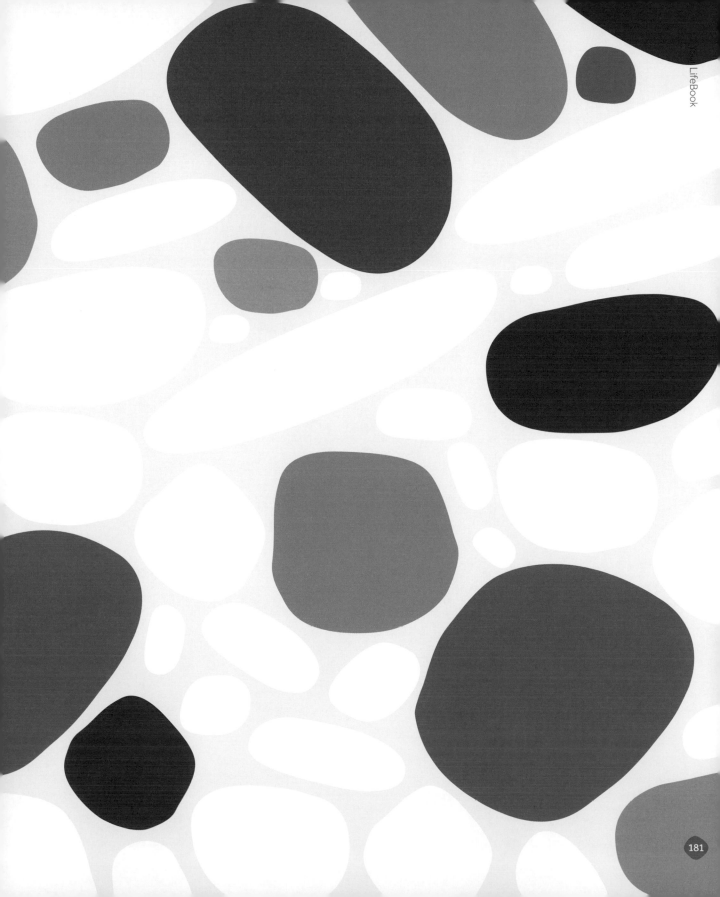

In an age where we barely have time to think you might find it curious that I am actually asking you to eat every three hours.

For over almost two decades now I have been recommending smaller feedings throughout the day and this simple Habit of Health stands out as being one of the most powerful in helping people create healthy weight management.

Many studies suggest that eating more frequently may offer benefits by decreasing hunger and food intake at subsequent meals. One study involving close to 2,700 women and men found that those who ate at least six times per day ate fewer calories, consumed healthier foods, and had a lower body mass index than those who ate fewer than four times over a 24-hour period.[1] Research has also shown that increased meal frequency has positive effects on cholesterol and insulin levels. In Part 2.2 in *Dr. A's Habits of Health, Your Blueprint: Safe Weight Loss and Health Gain,* I have provided a detailed explanation of all the benefits of smaller frequent meals. Some of the research over the last 10 years has challenged some of the benefits of eating frequent meals such as the effect on metabolism and the potential for overeating.[2] Yet, what I have found is if you learn the Habits of Healthy Eating System along with eating more frequently you have a proven system for long-term weight management.

We have discovered that sitting down to eating three meals a day in our modern world is very difficult. Eating so much food at a time is too much for many and the post-ingestion period creates slugginess. Also, waiting as many as six hours between meals can make you feel shaky, tired, and weak as they become hypoglycemic (low blood sugar). This is especially true in both prediabetics and diabetics as they do not handle fasting well.

On top of that we have found that those who avoid breakfast or wait too long between eating become over hungry and are then more likely to overeat. In fact, this is one of the reasons the popular trend towards fasting is so controversial as there are no long-term studies that show it is effective over time.[3] So we have used smaller feedings which we call fuelings throughout the day to ensure that your body has a constant source of healthy food to maintain energy and to keep the body in a balanced state of energy intake and utilization without overloading your digestion.

In addition, if you need to lose some weight to reach your healthy weight, we are able to insert three to five prepackaged fuelings along with the complementary whole food to adjust your total calories as needed so you are having six meals a day. This makes weight management in all phases (See Element 06, *Your Path To A Healthy Weight*) a breeze.

THE KEY TO REACHING AND MAINTAINING A HEALTHY WEIGHT IN OUR SYSTEM IS THE ABILITY TO EAT EVERY THREE HOURS.

One of the key strategies we will use throughout the next year is the idea of engineering an optimal day. We know that in order to help you transform your health and your wellbeing to reach all of your long-term goals, it will be all about your choices. And the more we can make better choices that support our journey and do them consistently every day, then we can automate these new behaviors into a series of Habits of Health.

We can strategize your long-term goals, but all you have available to you in terms of action is today.

As you will learn, our biological clock is no longer an effective device to run our day because of our modern, high-tech world, so we are going to build you a Habits of Health Clock.

The Habits of Health Clock is designed to build in routines and habits that serve you automatically to build more optimal days derived from the MacroHabits of Health which pave your path to optimal health and wellbeing.

In each appropriate Element, you will add MacroHabits, Habits of Health, and microHabits to improve your choices, and we will embed them into your day in a simple and convenient way.

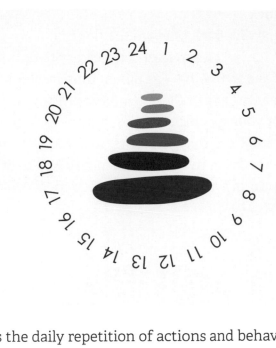

Remember, it is the daily repetition of actions and behaviors that will help you transform from your current state of health to your desired state of health and wellbeing.

You will notice that this is a 24 hour, 7 days a week, 52 weeks a year system that will build a new rhythm and create homeostasis for you over time. That means that your day will be integrated around what matters most to you in terms of your health and your wellbeing.

Habits of Health Clock

The eight-hour segment in dark blue are the hours you are enjoying high-quality sleep, which you will learn later is necessary to optimize your health, brain, mind, and wellbeing. The actual time can be adjusted to fit your chronotype (see Part 2.13 in *Dr. A's Habits of Health, Healthy Sleep and Unlimited Energy*) or your specific schedule, but the length of your sleep period should be pretty close to eight hours. You will see that there is an hour preceding your bedtime to transition from full on to off and in the morning to ramp up from sleep to being prepared for an optimal day.

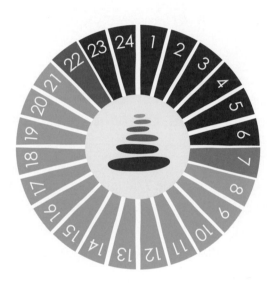

Fueling Schedule

At this point I have introduced you to your Habits of Health clock in advance of setting up your fueling schedule. Remember, you want to eat every three hours and should have your first fueling within 30 – 60 minutes of waking.

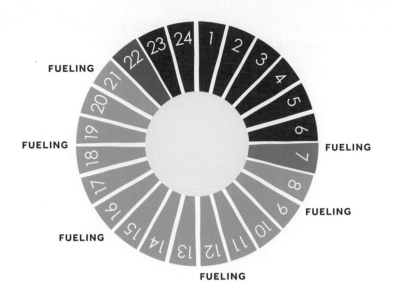

First Fueling:

Second Fueling:

Third Fueling:

Fourth Fueling:

Fifth Fueling:

Sixth Fueling:

The nice feature of the Habits of Healthy Fuelings is once you have adjusted your schedule to your particular lifestyle, you can use this new habit both in your weight loss as well as your health optimization. It is not like you need to vary the timing of your fuelings depending on what phase you are in.

Now let's look at how this new habit can be installed in a timely fashion using the Habits of Health Transformational cycle.

First, what cue will you use to eat every three hours?
(The Habits of Health App is ideal).

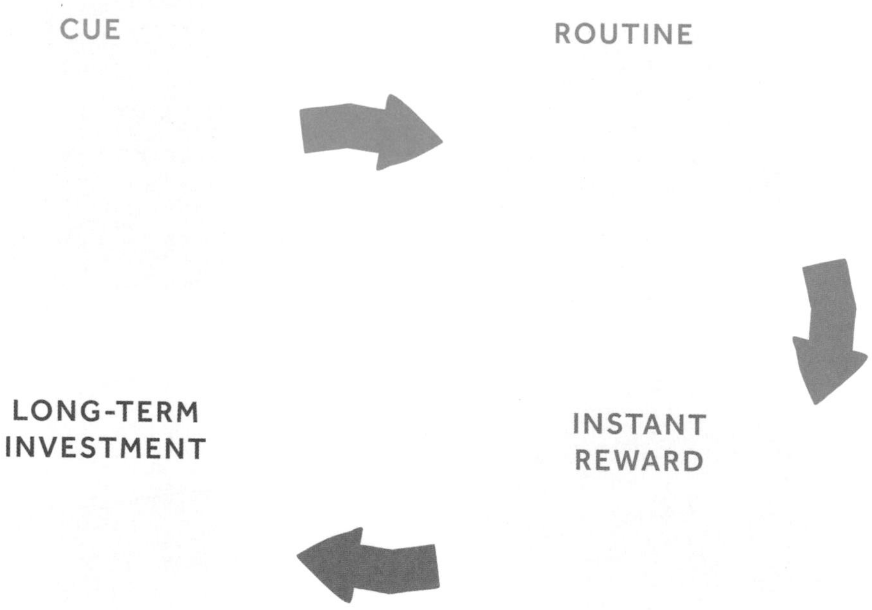

CUE

ROUTINE

LONG-TERM
INVESTMENT

INSTANT
REWARD

Describe what routine will you use to eat every three hours.
E.g. fuelings, location.

What is the instant reward you will receive from eating every three hours?
E.g. less hungry between meals, more energy, not as likely to overeat.

What is the long-term investment you will receive from eating every three
hours? E.g. better weight control, more productive at work, improving health.

Depending on what phase you are in or what plan you are using, which
we will discuss in the next Element, you will be eating either prepackaged
meals or healthy whole food fuelings in each of those six time periods.
As an example, on the Optimal Weight 5&1 plan®, which most of my clients
and patients choose, you will have a prepackaged fueling for five of your
fuelings and a lean and green meal for your sixth fueling.

This can be used at restaurants, while grocery shopping, and when traveling
because you will simply substitute it based on your current weight and BMI.
It just doesn't get any easier. It really sets you up for a pattern of healthy
eating for life.

Let's spend a moment to reflect on what we are learning and how it will
help you create a lifelong transformation and be an important part of your
weight management strategy:

Why is it important to eat every three hours?

Why is it important to have the Habits of Health clock to help guide your day?

What can you do to help remind you to eat every three hours until it becomes a habit?

Note: In addition to using the timer on your phone, the addition of the Habits of Health App will be very useful here. Not only will it help set up your schedule, but it will notify you when it is time to eat.

Now that you understand the importance and have decided to eat every three hours, let's jump to the next Element, which will help you decide what you will be eating!

Make sure you review all your notes and this Element often. Also, share it with your coach and spend time discussing how these possibilities will become a reality.

Notes to yourself:

Now that you have completed Element 08, *Learning To Eat Every Three Hours*, write down your thoughts guided by the following questions:

What does this Element mean to you right now?

What does this Element give you the opportunity to reflect on?

What actions are you going to take as a result of this Element?

I encourage you to connect with your coach, so you can share your thoughts and actions as soon as possible. Sharing your thoughts with your coach will help them become a reality. Make sure you review all your notes and this Element often.

1 *The Impact of Eating Frequency and Time of Intake on Nutrient Quality and Body Mass Index: The INTERMAP Study, a Population–Based Study* – Ghadeer S. Aljuraiban, Ph.D.; Queenie Chan, Ph.D.; Linda M. Oude Griep, Ph.D.; Ian J. Brown, Ph.D.; Martha L. Daviglus, MD.; Jeremiah Stamler, MD.; Linda Van Horn, Ph.D.; R. Paul Elliott, Ph.D. MBBS, FMedSci; Gary S. Frost, Ph.D.; RD Correspondence information about the author Gary S. Frost. Email the author Gary S. Frost of the INTERMAP Research Group.

2 *Nibbling versus Gorging: Metabolic Advantages of Increased Meal Frequency* – David J.A. Jenkins, M.D., Ph.D.; Thomas M.S. Wolever, M.D., Ph.D.; Vladimir Vuksan, Ph.D.; Furio Brighenti, Ph.D.; Stephen C. Cunnane, Ph.D.; A. Venketeshwer Rao, Ph.D.; Alexandra L. Jenkins, R.P.DT.; Gloria Buckley, M.SC.; Robert Patten, M.D.; William Singer, M.B., B.S.; Paul Corey, Ph.D. and Robert G. Josse, M.B., B.S. N Engl J Med 1989; 321:929 – 934.

3 • Skipping breakfast to lose weight makes you fatter and far more likely to raid the vending machine
   • Skipping meals changes the way brain recognises food
   • Makes calorie-laden treats such as chocolate much more tempting
   A recent study of the health and diet habits of 2,500 pairs of teenaged twins, siblings, or half-siblings showed that those whose family skipped meals were more likely to be obese or overweight. Duke Diet and Fitness Center Duke University.
   Skipping Breakfast results in Overeating Though out the Day "People who regularly skip breakfast likely have an overall unhealthy lifestyle," said study author Valentin Fuster, MD, Ph.D., MACC director of Mount Sinai Heart and editor-in-chief of the Journal of the American College of Cardiology. Br J Nutr. 2012 Jun;107(12):1823 – 32. doi: 10.1017/S0007114511005022. Epub 2011 Sep 29. Breakfast glycaemic index and cognitive function in adolescent school children. S.B. Cooper, S. Bandelow, M.L. Nute, J.G. Morris, M.E. Nevill.

ELEMENT 09:
HOW DO YOU USE FUELINGS TO REACH A HEALTHY WEIGHT?

Average time to complete: **1 week**

In Element 09, we will:

- Explore the value and simplicity of packaged fuelings when eating every three hours.
- Create a simple and convenient fueling plan for the weight loss phase of your journey.
- Understand the value and timing of eating whole foods.

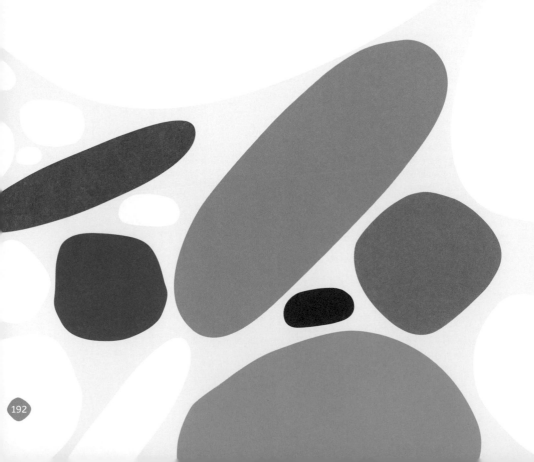

In the last Element, we discussed the importance of creating a habit of eating every three hours. In this Element, we will focus on what exactly you are eating every three hours.

One of the key obesity researchers, Danziger, once stated that if we could overcome the psychological and logistical barriers, we could eradicate obesity in a matter of months. That may be a bit of an exaggeration, but his point is well taken. And it is at the heart of the Habits of Healthy Weight Management strategic plan.

In terms of addressing the psychological aspects, as you have seen in the Elements you have already completed, we have spent a bunch of time going over managing our emotions, our thoughts, our choices, and our relationships to help you become the dominant force in your life by taking responsibility.

Here we are going to introduce a powerful way to overcome the logistical barriers to creating a healthy weight and eating pattern.

Eating something healthy every three hours that will optimize your nutrition and, at the same time, help you create healthy weight is asking most people to step way out of their comfort zone. They are not equipped with the knowledge or the skills to do it on their own.

I have found that for most people, including myself, having planned prepared meals is the key to success. But what is the best way of accomplishing this?

PACKAGED FUELINGS

Having our prepackaged meals to place in those three-hour fueling intervals has many advantages. (There are other brands available, but we are the only one that comes with a free coach, this Habits of Health Transformational System, and our amazing community of support.)

Important advantages and why I choose the OPTAVIA® prepackaged meals for our fuelings:

1. They are the best in class, provide all of the necessary vitamins and minerals, balanced proteins, and carbohydrates, and are relatively low fat.
2. The meals have amazing variety to avoid taste fatigue but, at the same time, their nutritional footprint is nearly identical. This allows them to be used in combination with a healthy lean and green to help create a mild fat-burning state and progressive healthy weight loss.
3. Their nutritional footprint creates the ideal state of metabolism because they are all low-glycemic, which turns off the metabolic switches that create fat storage. And the healthy protein source helps to protect your muscle and avoid eating saturated fatty sources of protein.
4. They are portable and easily prepared to overcome any logistical barriers, including traveling.
5. They can be used long-term to provide a solution to your every three-hour fueling when you are unable to cook or prepare a whole food meal as you move into the optimization and longevity phases.

You can see there are many advantages to starting your weight management with the prepackaged fuelings because they are easy, goof-proof, and extremely cost-effective.

While whole foods are better for you, our first area of focus needs to be getting down to a healthy weight.

Rest assured, our goal over time as you progress on your journey is to have most of your daily fuelings come from whole food. The problem is you probably have whole food available to you now, but has it been effective in helping you reach a healthy weight in a reasonable period of time?

For most, the answer is "no" simply because eating whole food does not teach you to pick low-glycemic carbohydrates, healthy proteins, and healthy fats in the right proportions necessary to lose weight.

And of course, coming back to the logistics, whole foods are often unavailable or too expensive, or people don't have the time or inclination to prepare them.

Instead, because we are rushed for time, most of us eat unhealthy processed food full of sugar, refined grains, and salt because they are convenient, cheap, taste good, and are everywhere.

So yes, we are going to teach you how to eat healthy for life, and most of that food will be whole food. Right now though we are going to start with baby steps and build the habits that will make your healthy eating transformation permanent.

Actually, with our lean and green, we are going to start your healthy whole food introduction right from the beginning, but we are going to do it at a simple, easy to do, and prepared pace. Our prepackaged fuelings provide a powerful tool to help do the healthy lifting as we start your weight loss journey. It is the first in a series of microHabits teaching you the necessary behavioral changes to carry you to a healthy weight and beyond.

Over time and in these next few Elements, I will help you to learn and use some simple tools to make your journey to healthy eating through fuelings a breeze.

If you decide to take on the whole learning curve at once, we will show you how to do that as well, but the rate of success will usually be lower.

Phase I: Weight Loss Phase

There are two general ways to use fuelings to reach a healthy weight. The first is using the prepackaged meals that I mentioned earlier. The second method is to prepare everything with whole food. Although this presents numerous challenges to overcome unless you have a solid understanding of nutrition; however, I will make these solutions available in Part 2.6 of *Dr. A's Habits of Health, Building Healthy Meal Plans for Optimal Health*.

The Optimal Health 5&1 Plan® has a long and successful history, and I have used it for the last 17 years as the most effective means to consistently help people lose weight in a safe and easy way.

It is really one of the first real ***microHabits of Health*** that I have utilized to help people of all backgrounds finally have a consistent, manageable way to lose weight. I have also found it the easiest way to help people overcome any challenges (logistics) in their current lifestyle. It's a fast, hassle-free, easy way to learn the Habits of Health of eating six meals every three hours.

You will lose weight quickly and safely. Also, as you feel better and have more energy, it creates what I like to call the teachable moment when you will be even more eager to learn the other habits necessary for success. It's a great catalyst and could not be easier.

It basically has three components:

1. You choose five prepackaged meals to use during the day
2. You prepare one lean and green meal (details below)
3. You use the Habits of Health Clock to space the six fuelings out over an every three-hour time period

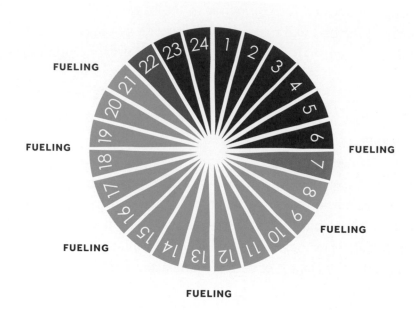

You pick where you want to have your lean and green during the day. Most people have it as their evening fueling with their family or as part of the rest of the family's prepared meal.

What is so amazing about this simple schedule is that once you have reached a healthy weight, you will simply substitute some of the packaged fuelings with whole food so you do not have to change your behavior. This leads to consistent healthy eating.

The Lean and Green

As I mentioned, one of the first things we added to the prepackaged foods was one meal using whole foods. The reason for this is to start training people to eat healthier in their food choices as well as maintaining their normal gut flora so that we are always stimulating a healthy gut.

The lean and green also makes sure that you are receiving healthy fat, which is important in maintaining absorption of fat soluble vitamins, normal digestion, and gallbladder function.

You will have a lean piece of meat, poultry, or fish along with a green vegetable or salad.

Write down some of the reasons we are using prepackaged fuelings to start our weight management journey.

Daily Schedule for Fuelings

One will be your lean and green. You can download copies at HabitsofHealth.com.

First Fueling: Lean and Green: (1 of the 6 fuelings)

Second Fueling:

Third Fueling:

Fourth Fueling:

Fifth Fueling:

Sixth Fueling:

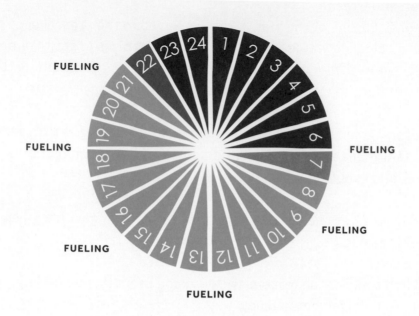

I would suggest that you take a couple of these daily fueling schedules and sit down with your coach and review them. For more information on lean and green, refer to the OPTAVIA® Guide which can be downloaded at OPTAVIA.com.

You now have an amazingly easy schedule and system to start gaining control over your weight and your health. As mentioned earlier, if for some reason you can not use the prepackaged fuelings, you can use the same schedule and use the fueling suggestions outlined in Part 2.6 in the Dr. A's *Habits of Health, Building Healthy Meal Plans for Optimal Health*. Yet almost everybody will find our Optimal Health 5&1 Plan® the easiest and most effective way to safely and consistently lose weight.

Now you understand the importance of eating every three hours. Make sure you review all your notes and this Element often. Also share it with your coach and spend time discussing how these possibilities will become a reality.

In the next Element we will address some of the important factors to pay attention to while you are reaching your healthy weight.

Notes to yourself:

Now that you have completed Element 09, *How Do You Use Fuelings To Reach A Healthy Weight?*, write down your thoughts guided by the following questions:

What does this Element mean to you right now?

What does this Element give you the opportunity to reflect on?

What actions are you going to take as a result of this Element?

I encourage you to connect with your coach, so you can share your thoughts and actions as soon as possible.

Sharing your thoughts with your coach will help them become a reality.

Make sure you review all your notes and this Element often.

ELEMENT 10:
THE KEY ROLE OF HYDRATION IN REACHING A HEALTHY WEIGHT

Average time to complete: **1 week**

In Element 10, we will:

- Discover some of the important factors to pay attention to while you are reaching your healthy weight.
- Realize the importance of water on your journey to Optimal Health.
- Identify the best ways to hydrate during weight loss.
- Provide you with the tools to plan and track your hydration as it develops into another Habit of Health.

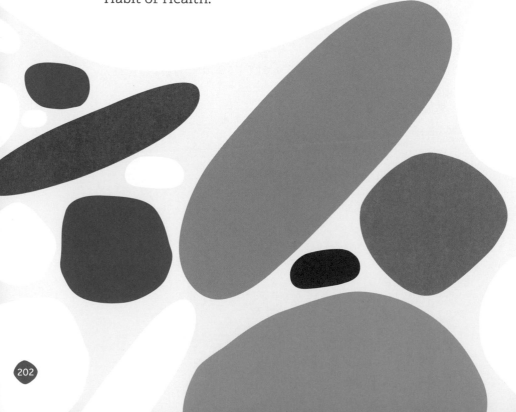

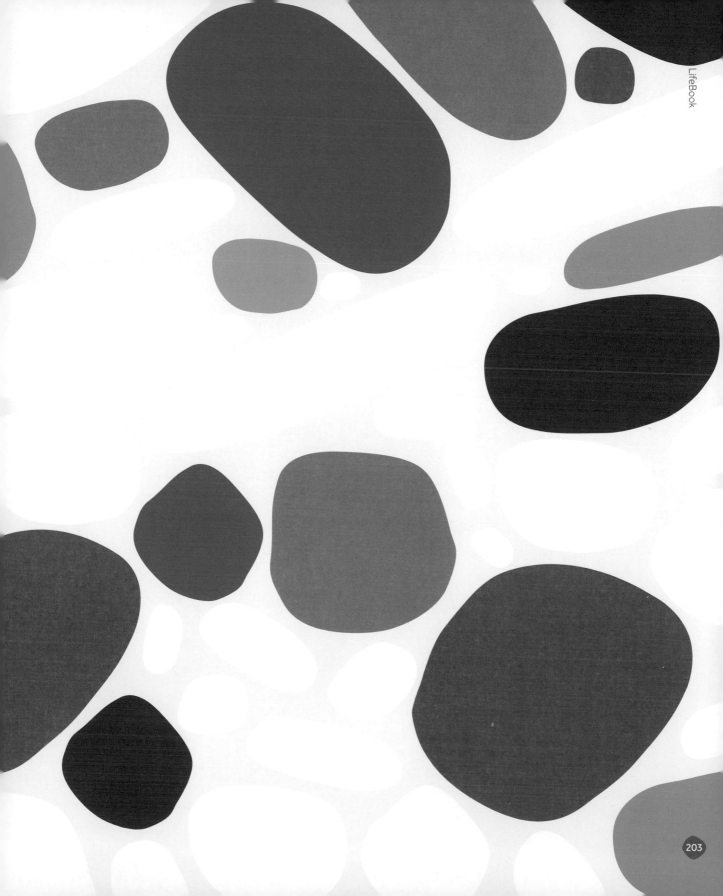

Water is a critical component of your body, making up between 55 and 60% of your weight.[1] Your body can't store water—unlike fat—so you need to replenish it often. That's why drinking eight (eight-ounce) glasses a day is a core Habit of Health.

Water plays a key role in supporting health, particularly during weight loss, when it helps remove toxins and other unhealthy substances stored in your fat cells. Being well-hydrated helps all your organs and systems function properly. In fact, every function in your body takes place in water. It's the solvent that moves nutrients, hormones, antibodies, and oxygen through your bloodstream and lymphatic system, and removes waste. And of course it's essential to your kidneys' ability to filter and eliminate metabolic byproducts and toxins. If you don't drink enough, your body is forced to recycle dirty water, diminishing the efficiency of every metabolic function.

What you may not realize is that we actually lose nearly 12 cups of water every day: two cups through perspiration, six cups through urine, two to four through breathing, and nearly one cup through the soles of our feet! And in high altitudes or dry environments, you lose even more, so you can get dehydrated in a hurry.[2]

How much water should I drink? It is recommended that you drink eight (eight-ounce) glasses each and every day.* This should be your guide unless you have a specific medical condition that requires you to restrict your fluid intake, such as renal failure or severe congestive heart failure, or if you've recently performed intense physical activity in a hot environment, in which case you should consume an electrolyte-enriched drink.

During Phase I of your weight loss plan, there are even more good reasons to make a conscious effort to drink your eight glasses a day.

Here are a few:
• It's calorie free, but helps you feel full and satisfied.
• It keeps you from overeating. Studies have shown that when we feel hungry, 30% of the time our bodies are actually signaling for water.[3]
• It facilitates the removal of toxins such as pesticides and preservatives from your cells.
• It prevents dehydration as your body eliminates excess salt and water from a diet of too much processed food.
• It minimizes or eliminates fatigue, lack of energy, headaches, and unclear thinking.
• It speeds up metabolism. A recent study showed that drinking two 8-ounce glasses of cold water increased metabolic rate by 30% for 90 minutes.[4]
• It helps your liver convert fat to energy.
• It compensates for the loss of glycogen stores as you lose weight.

* Author's note : The eight (eight-ounce) glasses is really an arbitrary number which is generally recommended to be a safe yet adequate amount.

OPTIMAL HYDRATION DURING WEIGHT LOSS

We know that proper hydration is critical for long-term optimal health and wellbeing. It affects not just our physiology but also our ability to think and allows our mind to function at the highest level.

We are going to take this very basic daily action and make sure you are building this key Habit of Health early on and placing it in your mason jar daily. As simple a task as it seems, 40% of Americans drink less than half of the recommended amount of water daily according to a 2013 public statement made by White House nutritional policy advisor Sam Kass.[5] This was based on the recommended daily consumption of water of approximately 64 ounces. Because most people struggle to drink a large quantity at one time, it makes sense to do this in eight-ounce increments throughout your waking hours.

In order to set this up, let's assess your current reality using our structural tension chart.

How many ounces of water do you currently drink on average per day?

ounces per day / current reality

CURRENT REALITY   **SECONDARY CHOICES**   **DESIRED RESULT**

If your desired outcome is 64 ounces (eight glasses of eight ounces each), a day of water and you currently are only drinking four glasses, it is important to work out what you can do to fill the gap.

These are the secondary choices you can make:

Use the Habits of Health App to remind you when to drink extra water.

Keep a large glass of water or water bottle nearby, including at your desk or in your car for whenever you leave home.

Use the OPTAVIA® Purposeful Hydration™ product to pick a morning, afternoon (twice), and an evening time to rehydrate.

What other choices can you make to get you up to the required 64 ounces?

What's the best source for my eight glasses a day?

Plain water is the best beverage for quenching thirst—it's cheap, calorie free, and contains no sugar, caffeine, or other additives. Tap water should be filtered first, however, to remove chlorine and other contaminants.

HEALTHY HYDRATION CHOICES BEYOND WATER

Below is a list of healthy choices to keep yourself hydrated. Teas, both hot and iced, have all kind of health benefits, but make sure you do not add milk, which inactivates the healthy phenolic compounds and—naturally—don't add sugar. Green tea, in particular, is full of health benefits: from decreasing inflammation and preventing cancers to improving your learning and memory.

Studies show many benefits of coffee due to its high level of antioxidants. They have proved that it decreases depression, reduces the risk of some cancers, and may help you live longer. It may also slow down cognitive decline, boost mood, increase stamina, and even protect against adult diabetes.[6]

And by the way, coffee and tea are not diuretics!

Coffee is a diuretic—it makes you go to the bathroom more often, so it must dehydrate you, right? Well, not so. Turns out that this idea dates back to a 1928 study, and it wasn't exactly rigorous research. Nonetheless, the results spread like wildfire and, ever since, caffeine has been considered a diuretic. Now, a recent study finds that coffee—and caffeine in other drinks— won't in fact cause dehydration.[7]

Infusers that are designed to provide additional vitamins, minerals, or other healthy supplementation are a great way to purposefully make sure your body is adequately hydrated throughout the day and evening. It's important that any infusers you use have minimal calories. As mentioned earlier, we have a purposeful hydration system that supplements as well as makes it easier to fulfill your habit of drinking eight glasses of water a day.

HEALTHY HYDRATION

- **Purified water**
- **Bottled water**
- **RO water**
- **Tea**
- **Coffee**
- **Infused water (calorie free)**

Pick which sources of hydration you are using currently or you are going to add to make sure you are getting your 64 ounces a day.

Note: Don't use thirst to guide your water intake! Thirst is a late warning symptom of dehydration. Waiting until you're thirsty to drink means that your body has been functioning at less than optimal efficiency for several hours.

How do I know if I'm not drinking enough? If you start feeling tired, have trouble thinking, develop a headache, or notice that your urine is darker than usual, these are late-stage signs that you need to drink more water! (Urine should be almost colorless unless you've just taken vitamins.)

UNHEALTHY CHOICES BEYOND WATER

One of the Habits of Disease is consuming sugary sodas, fruit drinks, and the many sweet beverages out there with added sugar or syrups and concentrates.

Half of the U.S. population consumes at least one sugary drink a day even when excluding fruit juice, diet soda, sweetened milks, and sweet tea![8] These sugary drinks can lead to diabetes and some forms of cancer. Each sugary drink you consume increases your risk of heart disease by almost 20%. It is estimated that 180,000 people a year lose their lives by consuming these sickening sweet elixirs![9]

The drinks on the list below not only stimulate insulin and drive glucose into the fat cells, worsening your weight issues, but will actually make it harder to stay hydrated!

In addition, alcoholic beverages also create a diuretic response and can aggravate dehydration. A good policy is if you are going to drink alcohol match each drink with a glass of water. And keep a restroom or bush in close proximity!

UNHEALTHY HYDRATION

- Fruit juices
- Sodas
- Almond, coconut, flax milks
- Diet soda
- Energy drinks
- Sports drinks
- Alcohol

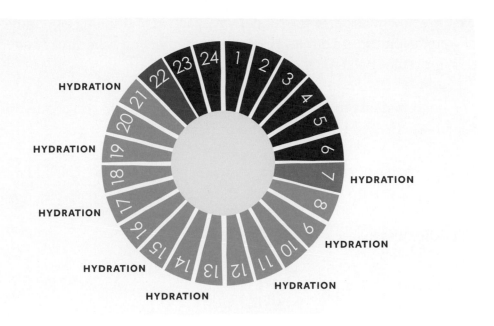

So let's conclude this chapter by purposefully adding eight times a day where we can make sure we are having a hydration break on our Integrated Habits of Health Clock. You can also use the clock to check each time you drink eight ounces or more of water to assess your current reality.
You can download copies at HabitsofHealth.com.

First Hydration:

Second Hydration:

Third Hydration:

Fourth Hydration:

Fifth Hydration:

Sixth Hydration:

Seventh Hydration:

Eighth Hydration:

We have now considered the fundamental action of drinking eight ounces of water eight times a day and evaluated whether you have already adopted this important habit or whether you need to work on it.

The habit installer in the Habits of Health App can help you create this valuable action and make it a Habit of Health for you.

What are some of the other things you are going to do to track and make sure we get you up to the 64-ounce threshold as soon as possible.

List other ways:

As we mentioned earlier, this habit is extremely important as your body starts shifting its metabolic machinery and storage to burn fat and empty your fat cells, which store toxins and other undesirable products. The best way to flush those from your system immediately is to make sure you are properly hydrated at all times.

Now you understand the importance of proper hydration!

Make sure you review all your notes and this Element often.

Also share it with your coach and spend time discussing how these possibilities will become a reality.

In the next Element, we will address how to start learning to eat healthy when buying food as you are zoning in on reaching your healthy weight.

Notes to yourself:

Now that you have completed Element 10, *The Key Role of Hydration in Reaching A Healthy Weight*, write down your thoughts guided by the following questions:

What does this Element mean to you right now?

What does this Element give you the opportunity to reflect on?

What actions are you going to take as a result of this Element?

I encourage you to connect with your coach, so you can share your thoughts and actions as soon as possible. Sharing your thoughts with your coach will help them become a reality. Make sure you review all your notes and this Element often.

1 *Percentage of Body Weight from Water* – H.H. Mitchell, Journal of Biological Chemistry 158.

2 *Clinician's Pocket Reference, 11th Edition.* Copyright © 2007 – Leonard G. Gomella. Published by The McGraw-Hill Companies.

3 *Physiol Behav* – 2010 Apr 26; 100(1): 22 – 32. Published online 2010 Jan 11. doi: [10.1016/j.physbeh.2009.12.026]. PMCID: PMC2849909 NIHMSID: NIHMS175763 PMID: 20060847.

4 *Water-induced Thermogenesis. Hunger and Thirst: Issues in Measurement and Prediction of Eating and Drinking* – J Clin Endocrinol, Metab. Richard D. Mattes, MPH, Ph.D., RD, 2003 Dec;88(12):6015 – 9.

5 That magic elixir is water, and some Americans just don't drink enough of it. Experts from the U.S. Centers for Disease Control and Prevention found in 2013 that 43% of adults drink less than four cups of it per day. This figure includes 7% of American adults who drink no water at all. Mar 7, 2016.

6 *The Impact of Caffeine on Mood, Cognitive Function, Performance and Hydration: a Review of Benefits and Risks* – C. H. S. Ruxton first published: 13 February 2008, www.doi.org/10.1111/j.1467 – 3010.2007.00665.x, Association of Coffee Consumption With Total and Cause Specific Mortality in 3 Large Prospective Cohorts. Rob M. van Dam, and Frank B. Hu originally published16 Nov 2015Circulation. 2015;132:2305 – 2315, Footnotes for Coffee, brewed from grounds, prepared with tap water, Source: Nutrient data for this listing was provided by USDA SR-21. Each "~" indicates a missing or incomplete value.

7 *The American Journal of Clinical Nutrition*, 2016, Mar 1; 103(3): 717 – 723, Pages 717 – 723, www.doi.org/10.3945/ajcn.115.114769, www.nutritiondata.self.com/facts/beverages/3898/2#ixzz5VHSBpNoD.

8 A Gallup poll reveals that 48% of surveyed Americans—nearly half!—drink soda on a daily basis. What's more, among those who drank soda, the average daily intake was 2.6 glasses per day.Jul 25, 2012.

9 *Sweetened Beverages and Coronary Artery Disease* – DeKonig Circulation 125(14)1735 – 1741, Wadeet al Sugary drinks linked to 180,000 deaths world wide CNN Health, 013/03/19//health.sugary-drinks.

ELEMENT 11:
HOW DO YOU EAT HEALTHY BEYOND FUELINGS?

Average time to complete: **1 week**

In Element 11, we will:

- Start learning to eat healthy when buying food as you are zoning in on reaching your healthy weight.
- Understand the importance of your lean and green meal.
- Discover how to create a new four-part shopping list that supports your Habits of Health transformation.

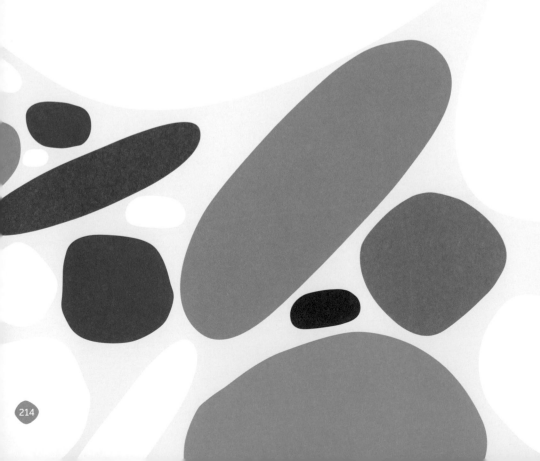

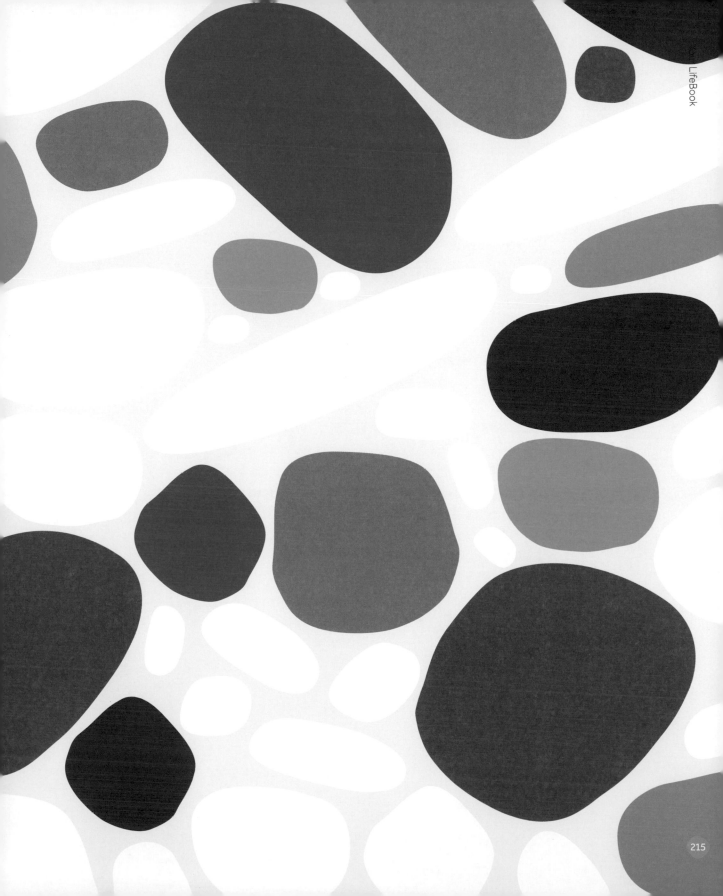

At this point, most of you are probably on your way to reaching a healthy weight using our prepackaged meals. You have chosen a strategy that is effective, easy to use, fits into your busy schedules, and is helping you to consistently lose weight and improve your health. I believe that fuelings are the easiest way to enter the path to optimal health.

This is also allowing you to start building new Habits of Health that are supportive not just during your weight loss, but they will also form a permanent part of your new automated way of making healthier choices.

Most importantly, the fuelings are providing you with a balance of high-quality protein, complex carbohydrates, probiotics, and 24 vitamins and minerals to protect your body and help you feel full and satisfied. And because they give you a scientifically determined dose of energy—between 90 and 110 calories per dose—they make it much easier to control your energy intake. So we have turned you into a fat-burning machine as you lose weight safely and effectively.

Our goal goes way beyond reaching a healthy weight and extends all the way to optimal health and wellbeing.

In order for that goal to become a reality, I am going to help you develop a complete healthy eating strategy to support you for the rest of your life, including advice on how to choose groceries, select from a restaurant menu, and cook a quick, low-glycemic meal. Fuelings can give you just the boost you need to get started on your journey to permanent weight loss and optimal health—just as I did.

If you are currently in Phase I and focused on reaching a healthy weight you are probably eating one lean and green meal a day. (Unless your needs require you to eat more than one.)

THE IMPORTANCE OF YOUR LEAN AND GREEN

Think of this meal as your training wheels to making healthier food choices.

At this point, all of your other meals are coming from our prepackaged fuelings unless you are preparing all your fuelings yourself.

A great way to build your new story and start to dramatically change your long-term weight management is to use your lean and green as the first *microHabit* of healthy eating for life.

We are removing all the unhealthy store-bought processed food from your diet and are now helping you make relatively simple healthy food choices. We will build on this so by the time you have reached your healthy weight, most (if not all) of your food choices that you make at the store and when you are out at restaurants will be healthy ones.

This approach also allows your body to continue to use all of its digestive functions, including enzymes, bile release, and the breakdown live food, so that your body doesn't miss a beat!

Let's review what you are eating and how to make great choices when at the store.

SHOPPING FOR YOUR LEAN AND GREEN

If you haven't had much experience selecting healthy proteins and vegetables, you may want to take a bit of time to ask the butcher or produce department for help. I learned a large amount just by asking store employees which items were fresh, healthy, and locally produced. Once you have it down, you should be able to get your weekly shopping done in no more than 15 minutes.

Your shopping list should include selections from these four major groups:

1. Lean protein
2. Healthy fats and oils
3. Green vegetables and salad
4. Healthy snacks and condiments

During Phase I, or the weight loss period, you will not be eating fruit or grains. We will add these during transition and beyond. Let's actually write down what choices you are currently making in each list and look for opportunities to improve.

1. Lean Protein

Shopping for protein is a great opportunity to try out new food sources, flavors, and recipes, and to learn a very specific Habit of Health. By choosing the leanest meats, experimenting with meat alternatives, and increasing your variety of fish and seafood, you're lowering and even eliminating unhealthy fats while adding healthy omegas to create a powerful, nutritious meal. To keep that fat content low, you'll be grilling, baking, broiling, or poaching your selections. And to make it easier for you to choose the leanest options, I've devised a color-coded system that takes you from lean (light green) to leanest (dark green). Here's a rundown of your Lean and Green protein sources.

Seafood

When you eat fish, you're choosing a great protein source and significantly reducing your risk of disease. Eating fish one to three times a week is an important Habit of Health and can have a profound impact on your wellbeing over time. In fact, one serving of fish a week may reduce your risk of fatal heart attacks by 40%![1]

What seafood do you currently choose?

What adjustments can you make to your choice of fish and shellfish using the diagram below?

LEAN (>9g FAT) 5 OZ PORTION; NO ADDITIONAL FAT SERVINGS	LEANER (6 – 9g FAT) 6 OZ PORTION; ADD ONE ADDITIONAL FAT SERVINGS	LEANEST (6g FAT) 7 OZ PORTION; ADD TWO ADDITIONAL FAT SERVINGS
• Salmon • Tuna (bluefin steak) • Farmed catfish • Mackeral, herring	• Swordfish • Trout • Halibut	• Cod, flounder, haddock, orange roughy, wild halibut, grouper, tilapia, mahi mahi • Tuna (yellowfin) canned in water • Wild catfish • Crab, scallops, shrimp, lobster

Meat and Poultry

It's important to lower your consumption of red meat and eat more fish, white-meat poultry (skinless), legumes such as beans, and low-fat or non-fat dairy. But if you're like me and once in a while need that savory taste of meat, just minimize the amount of saturated fat so you can enjoy this great protein source and still stay healthy.

What meat and poultry do you currently choose?

What adjustments can you make to your choice of meat and poultry using the diagram below?

LEAN (>9g FAT) 5 OZ PORTION; NO ADDITIONAL FAT SERVINGS	LEANER (6 – 9g FAT) 6 OZ PORTION; ADD ONE ADDITIONAL FAT SERVINGS	LEANEST (6g FAT) 7 OZ PORTION; ADD TWO ADDITIONAL FAT SERVINGS
• Lean beef, beef steak, roast and ground beef • Lamb • Pork chop and pork tenderloin • Ground turkey or other 80 – 88% lean meat	• Breast or white-meat turkey or chicken without skin • Ground turkey or other meat: 95 – 97% lean	• Buffalo, elk, deer • Ground turkey or other meat: 98% or >

Meat Alternatives

If you'd like to eliminate meat from your diet, or just reduce the amount you eat, there are some great meatless options available. I recommend that you stick with the choices on the list, but if you do find an alternative you'd like to try, please make sure it contains no added sugar.

What meat alternatives do you currently choose?

What adjustments can you make to your choice of meat alternatives using the diagram below?

LEAN (>9g FAT) 5 OZ PORTION; NO ADDITIONAL FAT SERVINGS	LEANER (6 – 9g FAT) 6 OZ PORTION; ADD ONE ADDITIONAL FAT SERVINGS	LEANEST (6g FAT) ADD TWO ADDITIONAL FAT SERVINGS
• 3 Whole eggs (limit to once per week) • 15oz Tofu, firm or soft variety	• 15oz Tofu, extra firm • 2 Whole eggs plus 4 egg whites • Add 1 additional fat serving	• 14 Egg whites • 2 Cups egg beaters

2. Healthy fats and oils

One of the most important improvements in today's meal fueling systems is that they now ensure that users get the right amount of healthy fats. An adequate supply of fat helps your body absorb fat-soluble vitamins such as A, D, E, and K, and contributes to gall bladder health. Fats also help you lose weight by giving you a sense of fullness and adding texture to your meals.

Our focus in the weight loss phase will be on eliminating unhealthy fats while supplementing your diet with healthy omegas that can accelerate your journey toward optimal health. Having a good supply of omega-rich antioxidants is particularly smart now during the weight loss phase, when your body is unloading fat cells and unhealthy fat-soluble substances.

What healthy fats and oils do you currently choose? e.g. 1 ½ ounces of avocado.

What adjustments can you make to your choice of healthy fats and oils using the diagram below? (Remember to eliminate salad dressings with soybean oil, which is high in Omega-6.)

EACH = 1 FAT SERVING

- 1 teaspoon of canola, flaxseed, walnut, or olive oil
- Up to 2 tablespoons of low-carbohydrate salad dressing
- 5 – 10 black or green olives
- 1 tablespoon of reduced-fat margarine
- 1 ½ ounces of avocado

3. Green vegetables and salad

I love vegetables and salads. As you'll discover in the following chapters, I believe you just can't eat too many healthy fruits and vegetables (with very few exceptions) once you reach your healthy weight. During the weight loss phase, however, I'm going to ask that you avoid fruit, which can be extremely high in carbohydrates, and really focus on selecting moderate amounts of vegetables from the green areas.

When we talk about the vegetables you will eat during this phase, we're referring to nutrient-dense, low-glycemic carbohydrates that support your health while you lose weight. Some popular diets reduce carbohydrates to such a low level that they bring about a profound state of ketosis, accompanied by dehydration and metallic-fruity breath. I don't advocate that. Rather, this plan will create an efficient physiologic state of mild dietary ketosis, or what I like to call a fat-burning state. This allows you to burn fat while providing enough carbohydrates (around 80–85 grams per day)to maintain muscle and brain health. The list that follows is designed to create this ideal state for optimal weight loss.

What green vegetables and salads do you currently choose?

What adjustments can you make to your choice of green vegetables and salads using the diagram?

As you'll see, your choices are color-coded but this time based on the amount of carbohydrates they contain. Darker green selections give you fewer carbohydrate calories. So if you're having trouble getting into a fat-burning state or if your weight loss slows down, it's probably a good idea to confine your choices to the dark green group, while also reducing or eliminating condiments and making sure your salad dressings are low fat and very low carb.

HIGHEST CARBOHYDRATE SERVING SIZE = ½ CUP UNLESS OTHERWISE SPECIFIED	MODERATE CARBOHYDRATE SERVING SIZE = ½ CUP UNLESS OTHERWISE SPECIFIED	LOWEST CARBOHYDRATE SERVING SIZE = ½ CUP UNLESS OTHERWISE SPECIFIED
• Broccoli • Cabbage (red) • Collards or mustard greens (cooked) • Green or wax beans • Kohlrabi • Okra • Peppers (green/red/yellow) • Scallions • Summer squash, (crookneck/straightneck) • Tomato (red ripe/canned) • Turnips • Winter squash	• Asparagus • Cabbage • Cauliflower • Eggplant • Fennel • Kale • Mushrooms (portabello) • Spinach (cooked) • Summer squash, zucchini, and scallop	• Mustard greens (1 cup) • Collards, fresh / raw (1 cup) • Romaine lettuce (1 cup) • Endive (1 cup) • Lettuce, butter head (1 cup) • Celery • Cucumber • Mushrooms (white) • Radishes • Sprouts, alfalfa or mung bean • Turnip greens

From the list, select any combination of three servings each day. (One serving = 1 cup of raw salad greens or ½ cup of cooked or raw vegetables.)

4. Healthy snacks and condiments

Use condiments to add flavor and zest to your meals—just remember that they contribute to overall carbohydrate intake. We recommend reading food labels for carbohydrate information and controlling condiment portions for optimal results. A condiment serving should contain no more than 1 gram of carbohydrate per serving. You can enjoy up to three condiment servings per day.

What healthy snacks and condiments do you currently choose?

What adjustments can you make to your choice of healthy snacks and condiments using the diagram below?

CONDIMENTS

- ½ teaspoon of most dried herbs and spices
- 1 teaspoon balsamic vinegar
- 1 teaspoon minced onion, lemon/lime juice, yellow mustard, salsa, soy sauce
- Up to 2 tablespoons sugar-free flavored syrup such as Da Vinci® or Torani®
- 1 packet artificial sweetener such as splenda®
- Tabasco® (or other hot) sauce and red, white, or cider vinegar (feel free to use liberally)

OPTIONAL SNACKS

- 3 celery stalks
- 1 fruit flavored sugar-free popsicle
- ½ cup serving sugar-free Jello® gelatin
- Up to 3 pieces sugar-free gum or mints
- Two dill pickle spears
- 1/2 oz. of nuts: almonds 10 whole),walnuts (7 halves) or pistachios (20 kernels) Note: Nuts are a rich source of healthy fats and additional calories so choose this optional snack sparingly

So now you have your four-part grocery list and the entire inventory you need to restock your kitchen for Phase I using the fuelings. It couldn't be simpler but remember, it's a precise eating strategy that works best exactly as outlined. That means that for the best results, you must confine yourself to only the foods on these lists.

Many communities already have grocers that allow you to shop online like Clicklist™. Imagine totally eliminating the temptation and having your healthy food delivered directly to your home!

Actually put together your healthy grocery list here and you can download extra copies from HabitsofHealth.com:

1. Lean protein

2. Healthy fats and oils

3. Green vegetables and salad

4. Healthy snacks and condiments

Now that you understand the importance of learning to choose healthy options in your lean and green, we will shift to how easy it is to eat healthy for life! We will complete the healthy eating section in a future Element once you have reached your healthy weight.

Make sure you review all your notes and this Element often. Also share it with your coach and spend time discussing how these possibilities will become a reality. In the next Element, we will address how to start learning to eat healthy when buying food as you are zoning in on reaching your healthy weight.

Notes to yourself:

Now that you have completed Element 11, *How Do You Eat Healthy Beyond Fuelings?*, write down your thoughts guided by the following questions:

What does this Element mean to you right now?

What does this Element give you the opportunity to reflect on?

What actions are you going to take as a result of this Element?

I encourage you to connect with your coach, so you can share your thoughts and actions as soon as possible.

Sharing your thoughts with your coach will help them become a reality.

Make sure you review all your notes and this Element often.

1 *Seafood Long-Chain n-3 Polyunsaturated Fatty Acids and Cardiovascular Disease: A Science Advisory From the American Hexart Association* — Alice H. Lichtenstein, published 17 May 2018 Circulation. 2018;138:e35–e47.

ELEMENT 12:
OPTIMIZING YOUR SUCCESS IN REACHING A HEALTHY WEIGHT

Average time to complete: **1 week**

In Element 12, we will:

- Learn why timing is so important in terms of waiting before adding key habits of optimal health.
- Clarify some important guidelines.
- Describe why the system works the way it does.
- Start using a checklist for success.

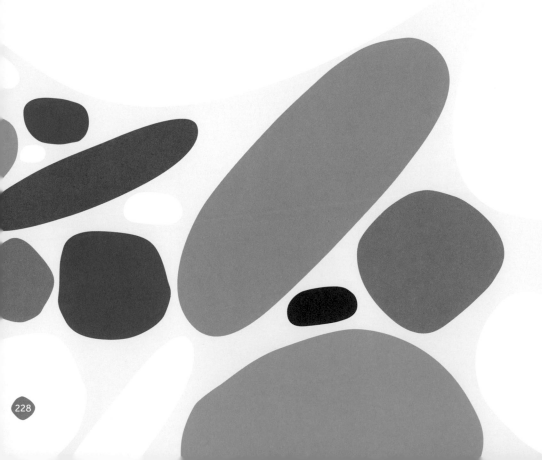

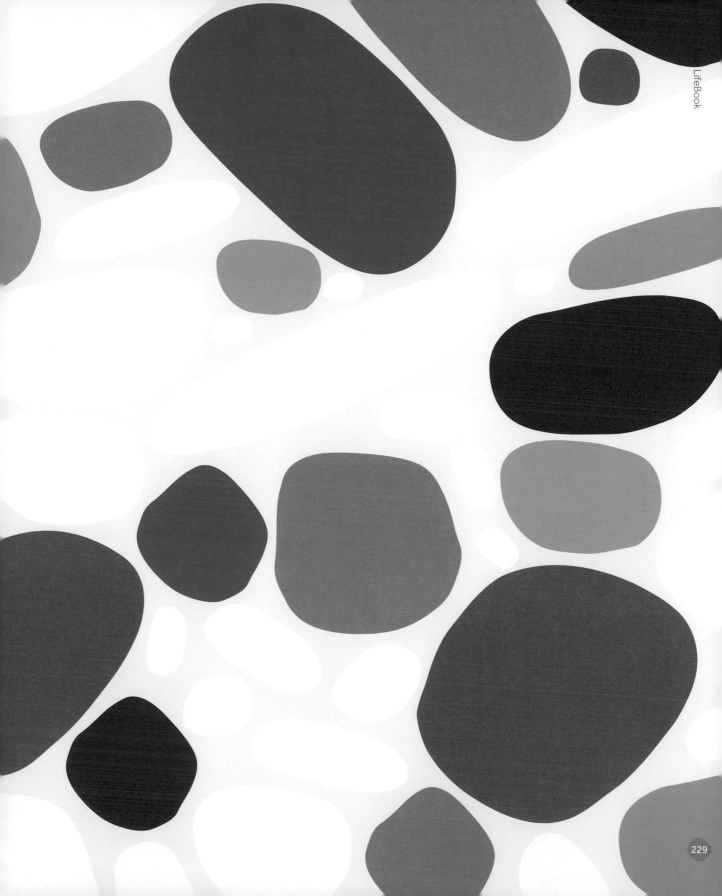

As you begin your journey to optimal health and wellbeing and primarily focus on reaching a healthy weight, there are a some important guidelines that may create some confusion for you. This is not what I want, so I am going to address them in this Element to make sure you understand why I am asking you to do what may seem counterintuitive to your overall success.

NO FRUIT OR EXTRA CARBOHYDRATES DURING PHASE I

No Fruit: While you are in Phase I and are using the prepared fuelings I ask you to not eat any fruit (or any additional carbs). We have always been told that fruit is essential for long-term health. It is absolutely correct—fruits is an amazing source of nutrients, antioxidants, and many other optimally healthy compounds. In the future, beyond Phase I, a healthy consumption of fruit will actually help you maintain your healthy weight and acts as a key component of our healthy eating system.

It is only during the weight loss Phase I that I ask you not to eat any fruit.

Why?

Whether you are using the prepackaged fuelings or preparing all of your fuelings on your own, understand that fruits has a considerable amount of carbohydrates which is mostly in the form of sugar. As a result, they have a relatively high-glycemic index and deliver a high carbohydrate load. This can take you out of the fat-burning state, which we are relying on to remove your excess visceral fat.

As you can see from the following diagram, during the state of Habits of Healthy Weight Loss, we have turned off the insulin pump by specifically avoiding excessive carbohydrates. As a result, the body is using fat as its fuel source to supplement beyond the energy and nutrition supplied by your fuelings and Lean and Green meal.

Habits of Health Weight Loss State Phase I

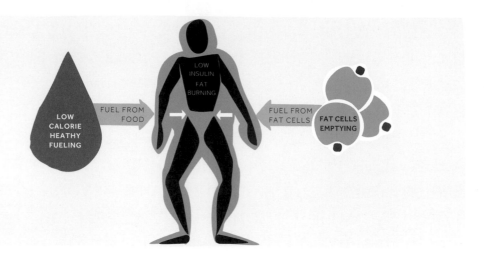

If you increase the carbohydrate level above a certain threshold, it will stimulate insulin secretion and shut down the fat-burning machinery.

Habits of Disease State

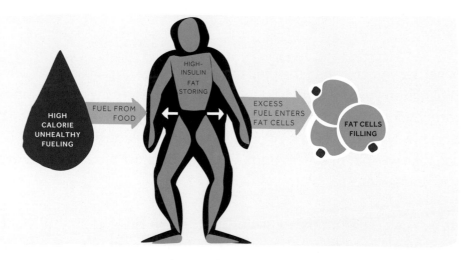

This is what happens when people inadvertently eat something with extra sugar. We ask you to completely eliminate eating carbohydrates and sugar-rich fruit only while you are in the weight loss phase.

Once you have reached your healthy weight and we have eliminated the excessive unhealthy fat, we will reintroduce fruit and recommend you fill a fourth of your plate with it at every healthy meal you have. You will then use our color-coded system to make sure most of the fruit you are eating is in the green zone to keep your insulin levels low, as depicted below:

Habits of Health Healthy Eating State Phase II and Beyond

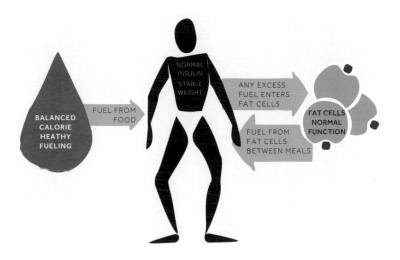

As you are settling into Phase I, it is important to do a review to make sure that you are not accidentally consuming a hidden carbohydrate source. This can slow down or even stop your weight loss now or in the future.

Check all of the things you put in your mouth for any additional sugar:

Morning Start e.g. brushing teeth, mouthwash, breakfast including coffee creamers, sweetners, vitamins

Daily Meals e.g. condiments, drinks

Others e.g. gum, candies, breath mints

Evening Leisure e.g. snacks, drinks

Eliminating these hidden (or not so hidden) sources of carbohydrates can be the difference between success and failure.

And don't worry because once you reach your healthy new weight, we will transition you to eat a variety of fruit using my color-coded plate eating system!

NO OR REDUCED EXERCISE DURING
THE FIRST THREE WEEKS OF PHASE I

How can eliminating or reducing the amount of exercise I do be a good thing as I start on this journey?

The Habits of Healthy Motion are a key MacroHabit in our system. It's one of those big rocks that we will be putting in the mason jar in the coming Elements.

It is much like the fruit guideline in that it's all about the timing.

When we switch your body over to a fat-burning state, it is important to optimize the conditions for success.

Your body is switching fuel sources and is not accustomed to using fat as its main energy source. Over a period of weeks, it will make that adjustment and we will add more activity to increase your motion. And, since we are dropping your daily calorie intake, if we do not go slow there is a chance that you will become hypoglycemic (low blood sugar) and not feel very well. In addition, if you create this state, the body releases hormones such as cortisol and epinephrine, which may actually slow down your weight loss.

If you have a great deal of weight to lose, a sudden increase in exercise places a high level of stress on your musculoskeletal system. Instead of risking injury, we encourage you to wait until you have lost weight and have begun to improve your stamina. Remember, our fuelings are providing the primary means of you losing weight in Phase I. In Phase II and beyond, the progressive motion and exercise will become a primary component in helping you maintain a healthy weight and optimizing your health and wellbeing.

So let's look at where you are in terms of your current activity level as you start the weight loss Phase I:

Currently Minimal Activity

In your case, you are probably excited that you are going to start losing your unhealthy fat without any initial need to increase your activity. In *Dr. A's Habits of Health* Part 2.2 and 2.3, we explain that our Phase I program focuses on the quantity and quality of the food you eat to put you in a fat-burning state.

Your work will start in earnest after the first three weeks, when we will increase your activity in baby steps as outlined in our system.

As your weight has decreased, I am sure you are feeling much better. Perhaps you've started adding more activity such as, using the stairs instead of the elevator, or taking the dog for a walk. If you've been in Phase I for a while, you may have started learning my progressive movement systems for sustainable exercise, as outlined in *Dr. A's Habits of Health* Parts 2.9 – 2.12 and Elements 17 – 18. Whatever your current level of physical ability, my plan is designed to give you an easy entry into the world of fitness. You've been hearing me talk about the relatively minor role exercise plays in weight loss. Well, that was true in the beginning of Phase I. But increasing your activity level becomes very important as you move from Phase I into Phase II and beyond. After the first three weeks of Phase I, your body is ready for increased motion. You're lighter, you have more confidence, you're physically healthier, you have the right motivation, you're in the process of installing and are in better command of the Habits of Health Transformational System. My NEAT and EAT plans for physical movement are doable and designed to fit your current level of health and fitness. Over time, these systems will put you on track for long-term success!

Currently Moderate Activity

A few years back, I spoke to a group of women at a local gym. They were all interested in reaching a healthier weight. As I explained how we would accomplish this they became noticeably anxious when I mentioned to them that we would want them to cut back their exercise for three weeks to mostly stretching and limited exercise that did not make them sweat. I asked them how long they had been at the gym and, on average, they had been there about two years. I asked them how long ago they started and how much weight they had lost. Most of them had lost a few pounds but had put the weight back on.

I first congratulated them on their success at establishing one of the Habits of Healthy Motion, Exercise (EAT), which we will discuss in the motion Elements ahead. I then explained how it is virtually impossible to lose weight consistently with exercise alone without diet modification. In fact, when women workout, they experience what's called "compensation". A state where you become so hungry that you have a tendency to eat more to make up for the calorie deficit. This explains why, despite their diligence, they were not losing weight as desired.

I then asked if they would follow my guidelines if I promised that they would see results, such as seeing the contours of their hard-earned muscles that were currently hidden by fat, in as little as three weeks.

They were more than pleased, and after the three or so weeks had passed, we started progressing them back to more activity.

As they slowly worked back to a full workout, I suggested they sandwich a fueling on either side of the workout. I recommended a shake before and a bar with a glass of water after the workout, especially as the body adjusts. In this group of moderate activity, we also taught them how to increase their activity throughout their day and not just when they are at the gym.

Currently Intense Activity

If you are in this group, the same rules apply as above. You will want to cut your exercise in half or more until your body acclimates. If you are training for a marathon or extreme games event, you should probably wait until after the event before going on our lowest calorie program. You can work with your coach to increase your calories by adding additional lean and green fuelings. Also, like the above group, it is important to sandwich a fueling on either side of the workout, especially in the beginning or if the workout is intense to avoid low blood sugar post-workout. If you are serious about not just losing fat but gaining muscle, it will be worthwhile to talk to a trainer who can explain the value of selective protein usage, such as branched-chain amino acids. Make sure you are adding the other Habits of Motion so you are working on your cardiovascular, endurance, and flexibility as well.

In summary, if you're inactive when you start the program, we'll begin increasing your motion as you start feeling better, losing weight, and feeling more energized. This will help you learn the Habits of Motion, which are critical to sustaining long-term weight control and optimal health and wellbeing.

If you are currently active, just cut it back until we get you into a solid fat-burning state and your body acclimatized. You can then slowly work yourself back to active at a rate that allows you to thrive.

For you hard-core enthusiasts that are into significant intense activity, move at a pace that allows your body to adjust so you lose that unhealthy fat and expose your underlying physique at a pace that is safe and effective.

What is your current level of activity?

In your first three weeks of adjustment, what are you going to do?

After the three weeks, write down how you are going to increase your activity.

WHY AM I EATING FUELINGS VERSUS WHOLE FOOD?

But isn't eating whole food better?

Yes, and we will get there as you learn the Habits of Health, but reaching a healthy weight is our first priority and the most profound change you can make to your health.

As we discussed in Element 09, *How Do You Use Fuelings To Reach A Healthy Weight?*, focusing on whole foods doesn't guarantee weight loss. There are many people who eat whole foods everyday and are obese. The secret is to understand how to use whole foods effectively and then the prepared fueling will be used when you do not have time or access to whole food. But we need to create success so you are in the game and getting healthier.

We are going to use our five fuelings along with a healthy lean and green as a plan because they are an easy, cost-effective, and safe way to start gaining health by losing weight. As you feel better, have more energy, and are sleeping better, you will start building the confidence in our system, in me, in your coach, and in yourself.

That creates the teachable moment where your motivation is higher and you are willing to go to work to learn the other necessary habits. None of which are more important than the healthy eating system that I will be teaching you shortly. It will give you full command over everything you eat and some great tools to make the job easier.

So yes, it's once again about timing. We start off using the fuelings in the 5&1 Plans to help you reach a healthy weight, which is the most important factor in our health. We then teach you in a series of *microHabits*, how to choose correctly at both the store and restaurants, and have full command over your weight management.

At that point you will be eating whole foods when it makes sense and the fuelings as convenient portable meals when you are short on time or if whole food is not accessible.

Please describe below why we use a combination of fuelings and lean and green in Phase I of our system.

Please describe below what role whole food and the fuelings now play in Phase I and how this will change over time. Discuss this with your coach.

We have now discussed the importance of timing and your current location on the path to optimal health and wellbeing.

Fruit, exercise, fuelings, and whole food are all critical components of your success, and their roles vary depending on which Phase you are in. Our system is designed to help you build a new story: one that will provide you a lifetime of health and wellbeing.

Fruit will be a core component for healthy eating for life but does not allow us to help you reach your healthy weight in a timely fashion because it keeps us out of the fat-burning state.

Avoid fruit in Phase I then, once you are at a healthy weight, begin to consume low and moderate glycemic fruit.

Exercise will be a key component of your Habits of Motion routine, but it needs to be avoided in the first three weeks as your body settles into using fat as its energy source.

Eliminate or reduce exercise during the first three weeks and then progress to increasing daily activity, eventually including robust exercise as you undergo the continuum of transformation.

We will teach you to make great healthy choices using whole food in your home-cooked meals and when you are out. We will also make the steps to eating healthy simple and strategic to help you reach optimal health and wellbeing. The fuelings will be primary during Phase I because of their power and design to help you reach a healthy weight. Once you have reached a healthy weight, they will become secondary to help provide healthy fuelings when the logistics of modern life do not allow the time or conditions to prepare or obtain a healthy whole food meal.

Checklist to Success

Eat one fueling every three hours. Don't skip meals even if you're not hungry. It's absolutely critical to fuel as scheduled; in fact, your weight loss may be slower if you don't.

Get some extra rest. You may feel a little tired during the first three days as your body switches on its fat-burning mechanism and gears up to use its stores of fat.

Drink eight (eight-ounce) glasses of water every day.

Eat slowly.

Stay busy and avoid sights and smells that remind you of food, especially during the first few days. Soon enough, your own energy stores will kick in and you'll feel more in control.

Use your support system. Call your coach, and if you don't have one yet, get one!

Connect with our community in person, online, and on video and conference calls. Ask your coach for more details.

Limit caffeine to no more than three servings a day. You may find that your body is more sensitive to the effects of caffeine, making this a great time to cut back on your daily consumption.

Avoid alcohol. It causes dehydration, throws you out of the fat-burning state you've worked so hard to achieve, and is a powerful appetite stimulant.

If you slip up, just get right back on track. But remember, it will take about two to three days after a slip-up to get back into a fat-burning state. (For some extra motivation, review Parts 1.3–1.5 in *Dr. A's Habits of Health* on making good choices.)

Make *Your LifeBook* your best friend. Print off tracking sheets. This is a great way to monitor your progress and help you focus.

Use *Dr. A's Habits of Health* and app to optimize your transformation.

Avoid exercise for the first three weeks. Or, if you do choose to exercise, reduce your usual amount by half.

How long you stay in this Phase I depends primarily on how much weight you have to lose and how long you take to lose it, as well as your target BMI. While your weight-loss goal can be whatever you've determined is healthy for you, there are some guidelines concerning body composition. Generally speaking, if your waist circumference is less than 37 inches (for men) or 31.5 inches (for women) and your BMI is less than 25, you're ready to transition to the healthy-eating phase.[1] In general, you should count on being in the weight-loss phase until you meet your goals and are able to maintain them for at least two weeks.

• If you have just a small amount of weight to lose, you'll transition to Phase II fairly quickly. Continue advancing through *Your LifeBook* Elements. You will also want to read the chapters on my healthy, low-glycemic portion-control system (Parts 2.4–2.7 in *Dr. A's Habits of Health*) before you begin transitioning in Element 14, because you'll be using much of that information as you learn to eat healthy for life. After that, you'll begin the progressive movement plan outlined in Parts 2.9–2.12.

- If you have a lot of weight to lose, you'll be in Phase I for a while. When the time comes, and you've reached your healthy weight, Part 2.8 will teach you about transitioning to Phase II. In the meantime, you should read the chapters on my healthy low-glycemic portion-control system (Parts 2.4–2.7) because you'll be using much of that information as you learn to eat healthy for life. In addition, once you've settled into a fat-burning state (after the first three weeks), you should start the progressive movement plan outlined in Parts 2.9–2.12.

However, your weight loss can vary depending on your gender and certain medical conditions that may slow down your weight loss, such as hypothyroidism and PCOS (polycystic ovary system).

I would review this material often as you are losing weight and creating health. Make sure you are taking some notes as you experience better health, and discuss how you are doing with your coach because understanding where you are on your journey and having support can make all the difference.

In the next Element, we will give you a simple way of evaluating your days one at a time because your transformation occurs one day at a time. Our goal is to make small incremental improvements one day at a time.

This will give you more optimal days which will be created by the Habits of Health in a series of *microHabit* installations. Over time you will become as healthy as you can be and experience thriving days of wellbeing. And since the goal is to get just one percent better each day, we need to evaluate, track, and make adjustments to get just a touch better each day. And if we are not, then explore why and amp up your support and maybe ratchet down the size of your *microHabits*. It doesn't matter because we are building your new story, and each day offers you an opportunity to be open, curious, and learn how to get better. But first we must have a way of checking how we are doing and develop a means of sharing it with our support team.

Notes to yourself:

Now that you have completed Element 12, *Optimizing Your Success In Reaching A Healthy Weight*, write down your thoughts guided by the following questions:

What does this Element mean to you right now?

What does this Element give you the opportunity to reflect on?

What actions are you going to take as a result of this Element?

I encourage you to connect with your coach, so you can share your thoughts and actions as soon as possible.

Sharing your thoughts with your coach will help them become a reality.

Make sure you review all your notes and this Element often.

1 These guidelines are based on World Health Organization and National Health and Medical Research Council recommendations.

ELEMENT 13:
TRACKING YOUR JOURNEY TO A HEALTHY WEIGHT AND BEYOND

Average time to complete: **1 week**

In Element 13, we will:

- Provide you with tools to assess how you are doing on a daily, weekly, and monthly basis.
- Measure your progress as you advance on your path to better health and wellbeing.

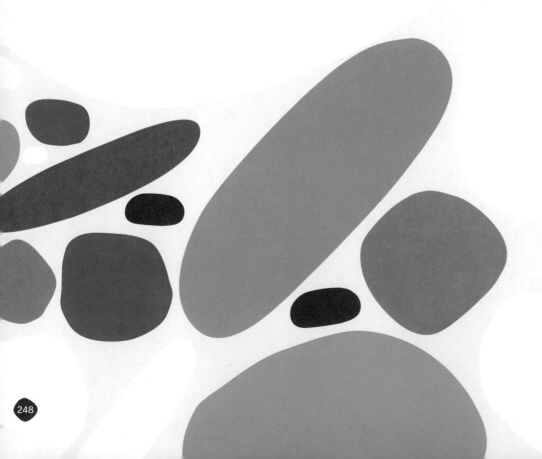

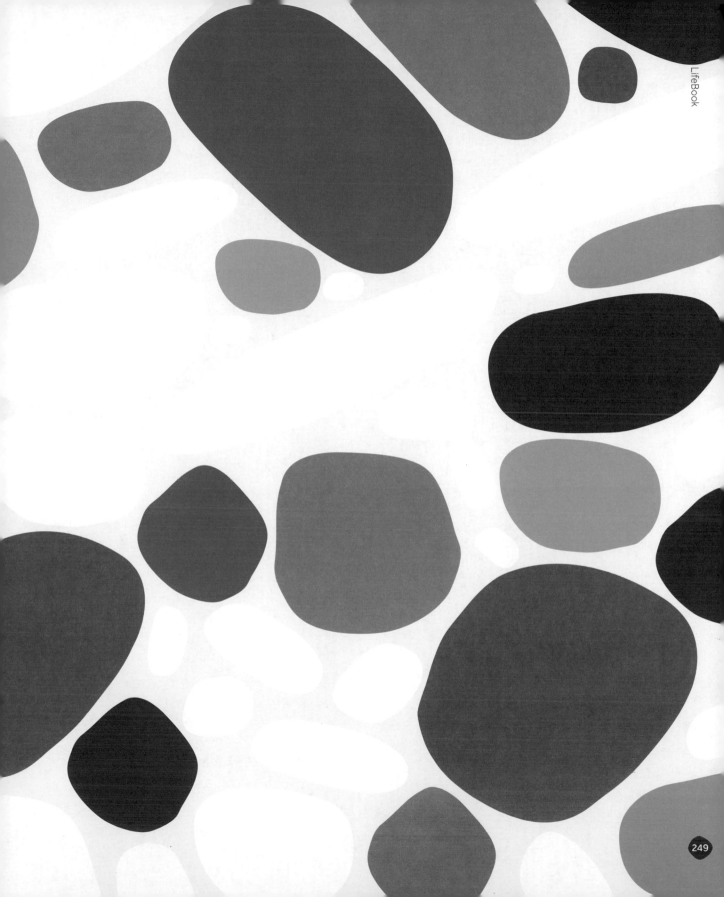

Your LifeBook is designed to help you understand the basics of what we will be using in terms of knowledge, skills, tools, and timing to create a solid foundation for optimal health and wellbeing for the rest of your life and put it into daily practice.

Elements 06 through 12 have focused on the installation of the first MacroHabit, which is your weight management. As you are advancing towards a healthy weight, we are simultaneously beginning the installation of the Habits of Health necessary to optimize and sustain your healthy weight throughout your life. As we discussed in Element 12, *Optimizing Your Success In Reaching A Healthy Weight*, if you have a lot of weight to lose, you will be on this portion of your journey for a while. If you only had a few pounds to lose or if your weight is not an issue, we have now equipped you with the skills and tools to stay at a healthy weight for the rest of your life.

In this Element, we are going to provide you with a means of assessing how you are doing on a daily basis. We will also focus on measuring your progress as you advance on your path to better health and wellbeing. Without these tools it becomes more difficult for you to assess how well you are adopting and advancing your habits to better serve your health and wellbeing. Also, by tracking both your consistency and your results, we can make corrections and adjustments and correct a deviation early rather than allowing you to ingrain a behavior or choice that is not providing the results we want.

You have heard about the 10,000 hours of practice that are required for mastery of a profession. As we mentioned earlier, this is a bunch of deliberate practice with proper feedback to make sure you are programming the right choices and behavior.

Pro-golfer Jack Nicklaus taught me a valuable lesson about deliberate practice several years ago when I was playing golf with a friend at a course where Nicklaus practiced. As my friend and I warmed up, we had the privilege of watching Nicklaus and his fellow pro-golfer Greg Norman practicing by targeting a flag about 80 yards away.

Although they were just getting started, the three dozen or so balls they'd hit so far were all within a couple feet of the pin. The tight grouping of balls on the rich carpet of the green was like an exclamation point showcasing the skill of these top professional golfers. Mesmerized by their precision, it was with reluctance that I left to tee off. As I hooked my drive into the sand trap and walked down the first fairway, I kept thinking how lucky these guys were to be so good.

We proceeded to play the first nine, and I hit one shot (out of 45) that was anything like as good as any of Jack's. The day was hot, and I was thirsty, so I headed back to the water fountain by the practice range. Imagine my astonishment when I discovered that Nicklaus and Norman were still there, still hitting the same shot. And every one of their hundreds of golf balls were within a few feet of the pin. They'd just spent two and a half hours in the summer heat practicing a shot they had already performed to perfection. It was a perfect example of making a secondary choice in support of a primary choice—in Jack's case, to be the best golfer in history. These guys created excellence by spending years and years ingraining a habit that becomes so automatic it would enable them to perform, even under intense pressure.

This is what we are doing with you as we begin ingraining these Habits of Health that will eventually become automatic. No matter what happens, you have the ability to make choices that support your optimal health and wellbeing and operate even when your willpower has left the building.

The key is to track the day you just had and to plan the day you will have tomorrow.

That way we can assess how you actually performed, celebrate your wins, and assess your mess-ups (you will have them, as humans we all do) so we can adjust and pick up ways to get better. It's not about perfect, it's all about being open, curious about how to improve, and growing. We can spot trends like breadcrumbs and look for what we can build on and what we can do a better job of avoiding. Your Habits of Health App tracks your consistent daily action by recording the days in a row as you build a new choice chain and install new behaviors. *Your LifeBook* builds an interactive advancing structure which allows you to fully immerse yourself in becoming an optimally healthy and vibrant human being.

Your daily log and checklist is our tracking mechanism to evaluate your progress daily in as little or as much detail as you want. I know you will want to know that several studies show that when we measure we perform at a higher level. Karl Pearson, a famous statistician and founder of mathematical statistics, said "That which is measured, improves". Like all of the Habits of Health, we will approach your daily tracking in small, doable steps or *microHabits* so you actually want to do it. It will also be a great way of sharing your journey with your coach. Remember you can only connect the dots looking backward from your days, not forward. We will use this daily log to track and accelerate your progress.

The strategic plan of the Habits of Health Transformational System is to make it easier to learn and install an effective set of habits that do not depend on willpower, but instead automated behaviors that support optimal health and wellbeing. The way we establish, monitor, and fortify this new lifestyle is by using the *Dr. A's Habits of Health* book, *Your LifeBook*, App, and this daily, weekly, monthly log.

We will develop this daily, weekly, monthly log in this Element and then provide you with a downloadable version you can print or fill out, along with a basic blank template that you can modify to fit your specific needs and adjust as you work through this year of healthy transformation.

You can also make your own and use this as a guide.

The key to this log and checklist is to let you know what you are currently committed to do every day. I am using the word "commitment" in a very specific way. Not as a statement of what I will do, but instead what I am doing.

What are your results? Your current weight, the steps you take in a day, the hours you are in bed, and how you actually act in stressful situations are the proof of what you are committed to doing presently.

This daily log and checklist will help you and your coach know what you are willing to work on at this point. It will show up as the consistent repetition, daily action, and time dedicated to focusing and getting better right now. The Habits of Health Transformational System and I are committed to making it easier for you to be healthy and to live well.

Taking full responsibility for yourself is the one thing that you must do that no one else can do for you. You must own what you eat, how you move, how you sleep, and how you handle stress by integrating your mind. You can not delegate your eating, moving, sleeping, and emotional management to the grocery stores, restaurants, government, or medical system.

At this point in *Your LifeBook*, I have only given you the habits that support your weight loss journey. In addition to implementing the other MacroHabits that we haven't unpacked yet, I would also recommend you start tracking your current habits so you can start assessing the healthiness of your current choices. It will be fun to watch how all your Habits of Health grow and support your journey during this year. I would highly recommend that you complete this during your Twilight Hour in the evening or during your Model morning.

This will take you around five minutes to fill out daily, or more if you write a lot of comments. This will show what is possible. You can download a blank one and customize it to your needs at HabitsofHealth.com.

MACROHABITS OF HEALTH DAILY LOG AND CHECKLIST

Date . . . .

Habits of Weight Management:

Goal Weight . . . . . lbs

Goal BMI . . . .

Goal Waist Circum . . . in

During Weight Loss

Daily Food Intake:

How Many Fuelings? . . . .

Every Three Hours? . . . .

Healthy Lean and Green

⬜ Yes ⬜ No

Cravings?

⬜ Yes ⬜ No

Hunger Level?

⬜ Low ⬜ Medium ⬜ High

Energy Level?

⬜ Low ⬜ Medium ⬜ High

These are typically done weekly:

Current Wt . . . . lbs

Current BMI . . . .

Current Waist Circum . . . in

Comments:

Habits of Healthy Eating and Hydration

Goal Weight · · · · · ·

Current Weight · · · · ·

BMI <25 · · · · · ·

Food Intake:

Fuelings?

◯ Yes ◯ No

How Many? · · · · · ·

Healthy Meals?

◯ Yes ◯ No

Low GI?

◯ Yes ◯ No

Healthy Fats?

◯ Yes ◯ No

Hunger Level?

◯ Low ◯ Medium ◯ High

Cravings?

◯ Yes ◯ No

Hydration:

64 ounces of water today?

◯ Yes ◯ No

How Much? · · · · ounces

Comments:

Habits of Motion:

Steps Today:

Activity level?
⬤ Low   ⬤ Medium   ⬤ High

NEAT Activities:

EAT Activities:

Workout (not for the first three weeks):

Comments:

Habits of Sleep:

In bed in time to get eight hours of sleep?
⬤ Yes   ⬤ No

How many hours did I sleep?

Energy level today
⬤ Low   ⬤ Medium   ⬤ High

Naps today:

Comments:

Habits of Healthy Mind:

Successfully Use Stop. Challenge. Choose.™ today:

◯ Yes ◯ No

How did you respond to the Challenge?

Did you set aside some quiet time for youself?

◯ Yes ◯ No

Did you meditate?

◯ Yes ◯ No

Did you spend some time reading an inspirational book or video?

◯ Yes ◯ No

Write down 1–3 things you are grateful for:

Comments:

Habits of Healthy Surroundings:

I connected with my support system and community today.

◯ Yes   ◯ No

How?

I talked to my coach.

◯ Yes   ◯ No

Did you improve your surroundings today to help with your health or wellbeing?

◯ Yes   ◯ No

Comments:

What three things will I do tomorrow to make my day more optimal?

1.

2.

3.

In addition to the daily log, we will want to track your weekly progress. Since we recommend that during your weight loss Phase I you only weigh yourself once a week because you will have daily fluctuations in your weight, it stands to reason that the choices you make will also vary. Daily repetition is the key to new habit installation, but the results you will experience will vary according to many factors. The weekly tracker allows us to measure trends and patterns in your habit installation without overly focusing on daily results. Over the rest of this year we'll be using the Integrated Habits of Health Clock to create more optimal days.

HABITS OF HEALTH WEEKLY TRACKER

Date . . . .

Goal Weight . . . . lbs
Goal BMI . . . .
Goal Waist Circumference . . . . in

Current Wt . . . . lbs
Current BMI . . . .
Current Waist Circumference . . . . . in

On a scale of 1–10 evaluate the progress you have made in the previous week using the progress ruler for each of the MacroHabits.

Progress Ruler

0	1	2	3	4	5	6	7	8	9	10

Back Slide   **No Progress**   **Excellent Progress**

Use the ruler to enter a number into each category for each week (three-month period)

Week	1	2	3	4	5	6	7	8	9	10	11	12
Weight Management												
Healthy Eating												
Hydration												
Motion												
Sleep												
Mind												
Surroundings												

Note: The idea here is to monitor whether we are on track, stalled, or moving in the wrong direction. The most important MacroHabit to track is the one we are working on, but a sudden backslide in another may be central to the lack of success in the one we are focusing on.

You can download the daily checklist and the weekly tracker from HabitsofHealth.com. I suggest you buy an inexpensive loose-leaf three-ring binder with a plastic cover that allows an insert. You can download a factsheet which will label your log and tracker. I suggest you keep it on your bedside permanently and after reviewing your current *Your LifeBook* Element and your App, transcribe the events of the day. I would use *Dr. A's Habits of Health* book for reference as well as to further your understanding.

In order to see your year of advancement and transformation, the monthly tracker below will document your progress on the path to optimal health and wellbeing.

HABITS OF HEALTH MONTHLY TRACKER

Month . . . .

Goal Weight . . . . lbs
Goal BMI . . . .
Goal Waist Circumference . . . . . . in

Progress Ruler

| 0 | 1 | 2 | 3 | 4 | 5 | 6 | 7 | 8 | 9 | 10 |

Back Slide   **No Progress**   **Excellent Progress**

Use the ruler to enter a number into each category for each month

Month	1	2	3	4	5	6	7	8	9	10	11	12
Weight Management												
Healthy Eating												
Hydration												
Motion												
Sleep												
Mind												
Surroundings												

I would review this Element again and discuss it with your coach to make sure you start logging and tracking your progress as you are creating your new story.

In the next Element, we will address how to transition from Phase I weight loss to Phase II, which focuses on learning how to eat healthy for life. Whether you are buying food to prepare at home or eating out, we are going to put you in charge. Your choices will support long-term weight management and help you generate optimal health and wellbeing now that you are zoning in on your healthy weight.

Notes to yourself:

Now that you have completed Element 13, *Track Your Journey To A Healthy Weight And Beyond*, **write down your thoughts guided by the following questions:**

What does this Element mean to you right now?

What does this Element give you the opportunity to reflect on?

What actions are you going to take as a result of this Element?

I encourage you to connect with your coach, so you can share your thoughts and actions as soon as possible.

Sharing your thoughts with your coach will help them become a reality.

Make sure you review all your notes and this Element often.

ELEMENT 14:
TRANSITIONING TO EATING HEALTHY FOR LIFE

Average time to complete: **2–4 weeks**

In Element 14, we will:

- Learn how to transition from Phase I of weight loss to Phase II, which focuses on learning how to eat healthy for life.
- Create a transition plan that works for you, because transition can be different for everyone!
- Empower yourself to make choices that will support long-term weight management and help you generate optimal health and wellbeing.

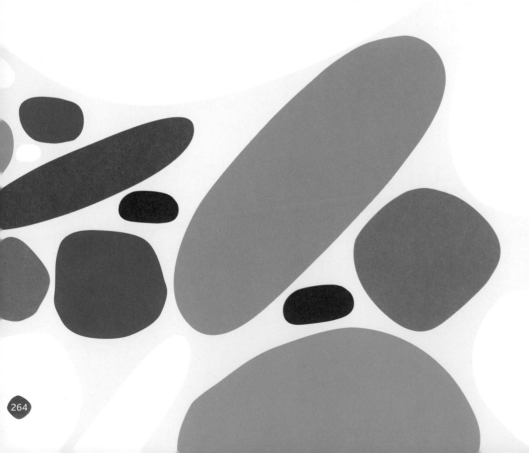

We have helped you reach a healthy weight as the first step on your journey to optimal health. We will now use the next two Elements to transition you from your weight loss regimen to mastery of eating healthy in all situations so you can sustain long-term weight management by introducing the knowledge, tools, and Habits of Health necessary to sustain an optimal weight throughout your life.

This Element is the transitional lesson from your weight loss regimen and will give you the ability to expand and add the full range of healthy food and shift your focus to healthy eating for your life. The amount of weight you lost will determine how long you will be in this transitional period and how much time it will take you to master this Element. And it's important to note that everyone transitions differently.

If you had a lot of weight to lose and you have been on this journey for a while your transition will be a little slower, but there is an advantage to this as you will have more time to study and absorb how to eat healthy and beyond. If you only had a few pounds to lose or if weight was not an issue, your transition will be quick. The good news is you have now have added to your skills and tools to stay healthy for the rest of your life. And your coach is still there to support you on this leg of your journey.

HOW DO YOU KNOW WHEN TO TRANSITION?

Let's review when Phase I, the weight loss Phase, ends and Phase II, your healthy weight Phase, begins.

As illustrated in the diagram below by the orange line when your BMI is <25, your waist circumference is <37 inches as a man or <31.5 inches as a woman.[1] If you are measuring your body fat (optional), the percentage is 18% as a man and 25% as a woman to be at a healthy weight by the numbers.

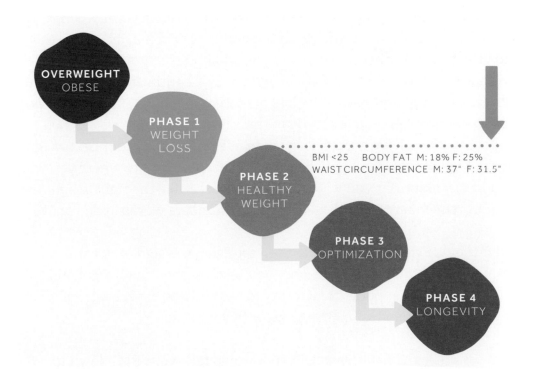

There is considerable research that supports these numbers as a reliable indicator of your risk for disease. It becomes quite low once you have reached this level of weight management.[1]

When you actually decide to stop losing weight and start transitioning is your choice. If you have a lot of weight to lose, you may think you will never get down to those numbers.

That belief is usually based on years of being overweight and previous attempts and failures to change. You may be hesitant to set what seems like such ambitious goals.

That's okay. The good news is that everyday you are in Phase I, you simply get up and focus on that day. Eventually you will reach a point when you are ready. It may be when you reach the numbers or it may be before then. And like all of our other *microHabits*, you will find that your body will continue to respond to our program and you will continue to improve your numbers. Each pound means the loss of more unhealthy fat. So you do not need to decide when you are ready to transition until you have reached the goal that you have chosen for yourself. If you were at your best weight back in high school or college, that will probably be close to where you will want to transition. Or you will just find what feels like the right weight for you. But remember the healthy targets and numbers we discussed above!

And if that weight freaks you out, then set a target weight you think is reasonable and then reevaluate once you have reached that target. Also, consult with your support community to hear others' experiences of when they transitioned and, of course, work with your coach.

What would be the healthy weight that would take your BMI down to under 25?

Your Current Weight?

Healthy Waist Circumference (WC)?

Your Current WC?

What are your thoughts on when you will transition?

Have you discussed this with your coach?

Premature Slowing of Weight Loss

If your weight loss slows way down or stops before you reach your goal, it may be because you are eating something off the plan (usually high GI carbohydrates) that takes you out of a fat-burning state.

You may be at a plateau, which can happen if your basal metabolic rate is low to start with and goes below the calories you are taking in on the program as you lose weight. Usually, picking only deep green choices in your lean and green can reverse that trend, but I have also found eliminating your snacks and being very careful with your condiments can get you back into fat burning. Consult with your coach and support network if that does not help.

Once you have decided on your goal weight and are getting close to your target weight, you will start planning for your transition.

Are you ready?

Have you talked to your coach?

TRANSITIONING

While you have been in Phase I, we have focused on decreasing your weight by eliminating the unhealthy extra fat in your body, which will dramatically improve your health and fitness. We have taught you a series of new eating habits that have lowered your total energy consumption and improved the quality of food you are now eating. We have specifically limited some of the foods you ate previously and reduced the total amount of calories to turn on the fat-burning state that eliminates the extra fat stored by your body.

You are now at a point where you have reached a healthy weight and have modified your body weight set point and accomplished our first major desired outcome. Read Part 2.8 in *Dr. A's Habits of Health, Healthy Eating for Life: Your Transition to Permanent Health,* for a detailed explanation of your body's set point but, in simple terms, you have increased the normal release of leptin to balance your hunger and minimize insulin secretion to avoid excessive fat storage.

Your body is much healthier and, by protecting your muscle from being catabolized (because we have flipped the metabolic switches to fat burning), your body composition has improved. In order to continue making progress, we need to transition your body to the full range of healthier foods that will allow you to eat more variety of meals and yet choose the foods that help support your long term health and weight. And we need to make sure we do not add too many calories or overstimulate insulin by adding high-glycemic foods in this process of transition from Phase I to Phase II.

Because you have lost weight, it's important that the total calories that you consume is reduced—you have lowered your total size, and we need to increase the set point that will allow you to gradually expend more energy. This is why it matters how much you eat: to keep the balance of the set point so you can compensate, increase leptin, reduce insulin, and prevent transitional weight gain.

The transition to your lifetime healthy eating strategy consists of two parts:

Part One:
Determining Your Total Energy Expenditure (TEE)
Adding calories until you reach your body set weight point
(calories in = calories out).

This is accomplished by keeping insulin at a healthy level and continuing leptin's job of feeling full working effectively.

Part Two:
Your Transition Eating Plan
Introducing a full range of foods to support optimal health and maintain your healthy weight.

Part One:
Determining Your Total Energy Expenditure (TEE)
Estimating how many calories you currently expend will keep you at a healthy weight. To start with let's figure out your body's set weight (BSW) point, which will keep your calories in/calories out balanced.

First, as we add more and more types of food back into your day, you will know you have your insulin/leptin in balance because you will not be hungry and you will have lots of energy. Secondly, we will watch your response as we add calories. The idea is to reach the point at which the number of calories you take in is equal to the number of calories you use. The best way to do that is to figure out how many calories you burn in the course of a day.

In other words, how many calories you should eat daily to remain where you have decided is your target weight. In order to have a starting point to guide us in how much you should eat, we will calculate your current total energy expenditure.

We are going to use a very simple formula to calculate approximately how many calories will keep your set point and your weight in balance. We will provide the more accurate and precise calculations for calculating your TEE online at HabitsofHealth.com.

Determining Your Total Energy Expenditure (TEE)

Want to figure out how many calories you need to eat in Phase II to keep those jeans fitting just right? The most common method is a simple formula to calculate your total energy expenditure, or TEE. Calculating your TEE as it is right now at your healthy weight will help us determine your optimal caloric intake during this phase. We'll work on increasing that number as we continue to add Elements around how you can increase your movement and exercise as part of our overall Habits of Health strategy and your new story.

Your TEE is determined by:
• Your basal metabolic rate (BMR)
• Your physical activity level (PAL)
• The thermic effect of the food you eat (TEF)

Together, these show us how quickly your body is burning the fuel you're taking in, day in and day out.

Let's begin by looking separately at those three components.

Basal Metabolic Rate (BMR) is the energy you use for your *basic bodily needs*. Even when your body is *at rest*, it's using fuel to breathe, grow, circulate your blood, adjust your hormone levels, repair cells, and perform other functions. Typically, BMR is the largest portion of the TEE energy equation. Because the energy required by these basic functions remains fairly consistent, this number doesn't tend to change much.

Physical Activity Level (PAL) is the energy you use when you move—playing tennis, walking to the store, chasing after the dog. You have control of this number and can change it quite a bit depending on the frequency, duration, and intensity of your activities.

Thermic Effect of Food (TEF) is the energy your body uses to process your food. Digesting, absorbing, transporting, and storing food all take energy—about 10% of the calories you use each day. For the most part, this number stays steady.

Calculating Your TEE

Now that you know what goes into your TEE, let's start figuring out your number. There are a couple of options available to help us, some more accurate than others. If you're not a math major or don't feel like getting out the calculator, you can start with a rough method to calculate your daily caloric needs. This initial number doesn't need to be exact, since it's only a starting point that you'll be adjusting as you monitor your weight throughout transition. See HabitsofHealth.com for a more elaborate calculation.

The easy way to calculate TEE

To find out your TEE using the easy method, use the following formula:

Your current weight (in pounds) × 11 calories = TEE (daily caloric need). This formula is based on a sedentary individual, so you'll need to adjust it as you step up your exercise, as follows:

Activity Level
Multiply your TEE by Your Current Activity Level:
- 1.2 (for light exercise)
- 1.5 (for moderate exercise)
- 1.7 (for heavy exercise)

For example:

$$162 \text{ lbs} \times 11 \text{ kcal/lb} = 1{,}782 \text{ kcal}$$
$$\times 1.2 = 2{,}138 \text{ kcal/day (TEE)}$$

I have found that it can be helpful to slightly underestimate your activity level above to ensure that you don't take in more calories than you are actually burning as you calculate your TEE.

Current TEE:

Your current weight . . . . . **x** 11 calories **=** . . . . . Your TEE

Now make the adjustment to add in your current level of activity.

Your TEE . . . . **x** Activity Level . . . . **=** . . Your Total TEE

Note: Make sure you are fairly conservative when selecting your current level of activity. Underestimate it so if you are off you will not have assigned yourself more calories than you are actually burning. 90% of the time, people overestimate their activity level and as a result start gaining weight during transition. You can always increase it later if you find you are losing weight. Also make sure you are working closely with your coach during this critical period.

Transition daily calorie intake (Your total TEE from above):
Write down this number here: . . . .

Phase I (weight loss) daily calorie intake:
On average, how many calories were you eating during the weight loss Phase I period? . . . .
(Usually 800–1,000 calories a day)

Transition Daily
Calorie Intake: . . . . **—** Phase I
Calorie Intake . . . . **=**

Estimate how many calories you will add during transition.
Adjust this up or down to keep your weight stable.

This is how many calories you will add. You will also track your weight and adjust this up or down to keep your weight stable.

Note: Your weight will increase a few pounds as you add back your glycogen stores and with it water. Do not worry as it will stabilize in the first week or so. Remember to recalculate this number as you track your weight over the next several weeks.

Now that you know how to calculate how many calories you will be adding as an estimate, let's look into how best we can add those calories and more healthy foods to your healthy eating plan.

Part Two: Your Transition Eating Plan

If you used the portion-controlled meal system exclusively during Phase I, you'll need to introduce new food groups as well as additional calories into your eating system. Read the next section about the process of transitioning from the packaged portion-controlled meal system to learn how to do this effectively.

Journal your weight. If you start to see your weight trending upward, check in with your coach and check in on your choices to see where you can improve.

You may gain as many as five pounds in the initial period during transition from rebuilding your glycogen stores and an increase in water retention, but this will subside as you increase your activity and refine your Habits of Healthy Eating over time.

If you have been using my healthy eating system to lose weight, you're already employing many of the principles of your permanent eating strategy and can skip the next section and go right to Transitioning to Your Permanent Eating System.

Transitioning from the Prepackaged Fueling Meals

If you've reached your healthy weight using portion-controlled meals, you need to add the full range of food groups back into your diet as well as calories. You're already used to preparing a healthy lean and green meal along with your fuelings, so this transition should be pretty easy for you.

We're going to introduce these new foods in a logical order that allows your digestive tract to become accustomed to them. Your starting point is five portion-controlled meals and one lean and green meal, for a total of 800 to 1,000 calories a day. For the first four weeks of your transition, you'll increase your daily caloric intake incrementally each week by adding one of the four food groups that you avoided during Phase I.

Below is the schedule we use at OPTAVIA® to transition from weight loss into maintenance:

• Week 1: additional vegetables
• Week 2: fruits
• Week 3: dairy
• Week 4: whole grains

By the end of week four, you will have added each of these four food groups and will be consuming approximately 1,350–1,500 calories.

TRANSITION

Once you've achieved your healthy weight, you're ready to make the transition to lifelong healthy eating. The transition phase gradually increases your calorie intake and reintroduces a wider variety of foods. The calories you need after transition to maintain your weight varies according to your height, weight, gender, age, and activity level. This six-week transition leads to an ultimate goal of fewer than 1,550 calories a day.

	TARGET NO. OF CALORIES	FUELINGS	LEAN & GREEN MEALS	ADDITIONS
WEEK 1	850 – 1,050	5	1	• 1 CUP (2 SERVINGS) OF YOUR FAVORITE VEGETABLES (ANY KIND)*
WEEK 2	900 – 1,150	4	1	IN ADDITION TO YOUR WEEK 1 ADDITIONS, ADD: • 2 MEDIUM SIZED PIECES OF FRUIT • OR 1 CUP OF CUBED FRUIT OR BERRIES (2 SERVINGS)
WEEK 3	1,000 – 1,300	4	1	IN ADDITION TO YOUR WEEK 1,2, AND 3 ADDITIONS, ADD: • 1 CUP OF LOW FAT OR FAT-FREE DAIRY (1 SERVING)
WEEK 4–6	1,100 – 1,550	3	1	ON TOP OF OUR WEEK 1,2, AND 3 ADDITIONS, ADD: • 4 – 6oz OF LEAN MEAT • AND 1 SERVING OF WHOLE GRAINS

*Fresh, or, if canned, unsweetened and packed in juice, not syrup. **Grilled, baked, poached, or boiled — not fried. ***Examples: 1 slice of whole-grain bread, 1/2 whole-grain English muffin, 3/4 cup of high-fiber cereal, 1/2 cup of whole-wheat pasta, or 1/3 cup of brown rice.

Here's how the first four weeks should look:
In this section, I refer to the color-coded healthy eating system that I will discuss in the next Element, which you will use to ensure that you are picking healthy choices. You can also read about it in Part 2.8 in *Dr. A's Habits of Health, Healthy Eating for Life: Your Transition to Permanent Health.*

Week 1: Add vegetables (850–1,050 total calories per day)
• Add any vegetable from the green section of the charts.
• You're now eating five fuelings, one lean and green meal, and one additional cup of vegetables.

Week 2: Add fruit (900–1,150 total calories per day)
• Drop one prepackaged meal.
• Add any fruit from the green section of the charts. (Fresh or frozen fruit is preferred, but canned may be used as long as it's not packed in syrup.)
• You're now eating four fuelings, one lean and green meal, one additional cup of vegetables, and two medium-sized piece of fruit or one cup of berries or chopped fruit.

Week 3: Add dairy (1,000–1,300 total calories per day)
• Dairy includes low-fat and sugar-free yogurt, milk, or lactaid product.
• You're now eating four fuelings, one lean and green meal, one additional cup of vegetables, two medium-sized piece of fruit or one cup of berries or chopped fruit, and one cup of low-fat or fat-free dairy.

Week 4: Add whole-grains (1,100–1,550 total calories per day)
• Drop one fueling.
• Whole grain choices include one slice of whole grain bread, ¾ cup of high-fiber cereal, ⅓ cup of whole-wheat pasta, or ½ cup of brown rice.
• You're now eating three fuelings, one lean and green meal, one additional cup of vegetables, one medium-sized piece of fruit or ½ cup of berries or chopped fruit, one cup of low-fat or fat-free dairy, and one portion of whole-grain starch.
• If you're exercising, add four ounces of lean meat, poultry, fish, or other protein.

Here is an example day:

Breakfast:
½ cup high-fiber breakfast cereal (over 5 grams of fiber per serving) with ½ cup skim milk and 1 cup fresh strawberries

Mid-morning:
Frothy Cappuccino Boost Fueling

Lunch:
4 ounces deli turkey; 2 cups salad greens with ½ cup diced cucumber, tomato, and green pepper (plus 1/2 tablespoons reduced-calorie salad dressing if desired)

Mid-afternoon:
Chicken Flavored & Vegetable Noodle Soup Fueling

Dinner:
4 ounces poached salmon with 1 cup green beans

Evening:
Decadent Double Chocolate Brownie Fueling with 1 teaspoon fat-free whipped topping

After the first four weeks, you will have introduced all four of the food groups you avoided during Phase I and will be eating approximately 1,500 calories per day. Over the following weeks, you'll continue to add calories until you reach your TEE, either by adding foods to one of your fuelings or to one of your meals using my color-coded portion-control system.

As an example, a woman whose target TEE is 1,900 calories means that she needs to add 400 calories over the next four weeks. An easy way to do this is to add 100 calories each week until she has reached the permanent healthy eating schedule outlined in the next Element.

Note: Also make sure you are working closely with your coach during this critical period.

In the next Element, we will introduce my healthy eating system, which will allow you to add calories in a progressive fashion and eat healthy and maintain an optimal weight for the rest of your life.

Don't Forget to Monitor Your Weight During Transition!
Your weight may fluctuate during transition as your body gets used to the additional carbohydrates, salt, and calories. Remember to monitor your weight vigilantly and adjust your calorie intake up or down if you fluctuate by more than a few pounds from your healthy weight. If you notice that you're gaining weight, cut back on calories a bit by recalculating your TEE and adjusting your intake accordingly. Give your body time to readjust its lower set point and be ready to catch yourself early!

Now that you are in transition, we will move into the final Element in weight management.

In the next Element, will introduce you to Dr. A's Healthy Eating System, which has a sustainable and satisfying methodology to allow you to duplicate the power of our fuelings in everything you consume.

Notes to yourself:

Now that you have completed Element 14, *Transitioning To Eating Healthy For Life*, write down your thoughts guided by the following questions:

What does this Element mean to you right now?

What does this Element give you the opportunity to reflect on?

What actions are you going to take as a result of this Element?

I encourage you to connect with your coach, so you can share your thoughts and actions as soon as possible.

Sharing your thoughts with your coach will help them become a reality.

Make sure you review all your notes and this Element often.

1 These guidelines are based on World Health Organization and National Health and Medical Research Council recommendations.

ELEMENT 15:
HOW TO EAT HEALTHY FOR LIFE

Average time to complete: **2 – 4 weeks**

In Element 15, we will:

- Introduce you to my healthy eating system.
- Share strategies for portion control, as well as quick and easy tools for healthy eating.
- Identify pitfalls and solutions to dining out.
- Provide you with a blueprint for sustainable success in managing your eating patterns for life.

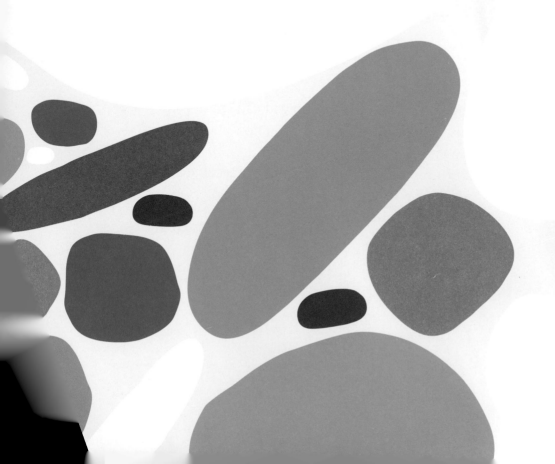

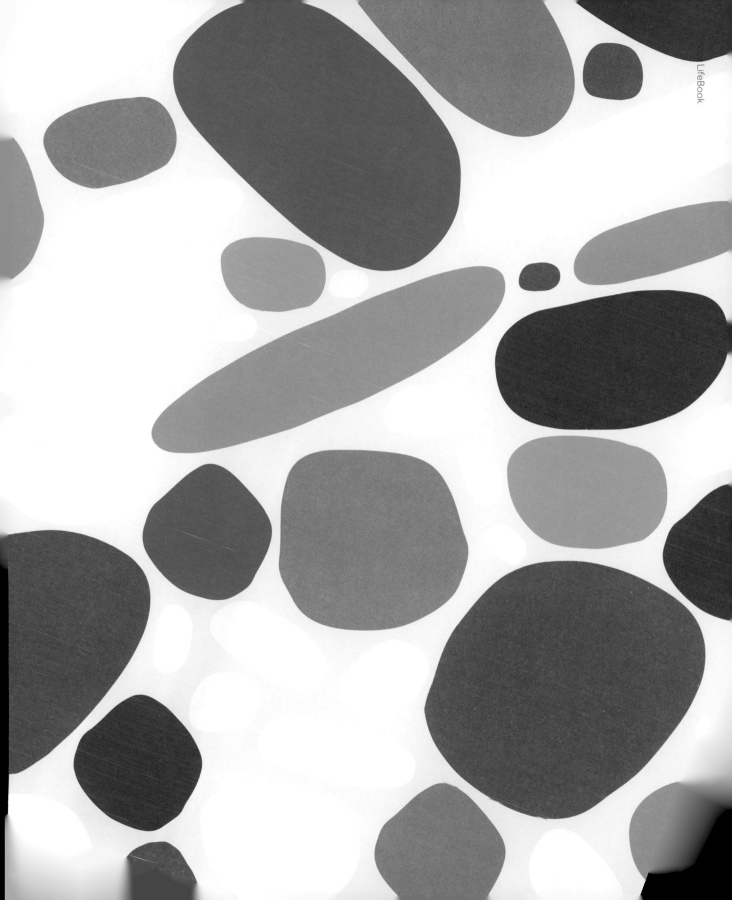

As we mentioned in the Element on timing, our goal is to initially use the prepackaged fuelings to help you lose weight safely and effectively in a goof-proof way. When they are combined with a lean and green, the fuelings are highly effective at producing predictable weight loss. Now that you are in transition, their role will change to being a convenient, fast fueling to overcome the times when healthy food is not available or you are limited on time.

The goal now is to make sure you have a system that will allow you to be in full control of your weight and your metabolic switches, but still be able to eat a large variety of whole foods that make up the full experience of modern life. This will be accomplished using my healthy eating system, which we will unpack now. There is a much more detailed description of my eating system in Parts 2.4–2.7 in *Dr. A's Habits of Health* which I highly recommend you read. In fact, in order to truly understand the benefits and master healthy eating, it's a must.

Here we will focus on the practical application of the system and refer you to the corresponding section in the *Dr. A's Habits of Health*.

My healthy eating system is designed to help you monitor and manage your energy intake while ensuring that you get a healthy, balanced diet. It's a simple visual system that teaches you the basics of portion size and the correct proportion of foods from our four designated major food groups: vegetables, fruits, proteins, and grains. We then provide a color-coded system for choosing food that has the highest value for optimizing your weight management and optimal health. It's so easy you can even use it in restaurants.

NINE-INCH PLATE SYSTEM FOR PORTION CONTROL (PART 2.4 IN DR. A'S HABITS OF HEALTH, DR. A'S HEALTHY EATING SYSTEM)

With the system, you'll use a nine-inch plate to help you judge proper portion size and proportions. If you don't already have a nine-inch plate in your kitchen, now is as good a time as any to go out and buy a few. Ideally, the plate should be shallow with just a small lip to prevent you from heaping it with too much food.

If you go online you'll notice that nine-inch plate systems are all the rage, which is pretty cool since they were non-existent when I wrote the first edition of *Dr. A's Habits of Health.* You can actually get a tracking app that connects with them. The bottom line is that I want you to have the easiest possible way to judge your portions and how much of each food group you are eating without major disruption in your routine and culture.

The harder it is, the less likely it is that you'll do it.

What plates have you chosen? This is an important first step in creating a visual image in your mind as well as a physical tool.

Back in Element 07, *Creating A New Leptogenic World,* we discussed the importance of plate color. How can that help with your visual image?

Take a look at the following diagram. I've simplified it into a four-component system that mirrors the way most people eat.

Our typical meal is made up of:
• healthy vegetables
• healthy fruits
• healthy protein (meat, chicken, fish, dairy, nuts)
• healthy grains (wheat, rice, oats, cornmeal, barley, or another cereal grain)

Each portion is 25% of total plate capacity. It's worth noting that although we designate 20–25% for the fruit and vegetable, as much as 50% can come from vegetables. As a general guideline I would avoid more than 25% coming from the fruit category.

Dr. A's Portion Control Plate System

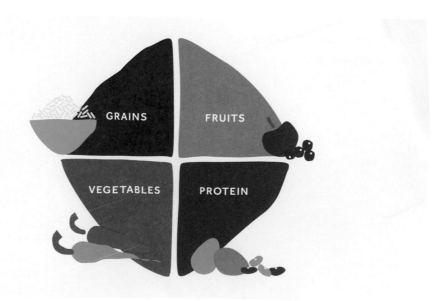

This breakdown gives you a healthy balance of nutrients in the right amounts to satisfy your hunger and burn fat. All you need to do is visualize this chart on your nine-inch plate, and plan your meals accordingly. As long as you maintain this ratio of grains, proteins, fruit, and vegetables, you can be sure that you're getting a healthy, balanced diet. In fact, we'll be using these proportions to build your long-term health plan—so you're already learning an important Habit of Health.

Before we move on, do you understand the difference between portion size and serving size?

Serving sizes are set by the U.S. Department of Agriculture. There are two serving size recommendations. The first is for a particular food—for example, a ½ cup of fruit. The second is the daily total recommendation for a healthy diet—for example, two cups of fruit for a 2,000 calorie diet. Portion is more commonly used to describe how much food is put on the plate in front of you. Portions may be larger or smaller than the serving size for a particular food.

Dr. A's Low-Glycemic Portion-Control System (CH10).

The practical system you're about to learn has three important benefits.

Can you name them? (Beginning of Part 2.4 in *Dr. A's Habits of Health, Dr. A's Healthy Eating System*).

1.

2.

3.

This simple, effective strategy has its own basic guidelines.

These are the most critical ones to understand at the beginning as you transition into long term optimization:

- You'll eat breakfast within an hour of awakening (30 minutes is ideal).
- You'll eat something every three hours.
- You'll have a healthy dinner.
- You'll eat only lower-glycemic carbohydrates in transition, then you can include light green.
- You'll gradually begin increasing your daily activity.
- You'll learn the key habits necessary to maintain a healthy weight, including support, monitoring, and reinforcement.

If you're not already familiar with the basics of healthy eating, don't worry. In Parts 2.5–2.6 in Habits of Health, I will show you how to shop for and plan great-tasting meals on your own, or you can simply follow my pre-planned menus that are on HabitsofHealth.com. I'll even make it easy for you to prepare foods at work or while traveling.

Your new healthy daily eating schedule starts with a solid breakfast and continues fueling you every three hours while you're awake with low-glycemic choices, including a healthy dinner. This plan helps keep blood sugar and insulin levels steady.

We are shifting your focus to the quality of the food you will be eating to support both your weight management and so that you will eat healthier food for life.

Our simple color-coded charts were developed to make it easy for people to master shopping for healthy proteins, starches, fruits, and vegetables. When combined with our easy visual portion-control system, this color-coded shopping system puts you well on the way to creating meals that help you lose weight and build optimal health.

The color-coded system has been extended to give you easy ways to make healthy choices in all of the food groups.

If You Stay in the Green You will Stay Lean (and Healthy).

LOW-GLYCEMIC FOODS FOR OPTIMAL HEALTH
(PART 2.5 IN DR. A'S HABITS OF HEALTH, CHOOSING WISELY:
DR. A'S COLOR-CODED SHOPPING SYSTEM)

The message couldn't be simpler: staying away from refined sugar and flour while, instead, focusing on eating low-glycemic carbohydrates and healthy foods is the best way to lose weight and create health.

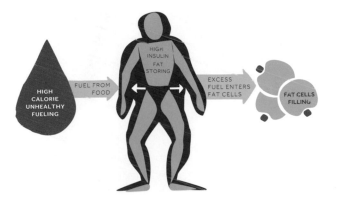

If we move people away from the ultra-processed western diet and unhealthy carbs, we can turn off insulin so the body stops behaving like a fat storage depot.

The system I developed takes all of the confusion out of shopping and ordering at restaurants.

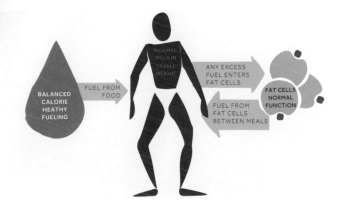

Here are your rules of thumb for foods that contain carbohydrates:
- Dark green = lowest glycemic (the best foods for weight loss and optimal health)
- Light green = moderate glycemic (foods to be eaten in moderation)
- Light orange = higher glycemic (foods to be eaten only rarely)
- Red = toxic (foods to be avoided at all costs)

Color Code for Glycemic Index

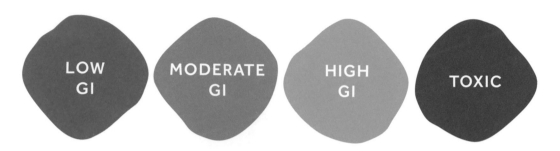

LOW GI   MODERATE GI   HIGH GI   TOXIC

As you experienced in Phase I or during your weight loss, your healthy eating selections in your lean and green came from the dark green charts. These foods are highly effective at turning off your insulin and fat storage and will facilitate reaching and maintaining an optimal weight. The light green charts list foods that are healthy but were used sparingly in the first phase of our journey. Foods on the orange chart should be used with care, and only after you've reached optimal health. And any food that is in the red is directly damaging to your health and should be eliminated completely from your diet forever. However good they taste, they are just not worth it.

And of course, the prepackaged low-calorie fuelings are designed specifically to provide a high-quality, low-glycemic choice, and are always an excellent way to obtain a nutrient-dense, calorie-friendly fueling or meal. They are always designated dark green.

The charts are available for download on HabitsofHealth.com and also are in *Your LifeBook* and the Habits of Health App.

THE ELEMENTS OF EATING HEALTHY: LIVING IN THE GREEN

The charts that follow are designed to steer you toward foods that rev up your health. Think of them as the octane-disclosure sheets at the gas pumps. Watch your engine's performance improve as you switch from regular gas (the low-octane, nutrient-poor foods you're eating now) to premium (functional foods that are nutrient-dense, highly efficient fuels that turn down your insulin pump and turn on fat burning).

As you shop, remember to visualize your nine-inch plate, with its divisions based on the proper proportion of foods for optimal health and weight loss. You'll need to have plenty of vegetables and fruits on hand, as well as lesser quantities of healthy complex starches and lean proteins to create healthy, delicious meals.

Your Nine-Inch Plate Divided into Food Types

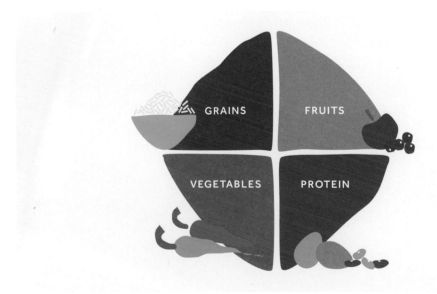

Dr. A's Healthy Eating Plate System for Life

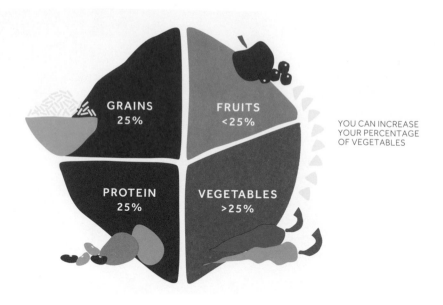

When you're shopping, think about the meals you're planning. A meal on your nine-inch plate should be made up of 50% vegetables and fruits, 25% protein, and 25% grain from my healthy food choices. Remember you can always add more vegetables and less fruit to the percentage, especially if your monitoring reveals you have gained a few pounds!

Vegetables and Fruits (Part 2.5 in *Dr. A's Habits Of Health, Choosing Wisely: Dr. A's Color-Coded Shopping System*)

(25 & 25 totalling 50% of Your Plate)

Make sure you read in Part 2.5 as to the benefits of eating healthy choices. Here we are focused on what you will actually select for yourself.

Vegetables and Fruits

- Berries
- Peaches
- Many More
- Apples
- Leaf Veggies

TRANSITION

Once you've achieved your healthy weight, you're ready to make the transition to lifelong healthy eating. The transition phase gradually increases your calorie intake and reintroduces a wider variety of foods. The calories you need after transition to maintain your weight varies according to your height, weight, gender, age, and activity level. This six-week transition leads to an ultimate goal of fewer than 1,550 calories a day.

	TARGET NO. OF CALORIES	FUELINGS	LEAN & GREEN MEALS	ADDITIONS
WEEK 1	850 – 1,050	5	1	• 1 CUP (2 SERVINGS) OF YOUR FAVORITE VEGETABLES (ANY KIND)*
WEEK 2	900 – 1,150	4	1	IN ADDITION TO YOUR WEEK 1 ADDITIONS, ADD: • 2 MEDIUM SIZED PIECES OF FRUIT • OR 1 CUP OF CUBED FRUIT OR BERRIES (2 SERVINGS)
WEEK 3	1,000 – 1,300	4	1	IN ADDITION TO YOUR WEEK 1, 2, AND 3 ADDITIONS, ADD: • 1 CUP OF LOW FAT OR FAT-FREE DAIRY (1 SERVING)
WEEK 4–6	1,100 – 1,550	3	1	ON TOP OF OUR WEEK 1, 2, AND 3 ADDITIONS, ADD: • 4 – 6oz OF LEAN MEAT • AND 1 SERVING OF WHOLE GRAINS

*Fresh, or, if canned, unsweetened and packed in juice, not syrup. **Grilled, baked, poached, or boiled — not fried. ***Examples: 1 slice of whole-grain bread, 1/2 whole-grain English muffin, 3/4 cup of high-fiber cereal, 1/2 cup of whole-wheat pasta, or 1/3 cup of brown rice.

Here's how the first four weeks should look:

In this section, I refer to the color-coded healthy eating system that I will discuss in the next Element, which you will use to ensure that you are picking healthy choices. You can also read about it in Part 2.8 in *Dr. A's Habits of Health, Healthy Eating for Life: Your Transition to Permanent Health.*

Week 1: Add vegetables (850–1,050 total calories per day)
• Add any vegetable from the green section of the charts.
• You're now eating five fuelings, one lean and green meal, and one additional cup of vegetables.

Week 2: Add fruit (900–1,150 total calories per day)
• Drop one prepackaged meal.
• Add any fruit from the green section of the charts. (Fresh or frozen fruit is preferred, but canned may be used as long as it's not packed in syrup.)
• You're now eating four fuelings, one lean and green meal, one additional cup of vegetables, and two medium-sized piece of fruit or one cup of berries or chopped fruit.

Week 3: Add dairy (1,000–1,300 total calories per day)
• Dairy includes low-fat and sugar-free yogurt, milk, or lactaid product.
• You're now eating four fuelings, one lean and green meal, one additional cup of vegetables, two medium-sized piece of fruit or one cup of berries or chopped fruit, and one cup of low-fat or fat-free dairy.

Week 4: Add whole-grains (1,100–1,550 total calories per day)
• Drop one fueling.
• Whole grain choices include one slice of whole grain bread, ¾ cup of high-fiber cereal, ⅓ cup of whole-wheat pasta, or ½ cup of brown rice.
• You're now eating three fuelings, one lean and green meal, one additional cup of vegetables, one medium-sized piece of fruit or ½ cup of berries or chopped fruit, one cup of low-fat or fat-free dairy, and one portion of whole-grain starch.
• If you're exercising, add four ounces of lean meat, poultry, fish, or other protein.

Here is an example day:

Breakfast:
½ cup high-fiber breakfast cereal (over 5 grams of fiber per serving) with ½ cup skim milk and 1 cup fresh strawberries

Mid-morning:
Frothy Cappuccino Boost Fueling

Lunch:
4 ounces deli turkey; 2 cups salad greens with ½ cup diced cucumber, tomato, and green pepper (plus 1/2 tablespoons reduced-calorie salad dressing if desired)

Mid-afternoon:
Chicken Flavored & Vegetable Noodle Soup Fueling

Dinner:
4 ounces poached salmon with 1 cup green beans

Evening:
Decadent Double Chocolate Brownie Fueling with 1 teaspoon fat-free whipped topping

After the first four weeks, you will have introduced all four of the food groups you avoided during Phase I and will be eating approximately 1,500 calories per day. Over the following weeks, you'll continue to add calories until you reach your TEE, either by adding foods to one of your fuelings or to one of your meals using my color-coded portion-control system.

As an example, a woman whose target TEE is 1,900 calories means that she needs to add 400 calories over the next four weeks. An easy way to do this is to add 100 calories each week until she has reached the permanent healthy eating schedule outlined in the next Element.

Note: Also make sure you are working closely with your coach during this critical period.

In the next Element, we will introduce my healthy eating system, which will allow you to add calories in a progressive fashion and eat healthy and maintain an optimal weight for the rest of your life.

Don't Forget to Monitor Your Weight During Transition!
Your weight may fluctuate during transition as your body gets used to the additional carbohydrates, salt, and calories. Remember to monitor your weight vigilantly and adjust your calorie intake up or down if you fluctuate by more than a few pounds from your healthy weight. If you notice that you're gaining weight, cut back on calories a bit by recalculating your TEE and adjusting your intake accordingly. Give your body time to readjust its lower set point and be ready to catch yourself early!

Now that you are in transition, we will move into the final Element in weight management.

In the next Element, will introduce you to Dr. A's Healthy Eating System, which has a sustainable and satisfying methodology to allow you to duplicate the power of our fuelings in everything you consume.

Notes to yourself:

Now that you have completed Element 14, *Transitioning To Eating Healthy For Life*, write down your thoughts guided by the following questions:

What does this Element mean to you right now?

What does this Element give you the opportunity to reflect on?

What actions are you going to take as a result of this Element?

I encourage you to connect with your coach, so you can share your thoughts and actions as soon as possible.

Sharing your thoughts with your coach will help them become a reality.

Make sure you review all your notes and this Element often.

1 These guidelines are based on World Health Organization and National Health and Medical Research Council recommendations.

ELEMENT 15:
HOW TO EAT HEALTHY FOR LIFE

Average time to complete: **2–4 weeks**

In Element 15, we will:

- Introduce you to my healthy eating system.
- Share strategies for portion control, as well as quick and easy tools for healthy eating.
- Identify pitfalls and solutions to dining out.
- Provide you with a blueprint for sustainable success in managing your eating patterns for life.

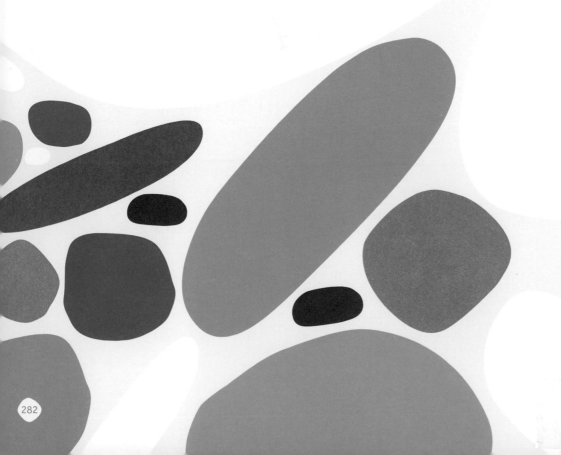

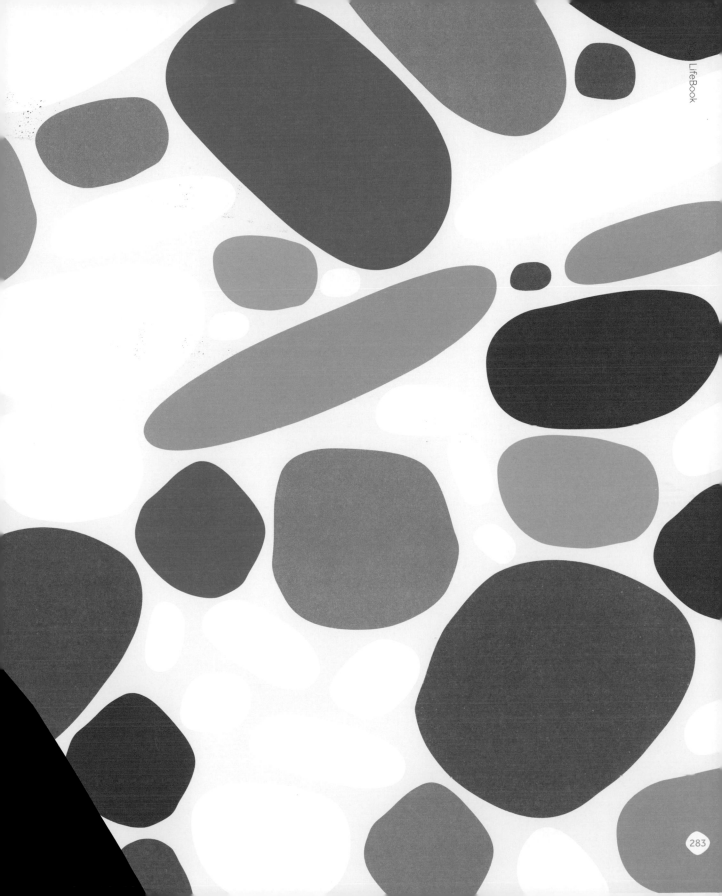

As we mentioned in the Element on timing, our goal is to initially use the prepackaged fuelings to help you lose weight safely and effectively in a goof-proof way. When they are combined with a lean and green, the fuelings are highly effective at producing predictable weight loss. Now that you are in transition, their role will change to being a convenient, fast fueling to overcome the times when healthy food is not available or you are limited on time.

The goal now is to make sure you have a system that will allow you to be in full control of your weight and your metabolic switches, but still be able to eat a large variety of whole foods that make up the full experience of modern life. This will be accomplished using my healthy eating system, which we will unpack now. There is a much more detailed description of my eating system in Parts 2.4–2.7 in *Dr. A's Habits of Health* which I highly recommend you read. In fact, in order to truly understand the benefits and master healthy eating, it's a must.

Here we will focus on the practical application of the system and refer you to the corresponding section in the *Dr. A's Habits of Health*.

My healthy eating system is designed to help you monitor and manage your energy intake while ensuring that you get a healthy, balanced diet. It's a simple visual system that teaches you the basics of portion size and the correct proportion of foods from our four designated major food groups: vegetables, fruits, proteins, and grains. We then provide a color-coded system for choosing food that has the highest value for optimizing your weight management and optimal health. It's so easy you can even use it in restaurants.

NINE-INCH PLATE SYSTEM FOR PORTION CONTROL (PART 2.4 IN DR. A'S HABITS OF HEALTH, DR. A'S HEALTHY EATING SYSTEM)

With the system, you'll use a nine-inch plate to help you judge proper portion size and proportions. If you don't already have a nine-inch plate in your kitchen, now is as good a time as any to go out and buy a few. Ideally, the plate should be shallow with just a small lip to prevent you from heaping it with too much food.

If you go online you'll notice that nine-inch plate systems are all the rage, which is pretty cool since they were non-existent when I wrote the first edition of *Dr. A's Habits of Health*. You can actually get a tracking app that connects with them. The bottom line is that I want you to have the easiest possible way to judge your portions and how much of each food group you are eating without major disruption in your routine and culture.

The harder it is, the less likely it is that you'll do it.

What plates have you chosen? This is an important first step in creating a visual image in your mind as well as a physical tool.

Back in Element 07, *Creating A New Leptogenic World,* we discussed the importance of plate color. How can that help with your visual image?

Take a look at the following diagram. I've simplified it into a four-component system that mirrors the way most people eat.

Our typical meal is made up of:
• healthy vegetables
• healthy fruits
• healthy protein (meat, chicken, fish, dairy, nuts)
• healthy grains (wheat, rice, oats, cornmeal, barley, or another cereal grain)

Each portion is 25% of total plate capacity. It's worth noting that although we designate 20–25% for the fruit and vegetable, as much as 50% can come from vegetables. As a general guideline I would avoid more than 25% coming from the fruit category.

Dr. A's Portion Control Plate System

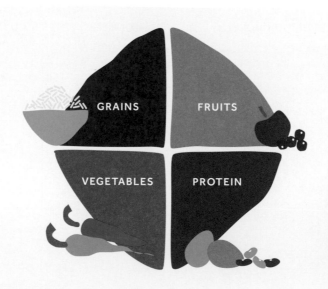

This breakdown gives you a healthy balance of nutrients in the right amounts to satisfy your hunger and burn fat. All you need to do is visualize this chart on your nine-inch plate, and plan your meals accordingly. As long as you maintain this ratio of grains, proteins, fruit, and vegetables, you can be sure that you're getting a healthy, balanced diet. In fact, we'll be using these proportions to build your long-term health plan—so you're already learning an important Habit of Health.

Before we move on, do you understand the difference between portion size and serving size?

Serving sizes are set by the U.S. Department of Agriculture. There are two serving size recommendations. The first is for a particular food—for example, a ½ cup of fruit. The second is the daily total recommendation for a healthy diet—for example, two cups of fruit for a 2,000 calorie diet. Portion is more commonly used to describe how much food is put on the plate in front of you. Portions may be larger or smaller than the serving size for a particular food.

Dr. A's Low-Glycemic Portion-Control System (CH10).

The practical system you're about to learn has three important benefits.

Can you name them? (Beginning of Part 2.4 in *Dr. A's Habits of Health, Dr. A's Healthy Eating System*).

1.

2.

3.

This simple, effective strategy has its own basic guidelines.

These are the most critical ones to understand at the beginning as you transition into long term optimization:

- You'll eat breakfast within an hour of awakening (30 minutes is ideal).
- You'll eat something every three hours.
- You'll have a healthy dinner.
- You'll eat only lower-glycemic carbohydrates in transition, then you can include light green.
- You'll gradually begin increasing your daily activity.
- You'll learn the key habits necessary to maintain a healthy weight, including support, monitoring, and reinforcement.

If you're not already familiar with the basics of healthy eating, don't worry. In Parts 2.5–2.6 in Habits of Health, I will show you how to shop for and plan great-tasting meals on your own, or you can simply follow my pre-planned menus that are on HabitsofHealth.com. I'll even make it easy for you to prepare foods at work or while traveling.

Your new healthy daily eating schedule starts with a solid breakfast and continues fueling you every three hours while you're awake with low-glycemic choices, including a healthy dinner. This plan helps keep blood sugar and insulin levels steady.

We are shifting your focus to the quality of the food you will be eating to support both your weight management and so that you will eat healthier food for life.

Our simple color-coded charts were developed to make it easy for people to master shopping for healthy proteins, starches, fruits, and vegetables. When combined with our easy visual portion-control system, this color-coded shopping system puts you well on the way to creating meals that help you lose weight and build optimal health.

The color-coded system has been extended to give you easy ways to make healthy choices in all of the food groups.

If You Stay in the Green You will Stay Lean (and Healthy).

LOW-GLYCEMIC FOODS FOR OPTIMAL HEALTH
(PART 2.5 IN DR. A'S HABITS OF HEALTH, CHOOSING WISELY: DR. A'S COLOR-CODED SHOPPING SYSTEM)

The message couldn't be simpler: staying away from refined sugar and flour while, instead, focusing on eating low-glycemic carbohydrates and healthy foods is the best way to lose weight and create health.

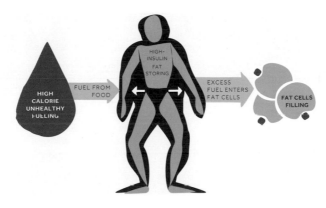

If we move people away from the ultra-processed western diet and unhealthy carbs, we can turn off insulin so the body stops behaving like a fat storage depot.

The system I developed takes all of the confusion out of shopping and ordering at restaurants.

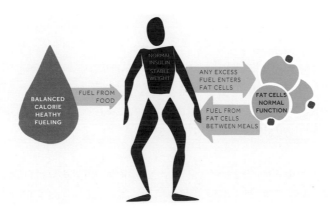

Here are your rules of thumb for foods that contain carbohydrates:

- Dark green = lowest glycemic (the best foods for weight loss and optimal health)
- Light green = moderate glycemic (foods to be eaten in moderation)
- Light orange = higher glycemic (foods to be eaten only rarely)
- Red = toxic (foods to be avoided at all costs)

Color Code for Glycemic Index

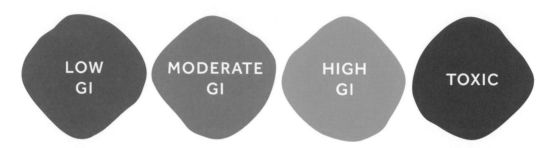

As you experienced in Phase I or during your weight loss, your healthy eating selections in your lean and green came from the dark green charts. These foods are highly effective at turning off your insulin and fat storage and will facilitate reaching and maintaining an optimal weight. The light green charts list foods that are healthy but were used sparingly in the first phase of our journey. Foods on the orange chart should be used with care, and only after you've reached optimal health. And any food that is in the red is directly damaging to your health and should be eliminated completely from your diet forever. However good they taste, they are just not worth it.

And of course, the prepackaged low-calorie fuelings are designed specifically to provide a high-quality, low-glycemic choice, and are always an excellent way to obtain a nutrient-dense, calorie-friendly fueling or meal. They are always designated dark green.

The charts are available for download on HabitsofHealth.com and also are in *Your LifeBook* and the Habits of Health App.

THE ELEMENTS OF EATING HEALTHY: LIVING IN THE GREEN

The charts that follow are designed to steer you toward foods that rev up your health. Think of them as the octane-disclosure sheets at the gas pumps. Watch your engine's performance improve as you switch from regular gas (the low-octane, nutrient-poor foods you're eating now) to premium (functional foods that are nutrient-dense, highly efficient fuels that turn down your insulin pump and turn on fat burning).

As you shop, remember to visualize your nine-inch plate, with its divisions based on the proper proportion of foods for optimal health and weight loss. You'll need to have plenty of vegetables and fruits on hand, as well as lesser quantities of healthy complex starches and lean proteins to create healthy, delicious meals.

Your Nine-Inch Plate Divided into Food Types

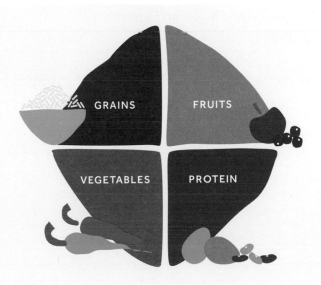

Dr. A's Healthy Eating Plate System for Life

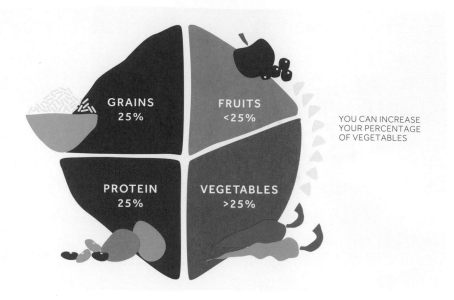

When you're shopping, think about the meals you're planning. A meal on your nine-inch plate should be made up of 50% vegetables and fruits, 25% protein, and 25% grain from my healthy food choices. Remember you can always add more vegetables and less fruit to the percentage, especially if your monitoring reveals you have gained a few pounds!

Vegetables and Fruits (Part 2.5 in *Dr. A's Habits Of Health, Choosing Wisely: Dr. A's Color-Coded Shopping System*)

(25 & 25 totalling 50% of Your Plate)

Make sure you read in Part 2.5 as to the benefits of eating healthy choices. Here we are focused on what you will actually select for yourself.

Vegetables and Fruits

- Berries
- Peaches
- Many More
- Apples
- Leaf Veggies

Healthy vegetable and fruit choices: A wide variety of vibrant foods including salads, crunchy raw vegetables, and nutrient-packed berries.

Proportion of your meal: 50% of your nine-inch plate between the two. Limit fruit to 25% but you can increase the vegetable percentage.

Portion size: About the size of a small paperback book of about 100 pages. However, green low-glycemic vegetables are so beneficial, you could probably even use a great big Tom Clancy book as your point of reference for judging the proper amount and still not overdo it!

Vegetable and Fruit Choices

Vegetables and fruits make up a whopping 50% of your meals, so it's especially important to select the lowest-glycemic varieties. The following charts are arranged from lowest glycemic (dark green) to moderate glycemic (light green) to high-glycemic (orange). If you see a red chart, avoid at all cost! Red can make you dead! (Okay, so it won't kill you instantly but predictably it will over time.)

	15 OR LESS				
VERY LOW GI	• Zucchini		• Arugula		• Broccoli
	• Spinach		• Asparagus		• Chives
	• Peppers		• Fennel		• Leeks
	• Onions		• Cucumber		• Celery
	• Mushrooms		• Cabbage		• Cauliflower
	• Lettuce		• Squash		• Chili peppers
	• Alfalfa sprouts		• Brussels sprouts		
	• Artichokes		• Bell peppers		
	20 OR MORE				
	• Eggplant	20	• Green beans	20	• Carrots (raw) 30
HIGH GI	**50 OR MORE**				
	• Peas	50	• Corn	65	• Carrots (cooked) 80
	• Taro	54	• Red beets (canned)	64	

Vegetables from the dark green charts have very little effect on blood sugar and insulin and should be used freely. In fact, if you find that you absolutely need a little something extra as you're settling into your new eating strategy, you can always select from this component. Celery is a great crunchy choice!

Make a list of your favorite vegetables in the dark green and light green for your shopping list Put a "g" next to the green choices and choose at least 75% from that group as you come out of transition to ensure you are not turning on insulin:

Fruit GI Chart

VERY LOW GI	30 OR LESS					
	• Olives	15	• Lemons	20	• Grapefruit	25
	• Avocado	10	• Raspberries	25	• Cherries	25
	• Limes	20	• Blackberries	25	• Tomatoes	30

LOW GI	50 OR LESS					
	• Apples	30	• Pears	35	• Apricots (dried)	35
	• Nectarines	30	• Strawberries	35	• Plums	35
	• Peaches	30	• Oranges	35	• Figs	40

HIGH GI	50 OR MORE					
	• Apricots	57	• Kiwi	50	• Pineapple	59
	• Bananas	60	• Grapes	53	• Watermelon	76
	• Blueberries	53	• Mango	51		
	• Cantaloupe	50	• Melon	60		

Make a list of your favorite fruits in the dark green and light green sections for your shopping list. Put a "g" next to the green choices and choose at least 75% from that group as you come out of transition to ensure you are not turning on insulin:

Protein
(25% of Your Plate)

Proteins
- Meat
- Fish
- Nuts
- Eggs
- Poultry
- Legumes
- Seeds

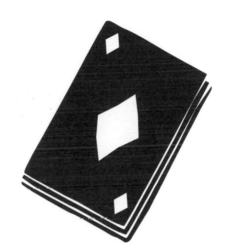

Proportion of your meal: 25% of your nine-inch plate.

Portion size: About the size of a deck of cards (after cooking).

Still Pick Green to Stay Lean and Healthy
The charts below don't list the glycemic levels for meat, fish, or poultry because the glycemic content for these foods is negligible. However, the charts do include the total fat and saturated fat levels for meats. To guide your choices for optimal health, just choose any fish from the charts or any meats that fall in the green area.

Fish and Seafood
When you eat fish, you're not only choosing a great protein source, you're also significantly reducing your risk of disease. Eating fish one to three times a week is an important Habit of Health and can have a profound impact on your wellbeing over time. In fact, one serving of fish a week may reduce your risk of fatal heart attack by 40%![1]

Note: Pregnant women and young children should limit their intake of fish to once a week due to the potential for high mercury content in some fish.

Healthy fish and seafood providing high levels of omega-3 fatty acids

FRESH FISH	CANNED FISH
• Atlantic and Pacific salmon • Smoked salmon • Atlantic and Pacific mackerel • Bluefin tuna • Oysters • Squid (calimari)	• Salmon • Sardines • Mackerel • Tuna (in water, canola, olive oil, tomato sauce or brine)

Seafood choices by fat content

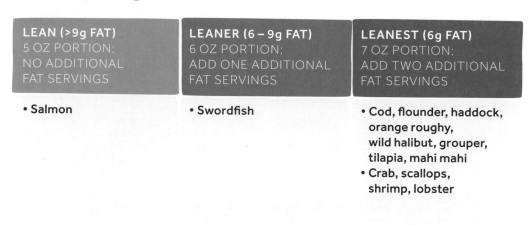

LEAN (>9g FAT) 5 OZ PORTION; NO ADDITIONAL FAT SERVINGS	LEANER (6 – 9g FAT) 6 OZ PORTION; ADD ONE ADDITIONAL FAT SERVINGS	LEANEST (6g FAT) 7 OZ PORTION; ADD TWO ADDITIONAL FAT SERVINGS
• Salmon	• Swordfish	• Cod, flounder, haddock, orange roughy, wild halibut, grouper, tilapia, mahi mahi • Crab, scallops, shrimp, lobster

Make a list of your favorite fish and seafood for your shopping list:

Meat

It's an important Habit of Health to lower your consumption of red meat. But if you're like me and once in a while need that savory taste of meat, just minimize the amount of saturated fat so you can enjoy this great protein source and still stay healthy.

Fat content of meat

	TOTAL FAT	SATURATED FAT
Buffalo, elk, venison	17%	7%
Pork loin	26%	9%
Round steak	27%	10%
Veal chop	39%	17%
Canadian bacon	41%	14%
Filet mignon	42%	16%
Sirloin steak	44%	16%
Flank steak	44%	19%
Lamb ribs	48%	22%
Spare ribs	52%	22%
Ground beef (very lean)	58%	23%
Sausage (beef)	80%	33%

Make a list of your favorite meat from the dark green and light green sections for your shopping:

Poultry
Chicken, turkey, and other forms of poultry are healthier choices than red meat.

Fat content of poultry

	SKIN?	TOTAL FAT	SATURATED FAT
Turkey breast		18%	6%
Chicken breast		24%	7%
Chicken breast	Yes	36%	10%
Turkey breast	Yes	38%	5%
Chicken dark meat		43%	12%
Turkey dark meat	Yes	47%	14%
Turkey sausage		50%	15%
Duck	Yes	50%	19%
Chicken dark meat	Yes	56%	16%
Cornish game hen	Yes	63%	28%
Turkey hot dog		70%	19%

Make a list of your favorite poultry from the dark green and light green sections for your shopping list:

A final piece of advice: free-range or organic poultry can help you avoid the antibiotics and growth hormones that are given to many commercially-raised birds.

Eggs (Part 2.5 in *Dr. A's Habits Of Health, Choosing Wisely: Dr. A's Color-Coded Shopping System*)

You should still limit your daily intake of dietary cholesterol to 200 milligrams—the amount in one small egg. There's no limit to the amount of egg whites you can eat, though, as long as they fit on the 25% of your plate devoted to protein.

On Shopping List: ⬤ Yes ⬤ No
Whites: ⬤ Yes

Legumes

This is a group that includes beans, peas, and lentils. Legumes are one of my favorite functional foods and probably my top pick for an all-around health food. A cup of legumes gives you 110–150 calories of the best fuel you can buy. Choose from any of the varieties in the chart for the protein portion of your meal—all are low-glycemic and do an excellent job of turning off your insulin pump.

Legumes GI Chart

VERY LOW GI	30 OR LESS						
	• Soy beans	18	• Chickpeas		• Lentils	25	
	• Edamame	20	(Garbanzo beans)	20	• Black beans	25	

LOW GI	50 OR LESS						
	• Lima beans	32	• Chickpeas	35	• Black-eyed peas	42	
	• Kidney beans	35	• White beans	35			

Make a list of your favorite legumes from the dark green and light green section for your shopping list:

A word about soy (Part 2.5 in *Dr. A's Habits Of Health, Choosing Wisely: Dr. A's Color-Coded Shopping System*)

One particularly amazing legume stands out: soy. Soybeans have twice as much protein as other legumes and provide nearly as many essential amino acids as animal protein but without all the saturated fat. They're a good source of calcium as well, making them a great alternative to dairy products. In addition, soy is full of naturally occurring isoflavones—phytonutrients that protect against cardiovascular disease and osteoporosis.[3]

In fact, I think so highly of soy that it's my top choice for the protein component of our portion-controlled packaged meals and fuelings are a great way to make using this healthy legume as your protein component a breeze!

When refined into soybean oil it loses my vote because it is full of omega-6 which is then inflammatory. And it is everywhere! (Look at your salad dressing).

Dairy Products and Cheese

Dairy products are not a necessary food group once we reach adulthood and, because they can wallop a lot of calories, I suggest you avoid them at least during weight loss. If you enjoy them, they can be a good source of calcium, protein, and other nutrients. They are the one protein source that can be quite high-glycemic. Remember, though, that a 1-ounce serving of cheese is a very small amount—about the size of two AA batteries.

Cheese with Calories per Ounce

Cottage	20	Soy	43
Ricotta	50	Feta	75
Mozzarella	90	American	94
Brie	95	Blue	100
Provolone	100	Gouda	101
Monterey jack	106	Swiss	108
Havarti	106	Jarlsberg	110
Parmesan	110	Colby	112
Cheddar	114		

Make a list of your favorite cheese for your shopping list (sparingly):

Seeds and Nuts: Your High-Octane Fuel Source GI Chart

VERY LOW GI	30 OR LESS					
	• Peanuts	15	• Sunflower seeds	15	• Hazlenuts	15
	• Brazil nuts	15	• Pecans	15	• Walnuts	15
	• Pumpkin seeds	15	• Almonds	15		

These health-giving, low-glycemic, protein-rich foods are also just chock full of healthy fats. Recent research indicates that walnuts may be even more important than olive oil in creating the health-boosting effects of the popular "Mediterranean diet."[2] But nuts and seeds are also extremely energy-dense, meaning that they pack a lot of calories into a small amount. Those calories can add up in a hurry—in fact, a serving size is no more than a handful.

Make a list of your favorite nuts and seeds for your shopping list:

Grains
(25% of your plate)

It may seem melodramatic, but it's true: your grain selections set the stage for success or failure. Starches come in a vast array of options. Sadly, most of the options developed and promoted by the fast-food and processed-food industries are bad for you. Healthy starches, on the other hand, are a nutrient-rich source of slow-burning fuel and long-lasting energy.

When looking at starches, it's essential to consider their position on the glycemic index. Most processed and prepackaged starches score high on the index, meaning that they deliver large amounts of carbohydrates and must be avoided. Instead, shop for healthy, low-glycemic starches using my color-coded system. This will act as your reliable guide in this vast and sometimes confusing food group.

Starches
- Breads
- Grains
- Rice
- Cereals
- Pasta

Portion size: about the size of a tennis ball

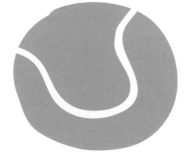

Cereals, Breads, and Pastas GI Chart

LOW GI	50 OR LESS			
	• Quinoa	35	• Buckwheat	45
	• Muesli (natural)	30	• Pasta (whole grain)	45
	• Rye bread	30	• Wholewheat bread (with bran)	45
	• Unrefined flour:		• All-bran cereal	48
	bread	40	• Sourdough bread	35
	pasta	40		

HIGH GI	50 OR MORE			
	• Oatmeal (from steel-cut oats)	58	• Corn flakes	70
	• Semolina (cream of oats)	60	• White bread (enriched)	71
	• Hamburger roll	61	• Bagel (white)	72
	• Couscous	65	• Dinner roll (white)	73
	• Cereals (refined)	70	• Kaiser roll (white)	73
			• Crackers	80

Commercial Breakfast Products GI Chart

LOW GI	50 OR LESS					
	• All-bran	34				

HIGH GI	50 OR MORE					
	• Frosted Flakes™	55	• Raisin Bran™	73	• Rice Krispies™	82
	• Special K™	56	• Bran Flakes™	74	• Crispix™	87
	• Nutri-Grain™	66	• Coco Pops™	77	• Shredded Wheat™	75
	• Fruit Loops™	69	• Corn Flakes™	77	• Wonder Bread®	80
	• Honey Smacks™	71	• Corn Pops™	80	• Oatmeal™ (instant)	82

Healthy starch choices: Bread, pasta, noodles, and breakfast cereals made from whole grains such as rice, oats, wheat, barley, and rye. Potatoes, though a vegetable, act more like a refined starch due to their high-glycemic and high-carbohydrate content.

Make a list of your favorite healthy grains for your shopping list:

Pasta, Potatoes, and Rice GI Chart

50 OR LESS					
• Wild rice	35	• Spaghetti		• Sweet potatoes	46
• Yams	37	(durum)	40	• Brown rice	50
• Spaghetti		• Basmati rice	50		
(whole wheat)	40				

MORE THAN 50					
• White pasta	55	• Potatoes		• Risotto	70
• Potatoes (with skin,		(mashed)	80	• Rice cakes	85
baked		• Potatoes		• Rice (precooked)	90
or boiled)	65	(instant mashed)	88		
• Potatoes (peeled		• French fries	95		
and boiled)	70				

Make a list of your favorite healthy pastas and rice for your shopping list:

Your grain (starch) choices can set you up for success or failure—low-glycemic, whole-grain starches are critical for optimal health, while refined and processed high-glycemic foods send your body into storage mode.

Remember, we are using grain and starch interchangeably to be able to use the tools presented in the My Plate System to guide you on healthy and unhealthy choices.

Unhealthy Grains (Starches): A Habit of Disease

What about the choice so many of us make to eat the starches that poison your body? Unhealthy starches, like the ones in the following chart, are convenient, inexpensive, readily available, and tempting, thanks to the food industry's heavy use of advertising. They fulfill a need for comfort and satisfy cravings and hunger for a short time. But they also rev up your insulin pump, turn on your fat-storage system, stimulate inflammation, and can lead to the myriad health problems that make up metabolic syndrome: the path to progressive poor health and disease. In the end, they leave you with nothing but fatigue, excess weight, more cravings, and poor health.

What's more, consuming unhealthy starches like these during Phase I of your weight loss will bring your fat-burning machinery to an abrupt halt for at least several days. Once you've reached a healthy weight, your body should be able to tolerate some of these foods on occasion. However, I recommend that you eliminate them permanently. You'll soon find that the meals I teach you to prepare using healthy starches will be just as convenient, taste much better, and bring you to a state of energy, vibrancy, and health.

Eliminating all ultra-processed unhealthy food filled with refined sugar and flours can have a dramatic positive effect on your health! Eating unhealthy starches like soda, French fries, candy, and doughnuts brings your fat-burning machinery to a halt.

Unhealthy starch and sugar choices

UNHEALTHY: HABITS OF DISEASE		
• Doughnuts	• Cookies	• French fries
• Sodas	• Candy	

Fats

Eating the right type of fats in the right amount can have a dramatic impact on your health and is an important component of our healthy eating strategy. The typical Western diet takes about 34% of its calories from fat: the vast majority from saturated, animal-based fat. According to the USDA, fat should make up between 25–35% of your daily caloric intake, with no more than seven percent coming from saturated fat.[3] It's no wonder that Western societies, who eat too much of the wrong fat, lead the world in heart disease, diabetes, obesity, and several types of cancer.

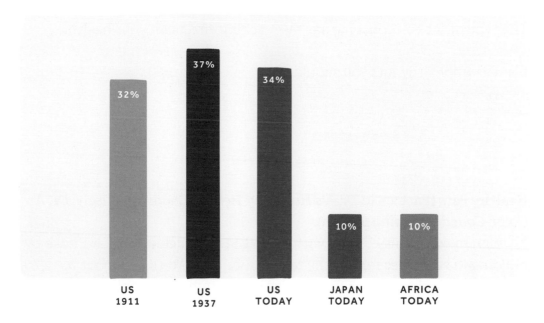

Take a look at the chart above, and notice how fat intake in the U.S. compares to other countries that have a lower incidence of these diseases.

Unhealthy Fats

Why does fat so easily lead to weight gain and disease?

- A gram of fat contains nine calories, which is more than double the calories in a gram of protein or carbohydrate.
- Combined with too many high-glycemic, processed carbohydrates, our bodies store fat calories at an accelerated rate.
- Calorie for calorie, fat is much less effective than protein or complex carbohydrates at satisfying your appetite and giving you a sense of fullness.

The type of fat you consume has far-reaching effects on your health.

List the unhealthy fats you should avoid:

Healthy Fats (Part 2.5 in *Dr. A's Habits Of Health, Choosing Wisely: Dr. A's Color-Coded Shopping System*)

My plan makes it easy to stay within the USDA guidelines for fat intake by building in strategies for healthy fat consumption. You'll get about 20–25% of your daily calories from fat, mostly through mono and polyunsaturated fats like those found in olive, canola, and flaxseed oils. You'll also consume small amounts of fat through fish, skinless white poultry, and healthy lean and wild meats.

It's worth noting however, that all fats and oils, while rich in health benefits, are a calorie-dense foods—with 120 calories in just one tablespoon. Therefore, they should be used sparingly, particularly during Phase I, when it's important to maintain a lower energy intake.

Top sources for healthy fat:

- Fatty cold-water fish, especially salmon
- Soybeans
- Olive oil
- Nuts, especially almonds
- Avocados, guacamole
- Flaxseed products

Cooking and Salad Oils

One benefit of oils high in monounsaturated fats is that when they're heated, they develop fewer free radicals than polyunsaturated oils. That means they're great for cooking. Note, however, that olive oil—my favorite healthy oil for just about everything else—cannot be used for high-temperature cooking because its low smoking point will cause it to smoke, impair flavor, and become degraded. So if you're really cooking, coconut oil may be a better choice.

	OMEGA TYPE	MONO-UNSATURATED	POLY-UNSATURATED	SATURATED
Olive	0–9	75%	8%	17%
Canola	0–6, 9	55%	38%	7%
Sesame	0–6, 9	39%	43%	18%
Coconut	0–6	34%	45%	21%
Corn	0–6	20%	66%	14%
Soy	0–6	19%	65%	16%
Safflower	0–6	13%	79%	8%
Sunflower	0–6	11%	80%	9%
Peanut	0–6	5%	2%	93%

Make a list of your favorite healthy oils from the chart for your shopping list:

The Omega Fats: Omega-3, Omega-6, Omega-9 (Part 2.5 in *Dr. A's Habits Of Health, Choosing Wisely: Dr. A's Color-Coded Shopping System*)

Think all omegas are alike? Think again. There are different types of omegas, some healthy and some not so healthy.

Which ones are good for you?

Which ones should you avoid?

Fiber (Part 2.5 in *Dr. A's Habits Of Health, Choosing Wisely: Dr. A's Color-Coded Shopping System*)

You've probably heard that fiber is an important part of a healthy diet. But the different types of fiber can be a little confusing. Here's a guide so you can be sure to include both types in your daily food choices. (There are about 3 grams of fiber per cup or piece of the foods listed below.)

Soluble fiber dissolves in water. Its benefits to your body include slowing the breakdown of complex carbohydrates and helping to reduce blood sugar. When you eat it in large enough quantities, it can help lower cholesterol as well.

Good sources of soluble fiber: grains such as rye, barley, and oats; vegetables and fruits; legumes.

Insoluble fiber doesn't dissolve in water and is not absorbed or digested by the body. But it does reduce hunger (it's filling!), helps keep your gastrointestinal tract clean, and aids regular bowel movements by pulling water into the colon.

Good sources of insoluble fiber: brown rice; whole wheat breads and cereals; seeds; fruit and vegetable skins; legumes.

Prebiotics, Probiotics, and Polyphenolic Compounds

Our digestive tract is extremely important for our overall health. The gut microbiome is made up of over a trillion microorganisms and is responsible for maintaining the integrity and health of our intestinal lining. With a proper diet, the bacteria produce more fermentation, which helps to nourish the gut flora.

So what can we do to improve gut health?

Polyphenols, like curcumin which is found in the spice turmeric and used in curry-based foods—can actually enter the bloodstream to have an anti-inflammatory effect on the whole body. Eating whole plant foods and live fermented products can really improve gut health. Great sources of probiotics come from several sources that most people do not eat that often. Fermented pickles (not those made with vinegar) such as sauerkraut, kimchi, and kefir are all great sources, along with live cultures of yogurt.

Topping It Off with Herbs and Spices (Part 2.5 in *Dr. A's Habits Of Health, Choosing Wisely: Dr. A's Color-Coded Shopping System*)

Herbs and spices are a great way to enhance flavor without adding calories, fat, or other unhealthy substances. And many do much more than that as they actually help you lose weight while providing particular health benefits.

Try these great choices:
- Toss foods with a simple mixture of sea salt, black pepper, olive oil, and vinegar.
- Add red pepper to an egg-white omelet to decrease hunger and increase your metabolism.
- Add a pinch of turmeric to add a hint of mustard flavor and reduce inflammation.
- Don't forget garlic, cilantro, parsley, and basil, which add so many flavors and have numerous health benefits

Save Your Salad with Salad Spritzers!

Too much dressing can turn a healthy salad into a calorie disaster. In fact, bottled dressings are often rich sources of saturated fat, calories, sodium, and added sugar which are all unhealthy for you. That's why salad spritzers are such a great invention. They deliver just one calorie per spray and help you to coat all of your yummy vegetables without all those calories.

An even better choice is to avoid processed salad dressings and instead use a drizzle of extra virgin olive oil with vinegar instead!

A Habit of Disease:
Polluting Your Body with Empty Calories from Processed Foods
Sugar and fat: the non-nutritive agents

The United States topped the list as the biggest eaters, according to calorie intake data released by The Food and Agriculture Organization in 2018. Americans eat an average of over 3,000 calories a day, according to the report. This is well above the U.S. Department of Agriculture recommendations. Amazingly, 40% of those calories come from refined, processed sugars and fats (primarily saturated animal fat). But when we fill up on calorie-laden fried foods and desserts, we leave ourselves very little room for the healthy, nutrient-rich foods our bodies need.

Where do our daily calories come from? Let's look at a breakdown.

Dietary Guidelines[4]

	DAILY CALORIE INTAKE	FAT CALORIES	SUGAR CALORIES	TOTAL FAT AND SUGAR CALORIES	REMAINING CALORIES
MALES	3,000	1,200 – 1,500	600	1,800 – 2,100	900 – 1,200
FEMALES	2,000	800 – 1,000	400	1,200 – 1,400	600 – 800

This means that the average male only needs 1,200 calories and the average female only needs 800 calories per day. And this should be from foods that contain nutrients!

This dramatic nutrient deficit is a major reason that many of us have a constant desire to eat, despite our ample caloric intake, and that means more cravings, more overeating, and excess weight. It's yet another Habit of Disease taking us down the slippery path to non-sickness and sickness at a breakneck pace.

A Habit of Health:
Choosing nutrient-rich foods

My healthy eating strategy ensures that you get nearly 100% of your calories from high-quality, nutrient-packed low-calorie meals and whole foods. Eating this way helps you feel pleasantly satisfied, protects you from the onslaught of nutritional pollution, and supports your goal of optimal health.

Legumes, including chickpeas, beans, soybeans, and lentils, are a wonderful alternative protein source. They are also low-glycemic, loaded with fiber and phytonutrients, and nutrient-dense with vitamins and minerals. I recommend eating them at least twice a week or more as your main protein source.

How many calories?

- ½ cup of legumes contain approximately 100–200 calories and are very low-glycemic.
- A 4-ounce portion of lean meat contains about 250 calories.
- A 6-ounce portion of skinless white-meat chicken contains about 300 calories.

CHOOSING RIGHT WHEN YOU'RE DINING OUT (PART 2.8 IN DR. A'S HABITS OF HEALTH, HEALTHY EATING FOR LIFE: YOUR TRANSITION TO PERMANENT HEALTH)

Going out to eat has become a way of life. I certainly look forward to dining out with family and friends. After all, everyone needs an occasional hassle-free evening, pampered by great service, with nothing to prepare or wash. You can make this indulgence a healthy one as long as you control your nutritional intake by following a few important guidelines.

Watch for Pitfalls

Look at dining out from the restaurant's point of view. Restaurants are in the business of making money and keeping their customers happy so they can make more money. They want you to come back and bring all your friends. And fat, salt, and sugar sell.

A Habit of Health: Avoiding Fast Foods (Part 2.8 in *Dr. A's Habits of Health*)

How can I avoid being tempted by fast food restaurants?

The Restaurant Trap (Part 2.8 in *Dr. A's Habits of Health*)

How can I eat better when I go to a restaurant?

Choose Healthy Cooking Methods (Part 2.8 in *Dr. A's Habits of Health*)

How should I have them prepare my food when I go to a restaurant?

Keep Portions in Check

Restaurant servings are out of control. An occasional treat is fine, but if you eat out often, you need to develop an overall strategy for portion control. Here are a few tips.

- Visualize the divisions on the nine-inch plate.
- Order two appetizers instead of an entrée, such as soup and a dinner salad, or shrimp cocktail.
- Split a meal with your dining companion.
- Don't rely on the chef or waiter to serve you the proper amount of food. Surveys show that people generally eat everything that's put in front of them, whether they wanted it or not.[5]
- Ask for a leftovers container when you place your order. When your meal comes, eyeball your proper portion right away and put the rest into the box to take home.

Prepackaged Meals: The Healthy Fast Food—for Weight Loss and for Life. Scientifically formulated portion-controlled meals are a convenient choice for your three-hour fuelings, especially if you don't have a lot of time to prepare food. These convenient low-fat, low-glycemic foods are loaded with vitamins and minerals, offer a careful balance of protein and carbohydrates, and provide you with a specific dose of calories so you don't have to worry about calorie creep. And because our fuelings are completely portable, they help to ensure that you're getting a proper fueling when it's not otherwise feasible. That's why I've used them myself for over 17 years now. They really help me to get my five to six daily fuelings even if I'm in the midst of a busy lifestyle, traveling away from home, or just out and about and hungry. For more information on ordering your fuelings, see the resource list in the appendix in Habits of Health.

Quick and Easy Tools for "Automatic Eating"

In Part 2.6 of *Dr. A's Habits of Health, Building Healthy Meal Plans for Optimal Health*, I lay out a whole system for preparing and making amazing meals in a fashion that is as easy as the fuelings.

In fact one of my most important goals for you is to make preparing healthy foods as easy as stopping into a fast food restaurant.

For most of us, eating processed, microwaved, or fast food is an easy alternative to preparing meals that seem too hard, too time consuming, and leave us with a messy kitchen and a load of dishes. Cooking just doesn't seem worth it!

Please read Part 2.6 in, *Dr. A's Habits of Health, Building Healthy Meal Plans for Optimal Health*, to learn how to build healthy meal plans. You will also find a list of healthy snacks and a whole bunch of tools to help overcome the logistical problems of eating healthy.

Beginning Your Lifetime of Healthy Eating

You should now have a firm grip on the eating strategy that will support you for life. You understand the full range of healthy foods that will help you maintain your weight and set the foundation for optimal health. You've calculated your daily energy requirements and are starting to increase your caloric intake based on those calculations, as well as adding calories gradually according to the amount of weight you have lost.

As you learned in Phase I, you're eating every three hours and using my low-glycemic, portion-control system to keep a handle on your daily fuelings. You know how to use the system even when dining out, and you're savvier about avoiding the pitfalls of the restaurant environment.

It's not always easy to have a low-fat, low-glycemic, low-calorie meal on hand when you need it. That's why portion-controlled meals have been a lifesaver for many of my patients and others I've coached. As a high-quality, portable fast food, our fuelings are just about unbeatable. It's a great tool as you continue your journey. A recent study showed that simply by decreasing portion size and energy density by 25%, people were able to maintain their healthy weight.[6] And now, so can you. Combine your new understanding of portion control and energy density with your knowledge of healthy proteins, starches, vegetables, and fruit, and you will have the Habits of Health to support a lifetime of healthy eating.

You have a bulletproof system to help you eat healthy for life. In the next Element we will discuss how to protect yourself from the allure of ultra-refined unhealthy nutritional pollution.

Notes to yourself:

Now that you have completed Element 15, *How To Eat Healthy For Life,* **write down your thoughts guided by the following questions:**

What does this Element mean to you right now?

What does this Element give you the opportunity to reflect on?

What actions are you going to take as a result of this Element?

I encourage you to connect with your coach, so you can share your thoughts and actions as soon as possible. Sharing your thoughts with your coach will help them become a reality. Make sure you review all your notes and this Element often.

1 *Seafood Long-Chain n-3 Polyunsaturated Fatty Acids and Cardiovascular Disease: A Science Advisory From the American Heart Association* – Alice H. Lichtenstein, published 17 May 2018 Circulation. 2018;138:e35−e47.

2 *Effects of Walnut Consumption on Blood Lipids and Other Cardiovascular Risk Factors: an Updated Meta-Analysis and Systematic Review of Controlled Trials* – Marta Guasch-Ferré, Jun Li Frank, B Hu Jordi, Salas-Salvadó Deirdre, K Tobias, The American Journal of Clinical Nutrition, Volume 108, Issue 1, 1 July 2018, Pages 174−187, https://doi.org/10.1093/ajcn/nqy091.

3 www.cdc.gov Mean total fat intake for men (percent of kilocalories): 33.6% Mean total fat intake for women (percent of kilocalories): 33.7%.

4 health.gov, Food and Nutrition, Dietary Guidelines 2015–2020 Dietary Guidelines for Americans.

5 www.foodpsychology.cornell.edu/discoveries/92-clean-plate-club.

6 *What is The Role of Portion Control in Weight Management?* – B J Rolls, Int J Obes (Lond). 2014 Jul; 38(Suppl 1): S1−S8. Published online 2014 Jul 25. doi: [10.1038/ijo.2014.82]PMCID: PMC4105579PMID: 25033958.

ELEMENT 16:
DEALING WITH ADDICTIVE FOOD

Average time to complete: **1 week**

In Element 16, we will:

- Explore the danger of addictive food.
- Identify your personal susceptibility to these addictive foods.
- Reinforce the importance of using the portion control plate system.

HIGHLY REFINED PROCESS FOOD IS AN ADDICTIVE SUBSTANCE

10,000 years ago, it was highly advantageous when we could assume a food's health benefits by its beautiful color, overwhelming fragrance, and the sweet taste of the fruit itself.

Unfortunately, today our society is completely saturated with cues to signal tasty, sugary, salty, and easily obtained unhealthy ultra-processed food.

Everywhere you go, you are inundated with advertisements and enticing brands, pictures, videos, and access to highly processed, highly addictive food that is portable, cheap, and available for just about any occasion. During those times when you are under stress, having an emotional crisis, or just bored, it offers a quick fix by sugar-jolting your energy and providing immediate, short-lasting pleasure. In this Element, we are going to help equip you with a better understanding of why these toxic non-food substances should be treated much like you would cocaine or heroin. The Habits of Disease can create instantaneous pleasure but they will ultimately result in significant consequences to your health and wellbeing.

In Part 2.5 in *Dr. A's Habits of Health, Choosing Wisely: Dr. A's Color-Coded Shopping System*, I talked about the addictive nature of ultra-processed food. Please read the White Powder section in that chapter, because it may save your life!

The refined state of sugar and flour is everywhere.

Those powders form the basis not just for breads and buns, but for a huge variety of processed foods from cereals, crackers, and pizza dough to cookies, cakes, and ice-cream cones. As a result, the average American now eats 10 servings of refined grains each day. And, as we showed you in Part 1.1 in *Dr. A's Habits of Health, It's Not Your Fault That You're Struggling*, refined sugar is in everything. In fact, we are consuming an average of over 150 lbs of refined sugar and flour products a year.[1]

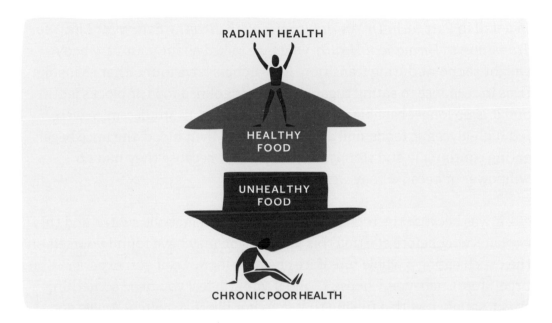

I talked about how the food industry is creating an addiction to this food, and by now you are probably tired of me talking about how bad these foods that make up the Habits of Disease are for you and your health and wellbeing.

Hopefully you are coming out of Phase I at the healthiest weight and the highest level of wellbeing you have had in years and realize this is as much due to eliminating toxic foods as it is about reaching a healthy weight. In fact, if you have sampled some of these toxic foods during your transition, you probably noticed that they make you feel bad.

I want to have this talk with you now as you work through your transition and on to eating healthy for life.

Avoid introducing ultra-refined sugar and flour into your diet at all costs! They are kryptonite and cause insatiable hunger and cravings, leading to addiction and loss of control!

Insatiable Hunger:

Leptin is the hunger suppressant hormone released by your fat cells that tells your brain you are not hungry anymore: Go get busy and build a hut, find a mate, do something to improve your survival. We went over its role in detail in Part 2.8 in *Dr. A's Habits of Health, Healthy Eating for Life: Your Transition to Permanent Health,* when we talked about your new body weight set point during transition. Researchers have found that as insulin rises in response to eating sugar and flour in refined food, it blocks leptin and it is no longer capable of suppressing hunger. In studies, mice were fed high-glycemic foods, and as insulin rose in their blood, the mice began eating continually and stopped moving. Was it because they had no willpower or because they were weak?[2]

No, it was because the refined foods flipped the metabolic switch and this explains why, before starting this journey, you may have found yourself on the couch eating a whole tub of ice cream at 10pm. So, if you experience an urge, Stop. Challenge. Choose.™ and if you still feel you need something sweet, satisfy it with a fueling that does not flip that switch. You've got this!!!!! It's biology, not psychology, although your Habits of Health will automate a healthy response over time!

Cravings and Addiction:

The second problem with refined sugar and flours is that they light up the brain just like cocaine and heroin. As we discussed in Part 2.5 in *Dr. A's Habits of Health, Choosing Wisely: Dr. A's Color-Coded Shopping System,* when subjects are placed in MRI machines designed to show areas of the brain that are activated after consuming sugar or refined flour, the subject's pleasure and reward center lights up like a firework display. The hyperactive area known as the nucleus accumbens releases large amounts of dopamine, which creates a pleasurable feeling and leads to the desire for more.[3]

This is why you may go out on a cold snowy night to get your favorite ice cream or eat a whole pizza or bag of potato chips.

And just like the continual use of a drug, if you continue to eat sugary and refined processed food, the brain adapts rapidly and starts to thin out the dopamine receptors because it senses that too much dopamine was released. As a result, the receptors down-regulate so now you lack the ability to feel the same level of pleasure unless you eat larger amounts to stimulate enough dopamine release.

In people who are more susceptible, it can create a state of lifeless, down, or even depressed feelings with a lack of energy between sugar rushes.

I may be describing how you felt before you started this journey, or maybe not. It depends on how susceptible you are to the addictive powers of sugar and refined flours.

Just like people have a varying degree of addictive potential to alcohol, the same is true with refined sugar and flour.

Susceptibility to Refined Sugar and Flour
Because refined, ultra-processed food lights up the pleasure centers of our brain, there is a degree of risk to all of us in this obesigenic world of processed food. But it is clear that some of us are at a much higher risk than others of being drawn into the dark web of sugar and refined flour addiction.

In one study, rats were exposed to a lever that they could push before a highly sugary food was released into a trough.[4]

Highly Susceptible Group (⅓) These rats loved the lever and would continually hit it even before the food was released.

Moderately Susceptible Group (⅓) These rats would come to the lever sometimes and sometimes they would not.

Low Susceptible Group (⅓) These rats would only come when food showed up.

Why does the lever help us understand the patterns of addiction? The highly susceptible rats fell in love with the lever, which is a strong cue that predicts reward. The cue actually becomes the reward and sets up a craving that is a powerful determinant of behavior.

How does this translate into our own lives?
Suddenly, a TV commercial stimulates you at a subconscious level to desire a dessert to the point that you will drive through a snowstorm to get it. Since our world is saturated with such cues, it is important that you are aware of your level of risk, so that you can be much more vigilant. Let's do a quick test to see which category you fall into in terms of addiction to sugar and refined flour. Just like the rats, humans also stratify into one of three general groups.

Habits of Disease Food Addiction Susceptibility Quiz

1. I find it difficult to control how much I eat:
- Rarely
- Occasionally
- Daily

2. I crash in the afternoon and have trouble waking up in the morning:
- Rarely
- Occasionally
- Daily

3. I have cravings for specific foods:
- Rarely
- Occasionally
- Daily

4. I suffer from moodiness, headaches, or fogginess:
- Rarely
- Occasionally
- Daily

5. When I only eat a moderate amount of food I am not satisfied:

◯ Rarely
◯ Occasionally
◯ Daily

6. I feel guilty after eating:

◯ Rarely
◯ Occasionally
◯ Daily

7. I spend a considerable amount of time thinking about food:

◯ Rarely
◯ Occasionally
◯ Daily

8. I eat even if I am not hungry because I crave a specific food:

◯ Rarely
◯ Occasionally
◯ Daily

9. I eat large amounts of food and feel powerless to stop:

◯ Rarely
◯ Occasionally
◯ Daily

10. I crave carbohydrates like pasta, bread, white rice, or deserts:

◯ Rarely
◯ Occasionally
◯ Daily

Score: . . . .

Low Susceptibility >6 Rarely
Moderate Susceptibility >6 Occasionally
High Susceptibility >6 Daily

This is an estimate of your susceptibility to the lure of sugar and refined flour. The more daily boxes you have ticked, the higher your risk.

If your score was high, then you want to avoid eating any sugar or refined flour processed foods now that you have reached a healthy weight. We have found that part of the higher susceptibility is genetically predetermined.[5] So just like alcohol, if you are at high risk, it is critical that you avoid sugary and starchy processed foods. A combination of genetics and environment puts you at risk. By adopting my healthy eating system and choosing only low-glycemic, green-coded foods, you can potentially keep your risk low. You can eat whole fruits, especially the lower GI deep green ones, but stay away from any processed fruits such as fruit juices or canned fruits with sugar added.

The whole idea is that through the Habits of Healthy Eating you will make good choices and avoid the need for willpower. Just say no to anything that is not in the green. You can eat an amazing array of healthy whole foods along with our prepackaged fuelings and keep the resulting hunger and cravings away.

If you have a moderate, or even a low susceptibility, still be cautious with any processed food that contains sugar and/or refined flour.

Review everything for hidden sugar and flour and look at the list in Part 1.1 in *Dr. A's Habits of Health, It's Not Your Fault That You're Struggling*, which describes all of the ways the food industry tries to disguise sugar.

Remember, if you can avoid stimulating the hormonal metabolic switches that stimulate insulin and allow leptin to signal you are full, your body will give you the proper advice. It is only when we start eating the food industry's ultra-processed food-like substances that we lose control. And by avoiding those sugar and flour substances, you will stop the wild surges of dopamine release that can create cravings leading to addiction and loss of control.

The Habits of Healthy Eating System will keep these two hormones in balance.

That is why you want to study and learn how to use the portion control plate system to avoid excessive calories and the color-coded charts to make sure you are avoiding high-glycemic foods. Study all of the parts on eating healthy in *Dr. A's Habits of Health* until you are clear on what it means to eat healthy for life. If in doubt, when you're hungry, grab a fueling, which ensures that you're getting a low-GI, portion-controlled meal.

By moving through Phase I and continuing to adopt my eating system, you can rewire your brain and it will become automated. During this period, we have up-regulated your dopamine receptors. If you are in the high susceptibility group, you are more likely to be sensitive to sweetness and refined flour products so you will want to avoid them to prevent a relapse into cravings again.

In addition, this is a great time to bring out Stop. Challenge. Choose.™ in full force for those times when you feel any emotional tension, extra stress, or other potential triggers.

A call out to your coach can also be helpful if you are having one of those weak moments. And use the Habits of Health App daily to help support you. Make a decision that nothing tastes as good as optimal health and wellbeing feels and stick to it.

Write down what you are going to do if you feel tempted:

Write down what else you can do to your surroundings to minimize the cues as we are rewiring your brain to be fully automated so it makes good choices:

You are well on your way to becoming the dominant force in your life. We have spent a considerable amount of time focusing on all aspects of eating for a very specific reason.

The world we live in presents a difficult environment for us to eat healthy on a daily basis. As I mentioned earlier, to overcome the psychological and logistical issues of our modern life, I have equipped you with a system, tools, skills, and access to a guide and a community. It has been said many times before that it takes a village to create a healthy eating environment, and now you are part of that community.

Practice daily and integrate all aspects of eating into your Integrated Habits of Health Clock. Leave nothing to chance: use your daily log and weekly and monthly tracker, and work with your coach and *Your LifeBook* to document your journey.

Remember that installing these habits allows you to have the freedom to continue to build optimal health and wellbeing without relying on willpower, which is ineffective by itself.

We have not focused a great deal on motion, increasing activity, or exercise during Phase I because our focus was on what is most effective in weight loss. Now that you are transitioning, you're probably feeling better, more flexible, and carrying around less weight and pressure on your joints. It is now time to shift our focus to motion. This wonderful world of movement will help you optimize your weight management and continue to build optimal health in your body and your mind.

Notes to yourself:

Now that you have completed Element 16, *Dealing With Addictive Food*, write down your thoughts guided by the following questions:

What does this Element mean to you right now?

What does this Element give you the opportunity to reflect on?

What actions are you going to take as a result of this Element?

I encourage you to connect with your coach, so you can share your thoughts and actions as soon as possible. Sharing your thoughts with your coach will help them become a reality. Make sure you review all your notes and this Element often.

1 www.dhhs.nh.gov

2 *Fat Chance: The Bitter Truth About Sugar* – Robert Lustig M.D., published by HarperCollins.

3 *Why Diets Fail* – Nicole Avena M.D., Eating high-sugar foods lights up your brain on an MRI "like a Christmas tree," Dr. Mark Hyman, M.D., founder and medical director of UltraWellness Center.

4 *A Behavioral and Circuit Model Based on Sugar Addiction in Rats* – J Addict Med. 2009 Mar; 3(1): 33–41. doi: [10.1097/ADM.0b013e31819aa621] PMCID: PMC4361030 NIHMSID: NIHMS669567 PMID: 21768998.
The Addicted Brain – Bartley G. Hoebel, Ph.D., Nicole M. Avena, Ph.D., Miriam E. Bocarsly, BA, and Pedro Rada, MD Scientific American 290, 78–85 (2004) doi:10.1038/scientificamerican0304–78.

5 *Dopamine-Based Reward Circuitry Responsivity, Genetics, and Overeating* – Stice, E., Yokum, S., Zald, D., and A. Dagher. 2011. Curr Top Behav Neurosci. 6: 81–93.
Reward Circuitry Responsivity to Food Predicts Future iIncreases in Body Mass: Moderating Effects of DRD2 and DRD4 – Stice, E., Yokum, S., Bohon, C., et al. 2010. Neuroimage. 50(4): 1618–25.
Activation Instead of Blocking Mesolimbic Dopaminergic Reward Circuitry is a Preferred Modality in the Long Term Treatment of Reward Deficiency Syndrome (RDS): a Commentary – Blum, K., Chen, A.L., Chen, T.J., et al. 2008. Theor Biol Med Model. 5:24. Review.
Anti-Obesity Effects and Polymorphic Gene Correlates of Reward Deficiency Syndrome – Blum, K., Chen, A.L., Chen, T.J. et al. 2008. LG839: . Adv Ther. 25(9): 894–913.
High-Dose Vitamin Therapy Stimulates Variant Enzymes with Decreased Coenzyme Binding Affinity (Increased K(m)): Relevance to Genetic Disease and Polymorphisms – Ames, B.N., Elson-Schwab, I., and E.A. Silver. 2002. Am J Clin Nutr. 75(4): 616–58. Review.

ELEMENT 17:
HOW DO YOU BECOME A PERPETUAL MOTION MACHINE?

Average time to complete: **1–2 weeks**

In Element 17, we will:

- Learn the importance of increasing your activity level.
- Discover new ways you can increase your activity level.
- Explore how the Habits of Healthy Motion can be a part of your new story.

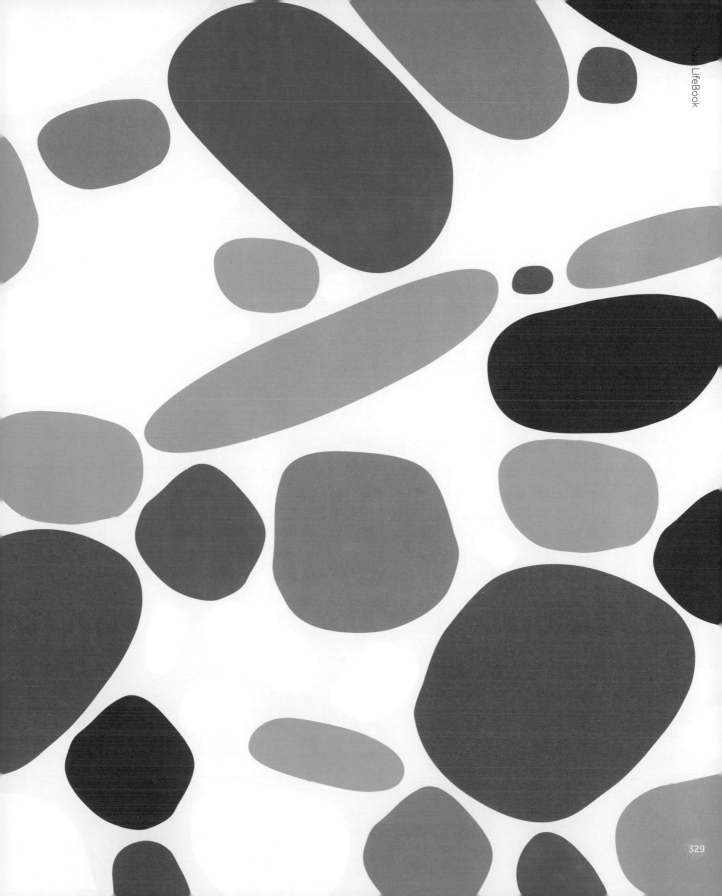

10,000 years ago we were in perpetual motion throughout our waking hours. It is estimated that we spent in excess of 3,000 minutes a week moving. Consider that if we move 300 minutes a week today, we are considered to be extremely active. How times have changed. And unfortunately, most are getting less than the 150 minutes a week recommended to prevent a steady regression to poor health.[1]

In this and the next Element, we will explore increasing your activity level with exercise as the ultimate, if not immediate, goal which is essential for disease prevention and creating optimal health. But exactly what that means day-to-day is different for everyone. As you'll have gathered by now, I firmly believe that the best way to integrate movement into your life is by using a plan that's tailored to your current state of health, activity level, and weight and progressing it to create strength, fitness, flexibility, and balance to last you for the rest of your life.

SEDENTARY LIFESTYLE: THE SITTING DISEASE

We have learned a lot from space travel. Our astronauts would leave to go in outer space, leaving the Earth's gravitational pull behind. A startling side effect following this relatively short time in space was that these incredibly fit humans would exhibit significant atrophy, loss of fitness, and other signs of aging in their physical health.

With the progressive sitting we do in our modern lifestyle, we are assimilating space travel daily as we are not moving against gravity. When I wrote the first version of the Habits of Health a decade ago, I stated that even for those that were exercising the standard three times a week that it was not enough activity to maintain (much less optimize) our health. A plethora of recent studies have validated that offsetting the negative effects of the sitting disease, which affects so many and leads to poor health, does indeed require motion all day long to compensate for the lack of activity even in those that exercise.[2] (See "The Mortality of Being Seated" Part 2.9 in *Dr. A's Habits of Health, Active Living: Inside and Out*). In fact, the innovative NEAT system that I created back then is now a highly recommended method to counter the ill effects of sitting on our health.

Do You Have the Sitting Disease?
At this point it would be really helpful for you to track the total time you are sitting during your waking hours:

You can make a list of all the things you do in a typical day and estimate how long you are sedentary, or you can actually use a stop watch to keep a running total of all the times you are sitting during the day.

Or JustStand.org has a sitting time calculator you can use to estimate your total sit time https://www.juststand.org/the-tools/sitting-time-calculator/

How many hours are you sitting?

A recent survey in juststand.org showed that 86% of all Americans sit all day. Daily sitting ranges from 9.3 hours on average to as high as 15 hours in some individuals.[3]

What can we do about it?

The Habits of Motion

My approach to physical activity takes a much broader outlook than exercise-focused plans do. It's based on creating habits of dynamic active living. We begin by stabilizing your healthy weight by gradually introducing the foundational principles of the Habits of Motion (without a lot of weight lifting and aerobics in the beginning). Throughout, we ensure that you're using the most efficient means possible to maintain your healthy weight. Fortunately, the most efficient way is also the easiest and safest way for you to start your movement plan!

I'm a firm believer in the motto, "You need to crawl before you can walk." My plan gives you time to build your foundation by assimilating some basic principles of physical activity. When you're ready, we'll move into some more advanced techniques, including weight lifting and aerobics. Throughout, we ensure that you are progressing at a pace that makes sense for you.

At the center of my plan is getting you to move your body like you did when you were a kid. Now that we're adults, life just seems to get in the way of getting out, playing, and having fun. Combine that with our terrible eating habits and sedentary jobs, and it's easy to see why we've just stopped moving. So we're going to start with baby steps, based on your current reality, and crawl our way back to energy equilibrium, fitness, and optimal health.

We'll start by looking at all the many little movements that make up your day, and put them to work for us. As I teach you the Habits of Motion, I'll be focusing on two major objectives:

1. Stabilizing your weight by increasing your energy expenditure, primarily through physical activity
2. Optimizing your health through carefully paced exercises

We'll accomplish our first goal by teaching you how to become more active, through movements centered round your job, your chores, your plans, and your activities. Even if you are currently exercising, I think you will find these next two Elements helpful in refining your perpetual motion and increasing your dynamics!

What's the difference between physical activity versus exercise?
You may think of the terms physical activity and exercise as one and the same, but I think it's important to make a distinction. Physical activity happens anytime your body's in motion. As you'll see later in this Element, that motion can be voluntary or involuntary. Exercise, on the other hand, is planned movement that's more vigorous and leads to improvements in overall fitness.

Activity and exercise have different roles in our system. Introducing each of them correctly and in the right sequence is critical to maintaining your motivation and ability above the activation threshold. This will make your new energy plan a permanent Habit of Health.

Habits of Motion Breakdown

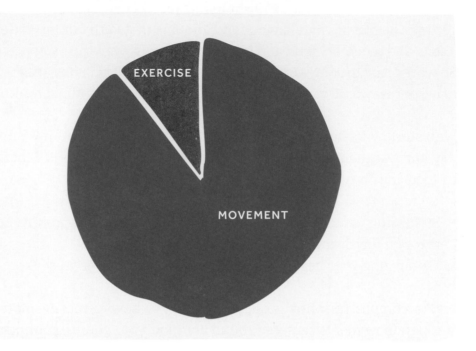

One big difference between exercise and physical activity is that exercise is generally done for a short period of time—usually just a few hours a week. Physical activity, on the other hand, can be integrated into your daily life in a much more organic and complete manner . Our main objective in increasing your activity is to put all your waking hours to work by tapping into the thousand different ways your body is active. We'll then start increasing your daily activity to serve your body's need for motion.

What is your current level of physical activity?
You can use the level you choose in Element 14, Transitioning To Eating Healthy For Life, to calculate your TEE:
- 1.2 (for light exercise)
- 1.5 (for moderate exercise)
- 1.7 (for heavy exercise)

How many hours a week do you currently exercise?

What do you do?

Summarize your current level of activity and fitness:

We are now going to continue your journey to optimal health and wellbeing with our system of healthy motion.

The Habits of Health System of Healthy Motion

In Part 2.9 of *Dr. A's Habits of Health, Active Living: Inside and Out*, I will explain in detail how our body uses energy and what we can do to increase that expenditure to help support your weight management as well as build strength, agility, flexibility, stamina, and overall optimal health and wellbeing.

What is important at this juncture is that the biggest improvement you can make in your total energy expenditure to help maintain a healthy weight and build optimal health is in your Physical Activity Level (PAL). As we previously discussed, PAL is made up of two parts: planned physical activity (what you probably think of as exercise) and the voluntary and unconscious movements you make as part of your everyday life. As we plan an activity program customized to your age, fitness level, and lifestyle, it's helpful to consider these two categories separately. One handy way to break it down is through the acronyms EAT and NEAT.

EAT and NEAT

EAT (Exercise Activity Thermogenesis) consists of the planned physical activities we perform in order to increase our energy expenditure and improve our overall fitness. It's what we do when we say we're "working out." These may range from the minimal task of going for a brisk walk to Herculean feats, like Chris Froome expending over 9,000 calories a day during the Tour de France. But despite all our talk of exercise today, for the vast majority of us, EAT is actually negligible. In fact, even exercise enthusiasts will find that EAT's contribution to daily calorie consumption pales by comparison to the power of NEAT. See the previous Habits of Motion Breakdown pie diagram.

NEAT (Non-Exercise Activity Thermogenesis) consists of the voluntary and unconscious movements we make as we go about our daily lives— by working, doing chores, and the combined effect of all our silly little motions. As I sit here writing, for example, I'm consuming extra calories just tapping my foot. It's easy, and it happened naturally as a result of getting into the beat of a great song on my phone. NEAT is highly variable, ranging from about 15% of total daily TEE in very sedentary people to more than 50% in people who are highly active.

We will devote the next Element to EAT and how it can be a gift to your health and wellbeing.

The rest of this Element will be dedicated to NEAT and how we can become a perpetual motion machine just like when we were kids.

DR. A'S HABITS OF HEALTHY MOTION
PART 1: NEAT SYSTEM

The NEAT System is designed for everyone. It's easy, it's effective, and you're already doing it— we're just going to make you NEATer!

NEAT is a bit like the story of the tortoise and the hare. By making small daily choices, you can win the race of weight management and set the stage for exercise at your own pace. My NEAT System adds motion to every aspect of your day but this is done gradually so that it won't seem like much effort at all. This makes it particularly helpful for people who aren't used to exercising, for those with a BMI (body mass index) above 30, or those with medical conditions (don't forget if you have a medical condition you need to be cleared by a health provider first). NEAT is a system you can do right now and continue doing into your 90s and beyond.

Just by making these little NEAT motions a part of your daily routine, you'll soon accomplish your primary goal of offloading a couple hundred calories each day, and that's going to help your energy management system function flawlessly indefinitely. Best of all, it's safe. There's no intense exertion involved (though we'll keep a close watch on your target heart rate just to be extra sure) and it's important that you feel comfortable and protected as you start creating a more mobile and fitter world for yourself. And now that you've lost some weight and are feeling better, you're ready to go!

Exercise and Your Heart:
The Benefits of Taking It Slow

It's a well-known medical fact that an unfit, sedentary lifestyle causes cardiovascular disease. Combine that with too much excess weight, and jumping too quickly into exercise can be a recipe for disaster. Although the risk is low, sudden death and heart attack are more likely to take place during exercise. That's why it's so important to ramp up slowly using the NEAT System and to continue monitoring your heart rate.[4] By the time you progress to the active exercising of EAT, your heart will be stronger than ever. Do, of course, consult with your healthcare provider as you increase your activity level.

You and NEAT

How many of the following things are you doing now?

Place a check mark if you are doing it.

At work:

○ Walking or biking to work

○ Parking far away from the entrance to work

○ Getting up several times an hour during each hour you are sitting

○ Using the stairs rather than escalator or elevator?

○ Using the restroom at the other end of building

○ Walking when in phone meetings

○ Holding walking meetings

○ Standing while on the phone

○ Having a tall core when sitting, standing, walking

What else are you doing to resist gravity at work?

What else are you doing to move more on the go?

At home:

○ Make your bed

○ Manually brush teeth

○ Use a shaker jar

○ Manually wash the dishes

○ Use a manual can opener

○ Use a manual broom

○ Use a hand rake for leaves

○ Hide the TV remote

○ Walk the dog

○ Have an after dinner passeggiata (leisure walk)

What else are you doing to resist gravity at home?

What else are you doing to move more at home?

On the go:

- Use a handbasket at the store
- Park further away
- Walk around the mall in bad weather
- Engage in outside hobbies at the weekends
- Do both outdoor and indoor sports
- Bicycle when possible
- Swim at a local pool or at home
- Walk in the woods or along the lake or beach

What else are you doing to resist gravity on the go?

What else are you doing to move more on the go?

In *Dr. A's Habits of Health,* I have taken all of the NEAT activities and organized them into six categories with names that all start S's. For those that like to track numbers, this will give you a way to measure the additional energy you are expending when you are engaged in these activities.

Managing NEAT: The Six S's of Success

The NEAT System helps you take control of your body's energy balance by harnessing the movements you make in the course of your daily activities—the way you move your body, for example, or the way your perform everyday tasks at work and at home. To help you keep track of these motions, I've divided NEAT into six categories that represent the movements and postures that typically fill our days. Together, they serve as a training system to help you transform NEAT into an integral Habit of Health.

The six NEAT categories:
- Stance
- Standing
- Strolling
- Stairs
- Samba
- Switch

These six categories cover the full range of muscle energy expenditure in your everyday life (outside of the scheduled exercises that make up EAT, that is). As part of this system, I'll teach you to track each one individually so that you know you're doing the most you can to increase your daily calorie burn. We want to make sure, especially in the beginning, that you're targeting behaviors from all six categories. For each of these categories you will want to read the corresponding explanation in Part 2.11 *Dr. A's Habits of Healthy Motion Part 1: NEAT System*. Online, at the HabitsofHealth.com, you can learn how to calculate the actual calories you expend. I will give you target goals which will allow you to avoid having to do the calculations.

Stance (Posture)

In fact, sitting is one of the best times to work on your posture and core axis alignment. Start by using a proper chair that helps you sit up straight. Now flex your stomach muscles and take deep, slow breaths.

What NEAT posture ideas can you add to your day?

At work: . . . .

At home: . . . .

MicroHabit: Add two additional minutes of focus on the core position per day.

Target Goal: 30 minutes of focus on the core position per day. An additional target is to use a balance ball chair all day at work. Download more charts at HabitsofHealth.com (1 month tracker).

NEAT MINUTES PER DAY	MON	TUE	WED	THU	FRI	SAT	SUN	TOTAL MINUTES PER WEEK
STANCE WEEK 1								
STANCE WEEK 2								
STANCE WEEK 3								
STANCE WEEK 4								

Standing

In merely moving from sitting to standing, you can substantially increase your energy consumption. When you stand, you begin to use weight-bearing NEAT. And one of the great advantages of weight-bearing NEAT is that the heavier you are, the more calories you expend. That's good news, because it means that if you're overweight, you can start off slowly and still receive the benefits of increased movement.

What NEAT posture ideas can you add to your day?

At work:

At home:

MicroHabit: Add 10 additional minutes of standing per day.

Target Goal: Two hours of standing per day. Download more charts at HabitsofHealth.com (1 month tracker).

NEAT MINUTES PER DAY	MON	TUE	WED	THU	FRI	SAT	SUN	TOTAL MINUTES PER WEEK
STANDING WEEK 1								
STANDING WEEK 2								
STANDING WEEK 3								
STANDING WEEK 4								

Strolling (Walking)

When I talk about walking in terms of NEAT, I'm referring to anything outside of a formal walking program. That includes going to the water cooler, delivering a memo to your boss, or shopping for that new dress at the mall. Remember, the point of NEAT is that it takes place within your normal routines.

What NEAT walking ideas can you add to your day?

At work:

At home:

MicroHabit: Add 100 additional steps per week.

Target Goal: At least 10,000 steps per day (a mile is about 2,000 steps). Download more charts at HabitsofHealth.com (1 month tracker).

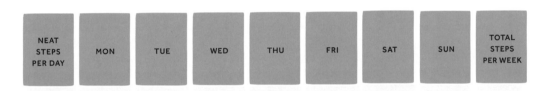

NEAT STEPS PER DAY	MON	TUE	WED	THU	FRI	SAT	SUN	TOTAL STEPS PER WEEK

STROLLING WEEK 1

STROLLING WEEK 2

STROLLING WEEK 3

STROLLING WEEK 4

Stairs

Stairs are a great way to accelerate NEAT. In fact, climbing just one flight of stairs is the equivalent of walking 100 steps. That means that climbing 10 flights of stairs gives you the same benefit as walking for half a mile.

What NEAT stairs ideas can you add to your day?

At work:

At home:

MicroHabit: Add one additional flight of stairs per week.

Target Goal: 10 flights of stairs per day. Download more charts at HabitsofHealth.com (1 month tracker).

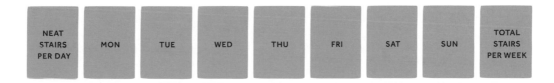

NEAT STAIRS PER DAY	MON	TUE	WED	THU	FRI	SAT	SUN	TOTAL STAIRS PER WEEK

STAIRS WEEK 1

STAIRS WEEK 2

STAIRS WEEK 3

STAIRS WEEK 4

Samba

Here, we're looking at the movement generated by your body's natural rhythm. What do I mean by that? Put on a song you like and watch what happens. You might start tapping your pencil or your foot or even singing as loud as you can.

What NEAT dance ideas can you add to your day?

At work: ·

At home: ·

MicroHabit: Add 10 additional minutes of music per day; work up to an hour or more of dance per week.

Target Goal: 90 minutes of music per day; one hour of dance per week. Download more charts at HabitsofHealth.com (1 month tracker).

NEAT MUSIC/ DANCE PER DAY	MON	TUE	WED	THU	FRI	SAT	SUN	TOTAL MUSIC/ DANCE PER WEEK
SAMBA WEEK 1								
SAMBA WEEK 2								
SAMBA WEEK 3								
SAMBA WEEK 4								

Switch

To switch means doing things by hand instead of by machine. That includes dishwashers, electric knives, snow blowers, remote controls, computers, and all the other automatic devices that steal from your energy-use account at an ever-growing pace. Your goal is to burn an extra 30 calories per day doing tasks by hand instead of using machines.

What NEAT saying no to machine ideas can you add to your day?

At work:

At home:

MicroHabit: Add one or two substituted manual tasks per day.

Target Goal: 10 substituted manual tasks per day. Download more charts at HabitsofHealth.com (1 month tracker).

NEAT TASKS PER DAY	MON	TUE	WED	THU	FRI	SAT	SUN	TOTAL TASKS PER WEEK
SWITCH WEEK 1								
SWITCH WEEK 2								
SWITCH WEEK 3								
SWITCH WEEK 4								

Tracking NEAT

The NEAT system includes a robust and comprehensive tracking and scoring system to help you measure your progress. The full breakdown of how to track your NEAT points and the calories you have burned is available online at HabitsofHealth.com, which is especially handy as you may need to print out extra tracking sheets as you fill yours in.

If you feel that tracking the NEAT increase is too detailed for you, it's okay to make your life more active in a more impromptu fashion. I want you to have fun and get into perpetual motion.

How often a day should I do NEAT activities?

Anytime you think about it. Just say no to machines. Also remember if you get up and move every 20 minutes, you dramatically lower your risk of heart disease—especially if you have a desk job.

You can set a timer on your phone, put up post-it notes to remind you, or drink a lot of water, which means you will have to get up more often.

See if you can turn yourself into a perpetual motion machine. Your body's 50 trillion cells need to sense motion in order to optimize your health.

Our Integrated Habits of Health Clock is a great way of thinking about how to install more and more NEAT activities into your waking hours. I use a timer on my phone and make sure I get up every 20 minutes from my desk to do five minutes of movement. It may be jumping jacks, burpees, or a trip to the kitchen for some water. Have fun with it, and treat yourself to a full clock!

It's worth taking a blank Habits of Health Clock, which you can download from the HabitsofHealth.com website, and start adding in more things you can do, so that you eventually fill it up with activity.

Perpetual Motion Machine

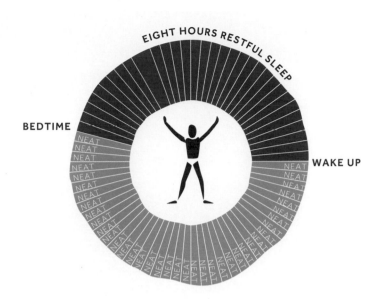

Moving Forward: From NEAT to EAT

By the end of the second month using my NEAT System, you'll be burning 200 more calories each day than you are right now, just by enhancing your normal, everyday activities. And that increase in energy expenditure means you'll be able to offset the natural decrease that occurs as you lose weight, which is the key to healthy weight maintenance! Just as important, you'll increase your flexibility, mobility, and total daily motion to make your whole body stronger.

Make sure you review all your notes and this important Element often. Also, share it with your coach and spend time discussing how these possibilities will become a reality and help you become the dominant force in your life.

Total extra NEAT month one:

Total extra NEAT month two:

Total extra NEAT month three:

This initial series of activities is the first step in your movement program for optimal health. Now, let's look at my scheduled exercise plan, beginning with walking, to help you prepare for your graduate degree in movement.

Notes to yourself:

Now that you have completed Element 17, *How Do You Become A Perpetual Motion Machine?*, write down your thoughts guided by the following questions:

What does this Element mean to you right now?

What does this Element give you the opportunity to reflect on?

What actions are you going to take as a result of this Element?

I encourage you to connect with your coach, so you can share your thoughts and actions as soon as possible.

Sharing your thoughts with your coach will help them become a reality.

Make sure you review all your notes and this Element often.

1 *Don't Just Sit There* – Katy Bowman, December 1, 2015.

2 *Too Much Sitting: The Population-Health Science of Sedentary Behavior* – Neville Owen, 1 Geneviève N Healy,1,2 Charles E. Matthews,3 and David W. Dunstan Exerc Sport Sci Rev. 2010 Jul; 38(3): 105 – 113. doi: [10.1097/JES.0b013e3181e373a2] PMCID: PMC3404815 NIHMSID: NIHMS229379 PMID: 20577058 3 www.juststand.org Sitting Disease.

4 *Sudden Death During Exercise Cardiology* – 1990;77(5):411 – 7. Amsterdam EA1.

ELEMENT 18:
EXERCISE IS YOUR GIFT TO YOURSELF

Average time to complete: **2–4 weeks**

In Element 18, we will:

- Discover my scheduled exercise plan to help you prepare for your graduate degree in movement.
- Position you to achieve the 3 core goals of the Habits of Motion System.
- Explore what a typical week of exercise will look like.

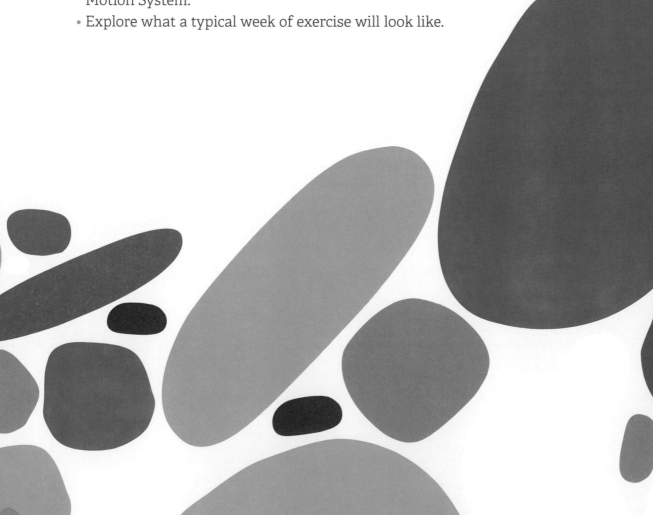

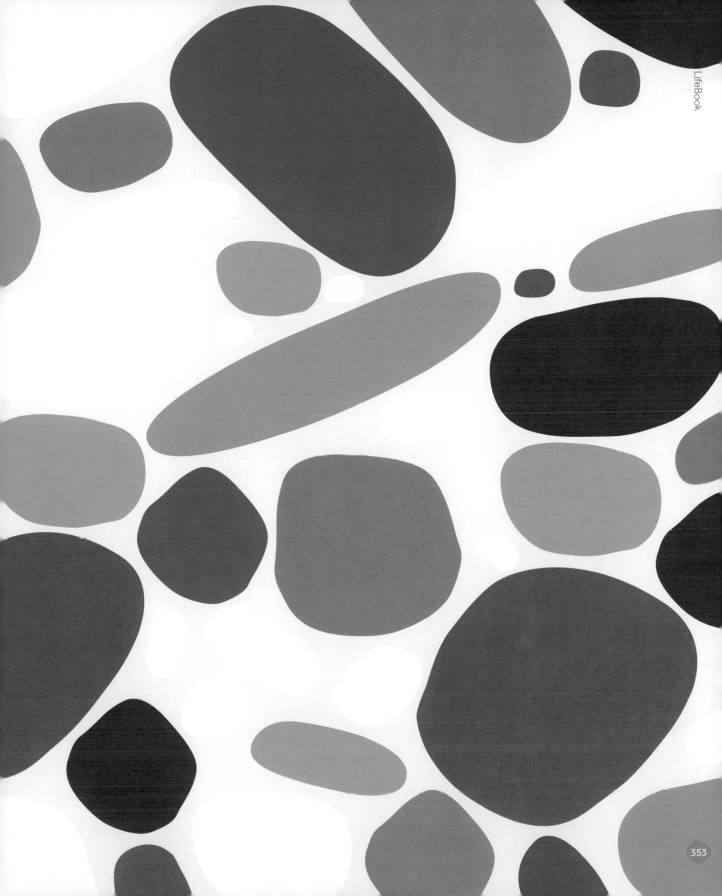

The NEAT System showed you how to burn an additional 200–300 calories a day without making major changes in your activity level or daily routine. You were able to put this user-friendly system to work right away to help maintain your weight, increase your flexibility and mobility, and build a healthier lifestyle.

But as you know, we have an even higher goal. We want to create optimal health. That's why you need the second part of my movement plan—the EAT System. Exercise Activity Thermogenesis helps you optimize your health through specific, regularly scheduled exercises that boost your energy expenditure and significantly improve your all-around health— from your heart and immune system to your mental aptitude and sex life. As a result, you'll work better, feel better (EAT can decrease your need for medication and arrest the progress of disease), and even live longer. In fact, EAT is our most important predictor of longevity.[1] It's the type of movement you don't want to rush into, but now that you're well on your way to a healthy weight and have increased your daily movement, it makes sense to add this powerful health-enhancing plan to your life.

I define Exercise Activity Thermogenesis (EAT) as any planned movement that's vigorous enough to improve overall fitness. Any activity performed deliberately to enhance the body's conditioning, ranging in intensity from a walk in the park to a triathlon. My philosophy is that it's best to incorporate activities of moderate intensity, based on the premise that you're going to use them until you reach the end of a full, thriving life.

And although the EAT System will take a bit of time out of your day, it's specifically designed to minimize your daily commitment by giving you the most effective results in the least amount of time possible.

How much time?

That's all it takes! 30 minutes a day of moderate activity for a lifetime of health and longevity. And that's because the NEAT System is already contributing the lion's share of your daily energy expenditure through your 10,000 steps a day and the other S's. The EAT System builds on this foundation by increasing your energy expenditure even more as you train and optimize your cardiovascular and musculoskeletal systems.

By adding EAT into the picture, you position yourself to achieve the three core goals of the Habits of Motion System:

- Increasing energy expenditure to create a consistent balance between energy in and energy out.
- Optimizing cardiovascular health so that your heart, lungs, and blood vessels can deliver enough oxygen to keep your cells functioning properly, especially your brain cells.
- Building a strong, healthy support system of bones and muscles to help you stay active, keep fit, and maintain a healthy weight.

The Three Progressive Levels of Exercise Activity Thermogenesis
The EAT part of our system is divided into three progressive levels which you will master at your own pace.

Level One: Walking and Fitness Program
Level Two: Resistance Program
Level Three: Boosting Your Workouts (High Intensity Interval Training)

Your current level of fitness will decide how fast you ascend through these levels.

Before we start, especially for those of you who have been rather sedentary in the past, we want to make sure you know the ground rules for protecting your body from injury and staying safe. The risk to your heart and brain are low, according to the research completed with cardiac patients, but we still want to start slowly and only after you have been evaluated by your healthcare provider.[2] Musculoskeletal injury is more likely if you overdo exercise and activity until your body has acclimatized to more strenuous activity.

- *Keep it slow.* Use slow, careful movements for weight training and other strengthening exercises. At the beginning, keep your heart rate at 50–65% of your maximum heart rate.

Maximum Heart Rate (MHR)

The highest number of times your heart can contract per minute during maximum physical exertion. To determine your MHR, subtract your age from 220.

For example, if you're 50 years old:

$$220 - 50 = 170$$
$$170 \times .50 \text{ (in other words, 50\%)} = 85 \text{ bpm (beats per minute)}$$
$$170 \times .65 \text{ (in other words, 65\%)} = 110 \text{ bpm (beats per minute)}$$

So, your target heart rate range is between 85 and 110 bpm (beats per minute) throughout your daily activity.

As you progress and begin to feel more comfortable, you can aim toward 65 or 75%, and eventually 85% once you're optimally fit.

What is your maximum heart rate?

220 - · · · · · your age = · · · · · Your MHR

Your MHR X .50 = · · · · · · · · · Your starting low end

Your MHR X .65 = · · · · · · · · · Your starting high end

Target Goal

Your MHR X .85 = · · · · · · · · · Optimal fit HR goal

• *Stretch it out.* Help prevent injury by stretching your major muscle groups, preferably directly after your daily EAT activity. Add some extra stretching for a few minutes each day to keep your muscles flexible, improve your balance, and increase your range of motion.

• *Cool it down.* After each session, allow your musculoskeletal and cardiovascular systems to return to their baseline state.

Ready?

Let's start your EAT System, beginning with our EAT Walking Program.

LEVEL ONE: WALKING AND FITNESS PROGRAM

The EAT Walking Program (See *Dr. A's Habits of Health* Part 2.12, *Dr. A's Habits of Healthy Motion Part 2: EAT System*).

Since you're already walking as part of your NEAT System activities, adding this natural, low-impact, safe, and simple activity in a more scheduled version should be a breeze. All you need is proper clothing, comfortable shoes, and your pedometer, and you're on your way!

You may be wondering how the NEAT walking you're doing differs from the kind you'll be doing in EAT. Basically, while adding steps through NEAT helps you burn more calories, it's not intense enough to produce fitness. The EAT Walking Program, however, is designed with fitness in mind, so you get essential cardiovascular benefits. And because walking is convenient and easy to do, you're more likely to keep at it so it can become part of your long-term plan for sustainable health.

Creating Success with EAT Walking Program:
Where should you walk?

What is Forest Bathing and how can it help you create better health?
(See Part 2.12 in *Dr. A's Habits of Health*)

What should you wear?

What shoes should you wear?

What is the level of walking that will support my cardiovascular health?

EAT Walking Program: Key Points as You Progress

Begin by walking 20 minutes a day, including five minutes for warm-up and five minutes for cool down. Try using this as a goal for your walking sessions: You can use either the amount of time or the number of steps to keep track.

Warm-up	5 minutes at 1 mph	(about 160 steps)
At pace	10 minutes at 2 mph	(about 665 steps)
Cooldown	5 minutes at 1 mph	(about 160 steps)

This 20 minute session of around 1,000 steps (about a half mile) will consume approximately 50 calories if your BMI is 30.

- Add five minutes each week, or as much time as you're comfortable with.
- Work up to a brisk pace of around four miles per hour.
- Work up to around 20,000 steps per week by week ten (depending on your level of fitness and weight-loss goals).
- Your long-term goal is to walk for 30 minutes a day, five days a week.

To keep track of your progress, use the EAT Walking Program Daily Tracking Sheet which you can download at www.HabitsofHealth.com. Just enter your daily minutes, steps, miles, and calories burned in the appropriate boxes.

Note: Playing an active sport for an hour will add 8,000 to 10,000 steps

Picking Up the Pace: Advancing Your Program

The goal of the EAT Walking Program is to boost your cardiovascular and musculoskeletal health now and for years to come. It's a solid program that you can stay with for life just as it's outlined above, but you can also adapt the program to increase your level of fitness by adding hills, distance, and speed.

You can boost your workouts either by increasing the intensity or the duration of your movement. My 30 minute guideline is merely the baseline required to maintain fitness without cutting too much into your daily commitments. If you have time for more, that's great. You'll see that by increasing the intensity you will be more effective at burning fat. We will explore that in more detail a little later when we talk about High Intensity Interval Training (HIIT).

How are you going to pick up the pace? (See Part 2.12 in *Dr. A's Habits of Health*)

How can you boost your walking workout? (See Part 2.12 in *Dr. A's Habits of Health*)

As you step up your intensity, remember the basic principles of cardiovascular fitness:

• If you're unable to carry on a conversation, slow down.
• Keep your Rate of Perceived Exertion (RPE) below a six.
(See Part 2.12 in *Dr. A's Habits of Health*)

Once you've reached your EAT Walking Program goal of 20,000 steps per week (on top of the steps you're taking as part of the NEAT System) and have been walking five days every week for at least a month, you're ready to add the other essential component of the EAT System: resistance training.

LEVEL TWO: RESISTANCE PROGRAM

Does the thought of weight training conjure up images of sweaty, grunting meat-heads in tank tops spending hours at the gym lifting ridiculous levels of weight? This type of bootcamp workout is not only unnecessary, it's downright unsafe. It has no place in a sustainable health plan. It is important to start thinking of exercise as a gift you are giving yourself versus a chore for you to do.

And, in the transformational cycle, we talked a lot about the immediate benefit of exercise on your body and mind as well as the long-term benefits.

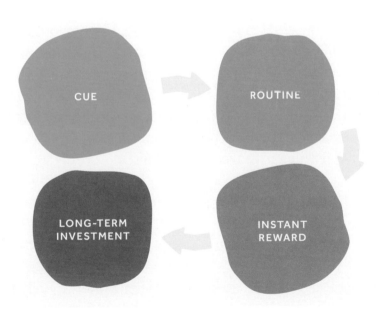

Make sure you note how you feel after you workout and write it down. It can have a positive effect on your mood, your focus and attention, your productivity, your performance, and your ability to use your imagination and create. Many have said that if we could bottle exercise into a pill it would be the most frequently prescribed medication. It can boost our energy levels, as well as increase our focus and attention, for up to 12 hours! A little bit like Ritalin and Prozac without the side effects!

Write down the instant rewards that you get when you workout:

Your EAT Resistance Program *(See Part 2.12 in Dr. A's Habits of Health)*
Most exercise programs try to do too much. They promise weight loss, cardiovascular performance, and muscle enhancement—and deliver none of these very effectively. Whereas the Habits of Health focuses on a variety of small daily choices to first create a healthy weight, then optimal health. We're not relying on exercise for weight loss. You're already doing that through the fat-burning healthy eating system. Energy expenditure is taken care of through the NEAT System, the EAT Walking Program covers cardiovascular health, and the EAT Resistance Program completes the picture by serving as a muscle and bone reconditioning program to help you retain your full range of movement for life.

In review, the NEAT Walking goal is 10,000 steps a day, which is all the movement that occurs in your work and leisure time 24 hours a day outside of your formal EAT walking program.

The EAT Walking Program is 4,000 brisk steps done intentionally five days a week as a routine resulting in an additional 20,000 steps a week! It is complemented with resistance training on the other two days, which we will discuss next.

The program I describe in Part 2.12 in *Dr. A's Habits of Health, Dr. A's Habits of Healthy Motion Part 2: EAT System*, is one I have used for years and it has kept me in great shape, but I am fine with you using whichever program works best for you because the best exercise program is one that you will actually do. You'll complete the EAT Resistance Program on the two days each week that you're not walking as part of the EAT Walking Program. Together, these two programs provide a complete cardiovascular and strength-training system in just 30 minutes a day.

What equipment are you going to use?
(See Part 2.12 in *Dr. A's Habits of Health*)

Are you going to join a gym? How about a trainer?
(See Part 2.12 in *Dr. A's Habits of Health*)

EAT Resistance Program *(See Part 2.12 in Dr. A's Habits of Health)*
Before you begin, make sure you've got the EAT Walking Program down and have been racking up 20,000 steps per week consistently for at least a month (average 4,000 steps 5 days a week).

Each EAT Resistance Program session works either your upper body or your lower body, along with your core muscles. Our major areas of focus are as follows:

Upper body
- core (upper)
- chest
- latissimus dorsi (back)
- shoulders
- arms

Lower body
- core (lower)
- thighs
- gluteals
- hamstrings
- calves

Note:

We want you to do what ever resistance training you feel comfortable with and will do at least two days a week.

Also consider using a trainer, which can be very helpful as you get started. There is information on how to pick one in *Dr. A's Habits of Health* Part 2.12. Remember, the best exercise is the one you will do. However, here I am giving you general guidelines to help you fit it into your busy schedule.

In the HabitsofHealth.com website we will outline exercises for each of the muscle groups, as well as coordinated stretches. I recommend starting with the level one exercises and only advancing once you can do both rotations at a Rate of Perceived Exertion (RPE) of two or less (See Part 2.12) And, of course, check with your healthcare provider before starting any exercise protocol.

Choose two days each week for your resistance workouts, leaving at least two days between sessions to let your body recover (I recommend doing the upper body session on Monday and the lower body session on Thursday).

Your Weekly Routine

Once you get going with the EAT Resistance Program, you'll complete two 30-minute sessions each week, consisting of:

1. A five-minute warm-up.
2. Five repetitions of five selected movements (a total of 10 minutes), followed by a rotation of five different exercises that work the same muscle groups.
3. A five-minute stretch of the muscles you've worked.

Let's break that down to get a better picture of what you'll be doing in each session.

Resistance Rotation: Two rotations of 10 minutes each

Challenge your muscles to grow healthier through short, intense workouts that stimulate all your muscle fibers. Strengthen your bones and build lean, efficient muscle—not bulk—through slow, focused movements that utilize the full range of motion.

- Choose a set of five exercises (one rotation).
- Begin each exercise with a slow consistent contraction (eight seconds), hold in place just before lock out (four seconds), then relax the muscle as you slowly return to your starting position (eight seconds)—for a total of twenty seconds per exercise.
- Immediately begin another repetition, for a total of five per exercise.
- Rest for 20 seconds before starting a new exercise.
- Follow with a second rotation using a different set of exercises that work the same muscles.

One Exercise Repetition

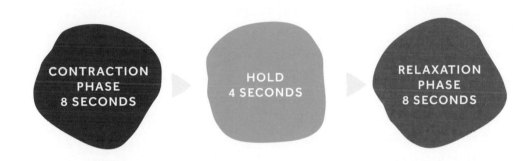

One exercise repetition: each 20 second repetition consists of a contraction phase, a holding phase, and a relaxation phase. You'll complete five repetitions for each separate exercise.

Stretching: Five Minutes
Spend five minutes stretching the muscle groups you've just worked to improve flexibility, increase your range of motion, and prevent soreness by encouraging your muscles to break down lactic acid (any soreness you do experience will decrease as your muscles get stronger and become reconditioned).

So, there you have the EAT Resistance Program—30 minutes of strength training to create a healthy musculoskeletal system and help you use more energy by:

• Boosting the calorie-burning capacity of all your NEAT and EAT activities
• Increasing your Basal Metabolic Rate (BMR) by adding muscle mass
• Burning energy even after your workout is done as your muscles replenish oxygen

To use the log:

• Write down the specific exercise you're doing for each muscle group.
• Note whether you're using your body alone without weights (B) or, if you're working with dumbbells, the amount of weight you're using. Refer to the Borg chart in Part 2.12 in *Dr. A's Habits of Health, Dr. A's Habits of Healthy Motion Part 2: EAT System* to calculate your Rate of Perceived Exertion (RPE).
• Before you begin, make sure you've got the EAT Walking Program down and have been racking up 20,000 steps per week consistently for at least a month.
• Choose two days each week for your resistance workouts, leaving at least two days between sessions to let your body recover. I recommend doing the upper body session on Monday and the lower body session on Thursday.
• Find a spot where you can focus without distraction, and use an exercise mat for support and cushioning. Take it slow—review each new exercise before you try it out; limit yourself to one rotation for the first week; and add new exercises slowly, letting your body become accustomed to the new movement.

Eat Resistance Program Training Log: Upper Body

MUSCLES GROUP	EXERCISE/LEVEL (LEVEL ONE, LEVEL TWO)	WEIGHT: BODY (B) OR POUNDS (LBS)	RATE OF PERCEIVED EXERTION (RPE)
ROTATION A			
CORE			
CHEST			
BACK			
SHOULDERS			
ARMS			
ROTATION B			
CORE			
CHEST			
BACK			
SHOULDERS			
ARMS			

Eat Resistance Program Training Log: Lower Body

MUSCLES GROUP	EXERCISE/LEVEL (LEVEL ONE, LEVEL TWO)	WEIGHT: BODY (B) OR POUNDS (LBS)	RATE OF PERCEIVED EXERTION (RPE)
ROTATION A			
CORE			
THIGHS			
GLUTEALS			
HAMSTRINGS			
CALVES			
ROTATION B			
CORE			
THIGHS			
GLUTEALS			
HAMSTRINGS			
CALVES			

These logs can be downloaded from HabitsofHealth.com in the EAT section.

How are the workouts progressing?

Share your progress with your coach.

Starting Your Program: Your First Day
Before you begin your first day, review the five exercises you'll be performing.

Go online to HabitsofHealth.com to watch the videos of the exercises. It's important you take it slow as you get comfortable with resistance training. For the first week, limit yourself to one rotation to give yourself time to master the five beginning exercises. Beginning in week two, add a second rotation to your routine, consisting of five different exercises that work the same muscle groups.

As with the EAT Walking Program, be sure to monitor your progress by entering each workout's data into a log. You'll find sample logs for upper and lower body rotations on the next page and also on the website at HabitsofHealth.com. Remember, for the first week limit yourself to one rotation.

LEVEL THREE: BOOSTING YOUR WORKOUTS

Six Options to Boost Your
EAT Resistance Workouts

As you become more physically fit the simplest way to advance is to increase the intensity, frequency, total amount of time, or decrease recovery time and I have provided some ways you can do this below. Additionally, in the next section, we will explore High Intensity Interval Training (HIIT). Checking with your healthcare provider as you advance your workouts is always recommended.

1. Increase Repetitions
Instead of performing five repetitions of each exercise, perform six to eight, while maintaining the 8-4-8 pattern (contraction-holding-relaxation) as well as your speed.

2. Increase Resistance
Increase the weight or resistance you use in each exercise by 10–15%, while maintaining the 8-4-8 pattern and your speed. You can accomplish this by using resistance bands and heavier dumbbells. Make sure your exercise ball is fully inflated to ensure the greatest balance challenge to your core. You'll also want to increase your own focus and effort of contraction.

3. Increase Sets or Rotations
Complete three rotations instead of just two. This will increase your EAT resistance workout time by about one-third, or ten minutes.

4. Decrease Recovery Time
Decrease the amount of time you rest between exercises from 20 seconds to ten seconds. Not only will this increase the demand on your muscle fibers, it will enable you to maintain an elevated heart rate throughout your resistance workout.

5. Increase Your Speed

Increase the speed of each repetition from 8-4-8 (contraction-holding-relaxation) to 4-2-4. You'll generate more force per repetition, which means you should also increase the resistance or amount of weight by 15–25%.

6. Maintain Muscular Contraction

Pay closer attention to keeping the contraction in your muscles, not your bones. It's common to "lock out" your joints during an exercise by straightening your elbows in a push-up or your knees in a squat, for example. This transfers the weight onto your bone structure and away from working muscles, and is not recommended. By avoiding "locking out", you increase tension and maintain a high-level of intensity throughout your repetitions.

Intensifying Your EAT Walking Workouts through Interval Training
We previously reserved the introduction of High Intensity Interval Training (HIIT) until the Ultrahealth™ section of *Dr. A's Habits of Health* book because of the conditioning that is required to perform this level of fitness. Recent studies and growing experience is showing that HIIT is highly effective at removing that stubborn resistant fat.[3] Once you have reached the level of fitness described below you might want to consider using at least some HIIT. High Intensity Interval Training is a time-efficient way to train your aerobic (cardiovascular) and anaerobic (muscle) energy-burning systems.

It's called interval training because it consists of short periods, or intervals, of high-intensity cardiovascular activity followed by short periods of lower-intensity cardiovascular activity. By alternating high- and low-intensity intervals, you intensify the metabolic challenge to your muscles, increasing the amount of calories burned in each 20-minute session. This can help prevent injury by keeping exercise time shorter and saving muscles from overuse.

Difference Between High Intensity and Low Intensity Intervals

- High-intensity interval: around 75–90% of your maximum heart rate (MHR), or a rate of perceived exertion (RPE) of around 7–9.

- Low-intensity interval: around 50–60% of your maximum heart rate (MHR), or a rate of perceived exertion (RPE) of around 5–6.

High Intensity Interval Training (HIIT) at Home

You can do this workout without any equipment. You just need some room where you can move around. Your perceived level of exertion will be greater than 7–9 which means it is important to rest between exercises every time. If you're just beginning, change the ratio of work to rest so that you're working for less time and resting for longer.

Routine One: Do each of these moves for 45 seconds, resting for 15 seconds after each exercise. Repeat this circuit twice.

1. Butt Kicks (45 secs)
- Stand with feet hip-distance apart.
- Kick your left heel to your left glute.
- Set your foot back down and repeat with your right foot. Continue alternating quickly for 45 seconds.

2. Jump Squats (45 secs)
- Stand with your feet slightly wider than hip-distance apart.
- Bend your knees and sit your butt back, keeping your chest upright.
- Jump up into the air as high as you can. Land softly and immediately lower into the next rep.
- Do as many reps as possible in 45 seconds.

3. Burpees (45 secs)
- Start standing with your feet hip-distance apart, and bring your palms to the floor.
- Jump your feet back so that you are in high plank, keeping your core tight and your hips lifted.
- Bend your elbows and do one push-up.

- Now jump your feet to the outside of your hands. As you stand up, explode upwards and jump as high as you can, bringing your arms overhead.
- Do as many reps as possible in 45 seconds.

4. *Mountain Climbers (45 secs)*

- Start in a high plank and draw your right knee under your torso, keeping your toes off the ground.
- Return your right foot to the starting position.
- Switch legs and bring your left knee under your chest. Keep switching legs as if you're running in place.
- Do as many as possible in 45 seconds.

5. *Alternating Side Lunges (45 secs)*

- Start standing with your feet together.
- Step your left foot out to the left. Keep your right leg straight. and bend your left knee.
- Step your left foot back to standing, and repeat, stepping out with your right foot this time.
- Continue switching back and forth.
- Do as many as possible in 45 seconds.

6. *Jumping Lunges (45 secs)*

- Starting standing with feet shoulder-width apart. Jump your left leg forward and your right leg back, and land in a lunge position.
- Jump up, and switch your legs in mid-air so that you land in a lunge with your right leg in front.
- Continue jumping back and forth, pausing as little as possible.
- Do as many as possible in 45 seconds.

Repeat the circuit twice.

Routine Two: Do each of these moves for 40 seconds, then drop into a forearm plank for 20 seconds after each exercise. Rest for one minute after each set.

1. Mountain Climbers (40 secs)
- Start in a high plank and draw your right knee under your torso, keeping your toes off the ground.
- Return your right foot to the starting position.
- Switch legs and bring your left knee under your chest. Keep switching legs as if you're running on the spot.
- Do as many as possible in 40 seconds.

2. Forearm Plank (20-sec hold)
- Start with your forearms and knees on the ground, shoulder-width apart. Elbows should be stacked underneath the shoulders, your forearms straight in front of you on the ground.
- Lift your knees off the ground and push your feet back to bring your body to full extension, so your body creates one long line.
- Keep your core tight and your hips lifted, and keep your neck in line with your spine.
- Hold for 20 seconds.

Rest for one minute.

3. Plank Jacks (40 secs)
- Start in a high plank.
- Keeping your core engaged, jump your feet in and out (like jumping jacks).
- If your wrists bother you, try this move on your forearms.
- Do as many as possible in 40 seconds.

4. Forearm Plank (20-sec hold)

Rest for one minute.

5. Lateral Plank Walks (40 secs)

• Start in a high plank with shoulders above your wrists and abs tight.

• Step your right foot and right hand to right side, then immediately follow this with your left foot and left hand. Take a few "steps" in one direction, then walk in the opposite direction.

• Do as many as possible in 40 seconds.

Rest for one minute.

Repeat the circuit twice.

How are your High Intensity Interval Training Workouts Progressing?

Are you burning more fat? Is your waist circumference and body fat percentage decreasing?

A WORD ABOUT BRANCHED-CHAIN AMINO ACIDS (BCAA)

As you progress the intensity of your workouts, you will most likely be exposed to BCAA supplements which have been shown to build muscle, decrease muscle fatigue, and alleviate muscle soreness.

These branched-chain amino acids are also called essential amino acids amino acids (BCAAs) because they can't be produced by your body and must be obtained from food.

There are three essential amino acids: leucine, isoleucine, and valine. These can be found in food and whole protein supplements.

Because most people get plenty of BCAAs through their diet, supplementing with BCAAs is unlikely to provide additional benefits. Obtaining your BCAAs from complete protein sources is more beneficial as they contain all the essential amino acids. Branched-chain amino acids are abundantly found in many foods and whole protein supplements. This makes BCAA supplements unnecessary for most, especially if you consume enough protein in your diet already.

BCAAs include many of the protein sources we have already discussed in healthy eating for life:

	SERVING SIZE	BCAAs
Beef, round	3.5oz (100g)	6.8g
Chicken breast	3.5oz (100g)	5.88g
Whey protein powder	1 scoop	5.5g
Soy protein powder	1 scoop	5.5g
Canned tuna	3.5oz (100g)	5.2g
Salmon	3.5oz (100g)	4.9g
Turkey breast	3.5oz (100g)	4.6g
Eggs	2 eggs	3.28g
Parmesan cheese	½ cup (50g)	4.5g
1% milk	1 cup (235ml)	2.2g
Greek yogurt	½ cup (140g)	2g

As you can see many of the protein-rich foods above contain high amounts of BCAAs. If you are consuming the above proteins in enough quantities, BCAA supplements are unlikely to provide additional benefits. I would discuss supplementation with a professional trainer or your healthcare provider.

Your Complete Habits of Motion System

To create and maintain optimal health, you need to be active every day. My Habits of Motion System is designed to make sure you get enough activity to keep your weight under control while moving you toward optimal health. You'll get most of this healthy activity through the NEAT System and the EAT Walking Program. The EAT Resistance Program takes you the rest of the way by helping you maintain your cardiovascular and musculoskeletal systems for the long-term. If you want to take it even further, a fitness trainer can help you create a more advanced program tailored to your goals (I've started using a trainer regularly myself), or you can use Level Three and boost your workouts and high intensity interval training as described above.

Now that you've put the Habits of Motion System together, let's take a look at the program in its entirety. Here's what a single week might look like once you're in the swing:

	NEAT SYSTEM	EAT SYSTEM	CALS BURNED
MONDAY	Walked four flights Walked to lunch	30 Minute EAT upper body	450
TUESDAY	Walked four flights Cleaned closet	30 minute EAT walk	425
WEDNESDAY	Walked four flights Washed car	30 minute EAT walk	375
THURSDAY	Walked four flights Raked lawn Washed dishes	30 Minute EAT lower body	450
FRIDAY	Walked four flights Walked to lunch	30 minute EAT walk	400
SATURDAY	Walked four flights Mall shopping Dancing	30 minute EAT walk	650
SUNDAY	Climbed stadium Upper deck	30 minute EAT walk	400

A Typical Week on the Habits of Motion System

By reviewing your activity and total calories burned for a week on the NEAT and EAT Systems, you can see how effective these activities are at upping energy expenditure without taking a lot of time from your day.

You now have the knowledge you need to take control of your energy management system. These Habits of Healthy Motion, combined with the Habits of Healthy Eating you've already learned, will have a dramatic impact on your journey toward your healthy weight and optimal health.

We're now going to look at an area of your life that's equally important but is all too often brushed aside in our time-starved world. Yet, nothing has the ability to age you faster or extend the quality of your life more than our next essential habit—the Habit of Healthy Sleeping.

Notes to yourself:

Now that you have completed Element 18, *Exercise Is Your Gift To Yourself*, **write down your thoughts guided by the following questions:**
What does this Element mean to you right now?

What does this Element give you the opportunity to reflect on?

What actions are you going to take as a result of this Element?

I encourage you to connect with your coach so you can share your thoughts and actions as soon as possible. Sharing your thoughts with your coach will help them become a reality. Make sure you review all your notes and this Element often.

1 *The Role of Exercise Capacity in the Health and Longevity of Centenarians* – Massimo Venturelli,a,b,c,* Federico Schena,a and Russell S. Richardsonc,d,e Perls T, Terry D. Maturitas. 2012 Oct; 73(2): 115–120. Published online 2012 Aug 9. doi: [10.1016/j.maturitas.2012.07.009 PMCID: PMC3618983 NIHMSID: NIHMS395602 PMID: 22883374 Understanding the determinants of exceptional longevity. Annals of Internal Medicine. 2003;139(Septmber 5 Pt 2):445–9.

2 *Exercise and the Heart: Risks, Benefits, and Recommendations for Providing Exercise Prescriptions* – Carl J. Lavie, MD, Richard V. Milani, MD, Patrick Marks, CEP, and Helen de Gruiter, RN Ochsner J. 2001 Oct; 3(4): 207–213. PMCID: PMC3116747 PMID: 21765739.

3 *Comparable Effects of High-Intensity Interval Training and Prolonged Continuous Exercise Training on Abdominal Visceral Fat Reduction in Obese Young Women* – Haifeng Zhang, 1 , 2 Tom K. Tong, 3 Weifeng Qiu, 4 Xu Zhang, 1 Shi Zhou, 5 Yang Liu, 1 and Yuxiu He 1, J Diabetes Res. 2017; 2017: 5071740. Published online 2017 Jan 1. doi: [10.1155/2017/5071740]PMCID: PMC5237463 PMID: 28116314.

ELEMENT 19:
HOW DO YOU CREATE HEALTHY SLEEP AND UNLIMITED ENERGY?

Average time to complete: **2–4 weeks**

In Element 19, we will:

- Focus on helping you optimize your sleep and energy management so that we are prioritizing your rest.
- Define why sleep is so important to you.
- Create a Twilight Hour to turn the day off.
- Create a Model Morning to start your optimal day.

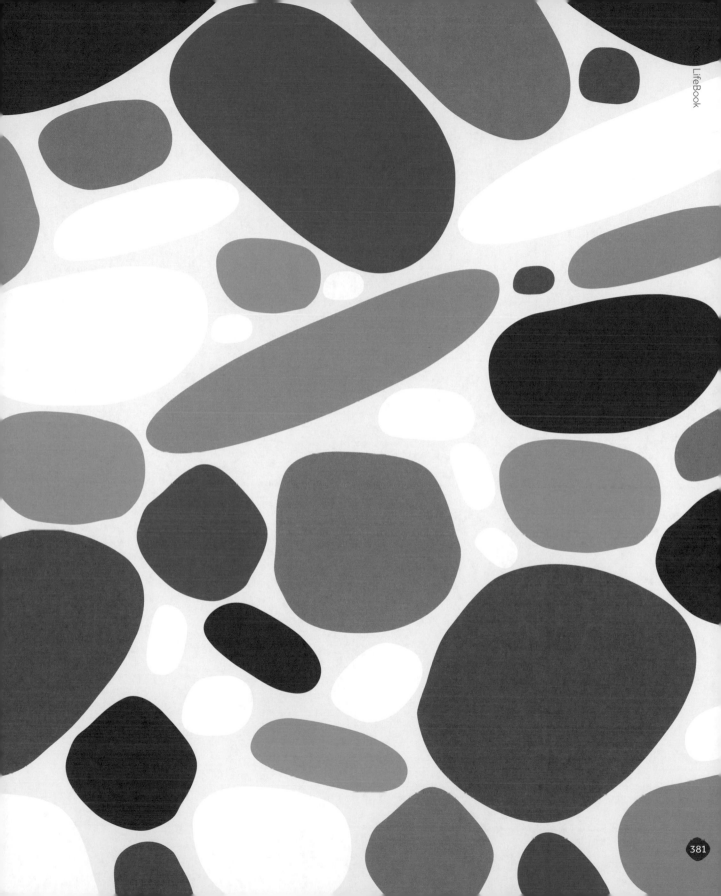

As a key physiological drive, the urge to sleep, much like hunger and thirst, plays an essential role in creating health and wellbeing. We are designed to live a third of our life in a state of unconsciousness, and yet modern life has reduced sleep for most into a luxury which fits in the cracks of our over-complicated lives.

And data shows our health and wellbeing are taking a significant hit as we ignore proper rest. The research gathered over the last decade is starting to uncover the key role that sleep plays in maintaining optimal health and the necessity of a good night's sleep to not only our health but our survival. One study, designed to test the vital importance of enough sleep, purposely deprived rats of sleep and the results were startling:[1]

All of the rats died within a month![2]

The role of sleep has an important roles in optimizing many of our systems from the inner workings of our immune system, to proper hormonal balance, to our emotional and mental health, to learning and memory, and even clearing toxins from our brain.

Research shows that people who have fewer than six hours of sleep had a higher likelihood of becoming obese. These are not very good odds if our goal is to optimize our weight management system.[3]

Besides being very tired, the consequences for those that do not prioritize this vital habit will find themselves winding up sick, overweight, forgetful, and depressed.

In this Element, we will focus on helping you optimize your sleep and energy management so that we are prioritizing your rest. We need to make sure you are optimally recharged every morning to have the resilience to power through whatever the day throws at you and thrive for the rest of your life.

Why is sleep so important to me? (See *Dr. A's Habits of Health* Part 2.13, *Healthy Sleep and Unlimited Energy*)

MY DESIRE FOR YOU

Adjusting your sleep and napping rituals will have you running on an optimum schedule and it will effortlessly support your energy and strength. It's the human equivalent of your smartphone's optimum status: five bars of service and 100% charge. These powerful habits will provide you with more energy, a better mood, better focus, and will supercharge your mojo!

Living in these times, it is our energy levels rather than our time management that really sets up the success we will have when installing our Habits of Health. When your energy and sense of wellbeing are high, you are in a position to begin your day on the right trajectory: early to rise, excited to be up and about, and ready for an optimal day. This is a highly engaged and productive day of accomplishing what is important to you which concludes with deep satisfaction. As the day drifts to its natural conclusion, it does so with a sense of calm and contentment and in anticipation of a night of restful deep sleep.

Doesn't that sound wonderful?

It is, and you will own this new and vital Element in your story. We will redesign your rituals and routines and install the new habits that will permit your body and mind's operating system to run at its highest efficiency to propel you to become the highest version of yourself.

Personally, everything in my life that has allowed me to flourish is predicated by starting each day with an incredible level of energy that makes the day a joy to live. And it is all set up by the quality of my sleep and supported by my naps when needed. It is my secret weapon.

HOW MANY HOURS OF SLEEP DO I NEED TO BE OPTIMAL?

The literature varies slightly depending on the study, but the consensus is you need at least eight hours of sleep every single night to be optimized. The range is seven and a half to nine hours.
The best way to find out is to measure what time you naturally awaken in the morning by the end of a long vacation (assuming you have not been partying excessively).

How many hours are you sleeping now on average?

Do you need an alarm to wake up in the morning?

How many times do you hit the snooze button?

Is it easier for you to stay up late or get up earlier?

Check which bird describes you:

Lark   **Easier to get up early**
Owl   **Easier to stay up late**

Installing Your Hours of Healthy Sleep Ritual into the Integrated Habits of Health Clock (See *Dr. A's Habits of Health* Part 2.13, *Healthy Sleep and Unlimited Energy*)

Meet the rest of the world start time

What time do you need to meet the world? This is the time when you need to first interact with others. It could be the kids, spouse, leaving for work, etc.

Comments

Model morning ritual awake time

If you are a lark, you may extend the morning ritual time longer than an hour, but you will then need to go to bed earlier by the equivalent amount of time to get your eight hours of quality sleep.

Comments

In bed time

Awake Time	−	In Bed Time	=	8 hours or your ideal (determined on vacation)

Comments

Have you decided what time you need to wake up and immediately get out of bed? After doing this, then count back eight hours. This is the time you must be in bed the night before ready to go to sleep when your head hits the pillow, (unless you are feeling frisky!).

Habits of Health Sleep and Energy Clock

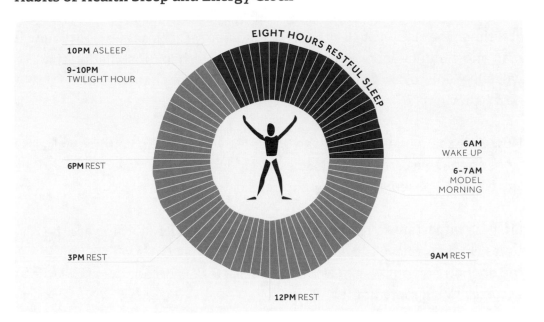

EIGHT HOURS RESTFUL SLEEP

10PM ASLEEP
9-10PM TWILIGHT HOUR
6PM REST
3PM REST
12PM REST
9AM REST
6-7AM MODEL MORNING
6AM WAKE UP

You have now set up the sacred uninterrupted time allotted for your Habits of Healthy Sleep, and we will now breakdown each component to customize for you.

Why is this so important?

Our circadian rhythm controls over 99% of our DNA, and 10,000 years ago natural light and a very simple lifestyle allowed it to function effectively.[4] Today with blue light, constant electronic connection, and complex schedules, it is no longer a reliable or terribly effective clock.

Our Integrated Habits of Health Clock is designed to create a reliable and specific schedule to reestablish adequate time, as well as a series of rituals, and habits that will allow you to once again thrive and create optimal health one day at a time.

Today is the only day we have control over. Building in this automatic clock will allow you to make this lifelong transformation one day and one habit at a time. The Habits of Health Sleep and Energy Clock shows how you will plan and conduct your own personalized 24-hour habit installation that will allow you to consistently mask the daily choices that will build new behaviors.

Now, let's zoom in and look at the two most vital areas in your biological clock so that we cannot only harness your energy and recovery but also set the pace and productivity for an optimal day.

First, it's important to realize that the evening and the morning are the times where we have the most control over our day. Once we are out of the door and on our way to work, our ability to control our own schedule becomes much more limited.

Most people spend all day tied to a schedule that is usually designed, directed, and accountable to someone else—a world in which you are not the central focus. If we look at our day, you can see how we have control over some of our time, as in the hours immediately surrounding and including sleep we have more potential control than any other area.

Work: 8 hours
8am – 3pm
Most of us have little control.

Non work: 8 hours
6am – 8am, 3pm – 10pm
We are mostly in charge but may have lots of commitments to manage.

Healthy Sleep: 8 hours
10pm – 6pm

Once you recognize the importance of sleep in making everything work, you can decide to have total control.

Evening Ritual and Twilight Hour

Since your evening ritual is what will set up those uninterrupted hours of healthy sleep, let's dive into how to create the best possible conditions to ensure great sleep.

Evening Ritual

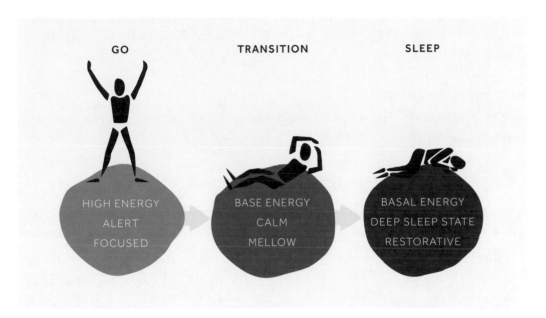

As you create your own personal transition you will need to put an intentional focus on finishing chores and work-related tasks, or resolving any family issues earlier in the evening. The closer you are getting to your hour before bedtime ritual, or twilight hour, the more mellow you will become. Dimming the lights and turning off the computer or putting on some soothing music are all helpful actions.

As you get better at planning your transition time, you will feel your *Go System* and stress level decreasing, thereby preparing you for the twilight hour to get your body ready for sleep.

What must I do to ensure my twilight hour is not interrupted each evening?

See HabitsofHealth.com to download a blank checklist you can fill in to make sure you finish all the necessary tasks before you start making time for you!

Twilight Hour Ritual

Below is an example of what a twilight hour—defined as one hour before you put your head on your pillow— might look like.

Example of a Bedtime Ritual in the Twilight Hour

1 HOUR	30 MINS	15 MINS	IN BED	HEAD ON PILLOW
All pets and children asleep	Out of bath or shower	Last minute entry in your LifeBook or journal	Use the restroom then get in bed	"I love you"
Run hot bath with salts, or shower	Loose-fitting lightweight clothes	Reading with bluelight suppression glasses	Pillows and sheets organized	Hug or goodnight kiss
Thermostat below 68°f	Self-care, teeth brushed and flossed	A few minutes of meditation	Prayer	Mind off
Clean up any clutter	Cool down starts	Deep breathing	Flip the switch	
All blue light off: Tv, computer, phone	Place chamomile, jasmine, lavendar on pillow and sheets	Gratitude	Cuddle, partner massage or foot-rub	
Take your medications		Room cold, dark and quiet		
Avoid any additional water intake other than a cup of tea		Sleepy-time tea		

If all of this seems a little bit over structured, that's because it is. If you do not have a plan and an allotment of time, life will get in the way and sabotage you!

Write down your Twilight Hour Ritual

1 HOUR	30 MINS	15 MINS	IN BED	HEAD ON PILLOW

Sleep Disruption

There are several potential things that can affect our sleep. There is a detailed discussion in Part 2.13 in *Dr. A's Habits of Health, Healthy Sleep and Unlimited Energy*.

Here, we want to evaluate if your behavior and habits are an issue and to what extent they affect you in order to stop them having a negative impact on your sleep.

Write down on a scale of 1–10 how much these may be affecting your sleep (10 being the most harm):

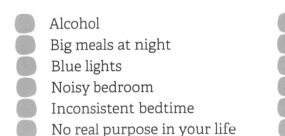

Do not see the value of sleep   Alcohol

Caffeine   Big meals at night

Exercising in evening   Blue lights

Messy bedroom   Noisy bedroom

Too much light   Inconsistent bedtime

Anxiety or mind racing   No real purpose in your life

Now put them in descending order and choose below which ones you are going to work on first and what you are going to do. Read Part 2.13 in *Dr. A's Habits of Health, Healthy Sleep and Unlimited Energy* for many ideas on taming these disruptors.

Next, we will set some times that you can insert into your integrated Habits of Health Clock to minimize the effects of some of these behaviors that you do not intent to fully stop.

Bright Line Curfews

In order to manage some of the behaviors and habits which may be having a negative impact on our sleep and energy, it is important to create bright lines. In legal jargon, bright lines are the boundaries we create and enforce by drawing a line in the sand of what can and cannot be done. They are lines that cannot be crossed. In terms of the behaviors listed below (such as drinking alcohol or caffeine), it is usually better not to do these if you want to be best prepared for sleep. But if we are unwilling to eliminate them at this time, we need to set hard curfews to help create a cue for the time we will stop this behavior in order to support our best sleep.

Here is an illustration that shows you when you should stop certain behaviors that can have a negative impact on the quality or quantity of your sleep.

Bright Line Curfews

HOURS BEFORE BED	
8 HOURS	Coffee
5 HOURS	All caffeinated products
4 HOURS	Exercise
3 HOURS	Alcohol and heavy meals
2 HOURS	Work and serious conversations
1 HOURS	Digital sunset
IN BED	Lights out

Note that in terms of highly caffeinated products like coffee, espresso, and others with over 50 milligrams (mg), these should be suspended eight hours before you expect to be in bed. All lower level caffeinated items should stop being consumed within five hours of sleep to make sure the level does not interrupt your induction into deep sleep.

Changing your bedroom sleep architecture

There are some things you can eliminate once that will have a profound effect on your sleep.

- Remove all electronics from bedroom:
  - TV
  - Cell phones
  - Blue lights
- Darken all clocks and other devices that emit light
- Use special glasses that block blue light or get special bulbs
- Make sure your temperature is less than 68 degrees (experiment between 62–68 to find the ideal temp for you). Write down what is best.

- Make sure you are not using a quilt which makes you hot. The idea is for your body to lower its core temperature to maintain ideal sleep.
- Also wear lightweight clothes for the same reason.

If you cannot avoid outside noises, get an air filter that can create ambient noise or invest in a sound device that creates natural sounds like the ocean surf or rainfall.

The Stress and Anxiety Factor

Research confirms that stress and anxiety are the number one causes of poor sleep.[5]

The following are some of the best and easiest ways to consciously calm your mind:

One: The easiest thing is to take control of your breath.
Discuss how you are going to add this into your day and rituals:

Two: Use Stop. Challenge. Choose.™ to shake off negative self-talk
or break the loop that you're obsessing over—it's non-productive.
Discuss how you are going to add this into your day and rituals:

Third: Take five to ten minutes to meditate and bring yourself back to the
present moment and into a calming state. Discuss how you are going to
add this into your day and rituals:

These can be used all day long to help you gain better control of your stress,
anxiety, and thoughts. With practice, you can enjoy a calmer mind overall.

Beyond that, you will, with practice, become a master of sleep, flipping that
switch, taking that centering breath, shutting your mind off, and entering
the right state totally prepared for sleep.

Now let's look how we can optimize the start of our day.

HOW DO YOUR MORNINGS START?

Do you wake up in the morning in a calm, relaxed, fully-invigorated state, ready to attack the day? If so, congratulations, you're ahead of the game.

For most, it is a little more like a fire drill: a hectic scramble filled with varying degrees of stress and chaos. For others, it feels like coming out of a coma with lethargy: a sense of clearing the fog and dreading the day.

As we are rushing to get ready for the day, our minds are plagued with inner thoughts of what we have to do, where we have to go, what we have to accomplish, and worrying that we are already running late.

Or maybe there is an unresolved issue with our partner or our kids?

Stressed and rushed or slow and unproductive, we are starting the day on the wrong foot, and it will make it difficult to create an optimal day.

Just like it was critical in the twilight hour to create a ritual, habitualizing a routine to align your biological clock to establish high quality sleep, the early morning ritual is equally important to establish the optimal physical and mental state to energize and power your day.

Morning Ritual

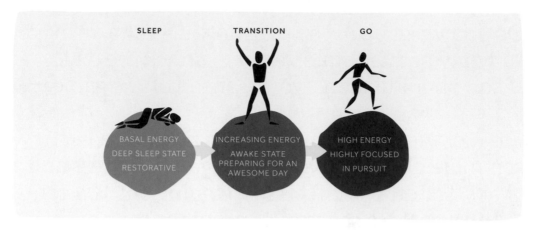

I like to think of the morning ritual as a model morning. It is the morning version of the twilight hour in the evening.

By planning and executing a specific routine or ritual in the morning, you are equipped to handle whatever the day throws at you. Our goal is to give you eight solid hours of sleep followed by a model morning that creates a whole transformation of your level of health and wellbeing.

Example of Ritual for Your Model Morning

AWAKE	CALM	DESIRED OUTCOME	MOTION	SELF-CARE	READY WORLD
I hour before facing the world	Meditate, prayer, reflect 1-10 mins	Focus on what is most important to me	Do 5-10 mins of activity	Shower	Off or in to work
Get out of bed	Deep breathe	Write down in Your LifeBook or journal 3 things I will accomplish today	Walking	Brush and floss teeth	Create an optimal day
Thermostat to normal	Gratitude		Exercise	Other personal hygiene	Fully conscious
Open all blinds to let in sunlight		Visualize your optimal day	Stretch	Fueling	
Use restroom		Possible 10 mins reading			
Weigh		Fuelings, motion, relaxation goals			
Drink glass or two of water					
Put on workout clothes					

If you give yourself just an hour from awakening until you have to start working with others or leave your home to go to work, you can prepare you mind and body for an optimum day.

Let's review this model hour:

Awake: First, it is important to adjust the time you go to bed so that in a relatively short time you will awaken without the alarm. When we wake up on our own instead of being prompted by an alarm, we seize control of our day, living on our terms rather than supporting the demands of someone else, such as an employer. I resented having to get up at 5am to go make my rounds every morning before surgery. I have used an alarm less than a dozen times in the last 15 years and wake up naturally, and it really starts my day off right.

But until you get that figured out, you can use a Natural Dawn Simulator Alarm Clock that will simulate the lighting in the morning and wake you gently. Once you are awake, get out of bed and do not use the snooze feature. This is critical to create the habit of starting the day every morning with eager anticipation. The next hour is going to be like Christmas morning, and you are going to give yourself a gift before you are available to others. Again, you have to work around family logistics to make this happen.

For those that use the snooze button, please note that this is a Habit of Disease. For some, this unhealthy habit may last over an hour. Research shows it does not count toward deep restorative sleep. And it sets up a negative precedent to start your day. If you want to break this bad habit, set your alarm clock the night before to the last possible time you can actually get up and make everything happen. Getting up immediately by necessity will help you break this habit in a hurry!

Open up the blinds or drapes immediately as the bright light will help your brain turn off any residual sleep chemicals and turn on awake chemicals. Increase the room temperature, go to the restroom, weigh yourself to record your current weight reality, and then put on your workout clothes which you have made conveniently available the night before.

Let's review this Model Morning Hour:

Calm: This is the period of time where you align your body and your mind to a state of peace, calm, and clarity of purpose. This allows you to reflect on why you are improving your habits and your relationships, as well as setting the right tone for your day.

Desired Outcome: Once you are centered and in control, you can start visualizing what your day will look like, what you will accomplish, and the priorities you will focus on. Depending on how much time you have, it's always good to read something that will help you with your personal or spiritual growth.

Also, make sure you are focused on your habit installation. The Habits of Health App can help you.

Motion: As we discussed in the section on motion, active movement will give you up to 12 hours of improved focus, mood, and energy. As little as 20 minutes is the equivalent of a dose of Ritalin and Prozac in improving your mental and physical state!

Self-care: This is when you conclude your model hour with a hot shower directed to your neck and back, as well as brushing and flossing your teeth. During this period, I visualize and smile as I anticipate an amazing day ahead of me as well as express gratitude for everything around me. Then I shave, dry off, and put on my clothes and—hey presto—I am ready to interact in an attractive and successful way with my surroundings.

And the final step is to prepare and fuel yourself with a high-quality first meal of the day.

Ready: At this point, I have preemptively prepared my thoughts, emotions, energy, priorities, and direction so I can have an optimal day.

Note: Contact with the outside world isn't part of this ritual. If you are using the recommended times of optimal sleep, this morning model will have you ready to interact with your family by 7am. I focus on my family and my dogs, but most importantly I have prepared myself with the model morning to create an optimal day for myself before I let the outside world in.

Now write down your own Model Morning:

Your Model Morning Ritual

AWAKE	CALM	DESIRED OUTCOME	MOTION	SELF-CARE	READY WORLD

Make Your Bed: It Starts Your Day off Right

Why is making your bed such a powerful way to start your day?
(See Part 2.13 in *Dr. A's Habits of Health, Healthy Sleep and Unlimited Energy*)

Depending on your individual needs, such as tending to your children and other family members or other early morning requirements, you can expand or shrink these 60 minutes to fit your obligations.

Developing Habits of Health and rituals that fuel the start of your day and having proper direction can change everything.

Your Optimal Day: Energy Levels

If everything went well and your evening ritual and twilight hour went off without a hitch, you should have had seven and a half hours or more of high-quality sleep. Your model morning will place you in the best possible position to have an optimal day. If you have installed the rituals and they are now your Habits of Healthy Sleeping, I will guarantee that you have increased your energy, and you'll be in great shape to create better health and wellbeing.

Unfortunately, it does not prevent you from occasionally having a bad night of sleep. Your child may be sick, a bad storm keeps you up, you do not feel well, or you just had a nightmare. And we all have times during the day where we become fidgety or drowsy and just need to take a break.

All is not lost. We have two different recovery methods: **passive rest** and **active rest**. Both are important to boost energy, re-establish alertness, create focus, and improve selective attention. First, let's spend a moment explaining how your waking hours have a rhythm that matches your nighttime REM cycles.

Our Rest and Energy Waves

It seems that within our waking hours we have 90-minute cycles called ultradian rhythms, which are similar to our nightly REM cycles.

The ultradian rhythm is the equivalent daytime cycle needed to have effective attention and focus.

During the day, we move from higher to lower alertness. When we need a rest, our body signals us with hunger, drowsiness, fidgetiness, or loss of focus. We generally override the bodies need to rest with caffeine, foods high in sugar, and simple high-glycemic carbs, and then our bodies— on their own—produce stress hormones like adrenaline, noradrenaline, and cortisol.

In the diagram below, the red area illustrates when these stress hormones are released and the effect they have on both our productivity and our health.

Ultradian Cycle

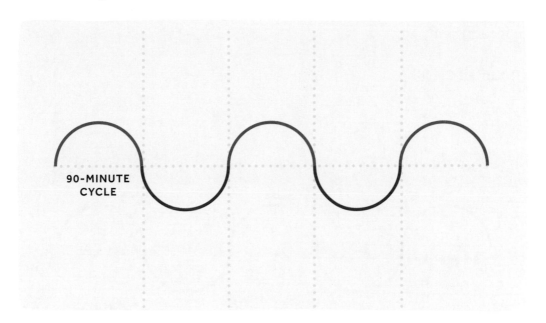

90-MINUTE CYCLE

For the next few days, take note of the changes in your energy level throughout the day. Note when you are the most alert and also when you are at your lowest level. Are you drinking coffee or tempted to eat sugary foods at certain times in the day?

Now, let's plan how you are going to recover and prevent these lows in the future.

We want to insert either **passive** or **active rest** periods into the red zones that you have identified above. The following illustration shows where to insert them:

Ultradian Cycle

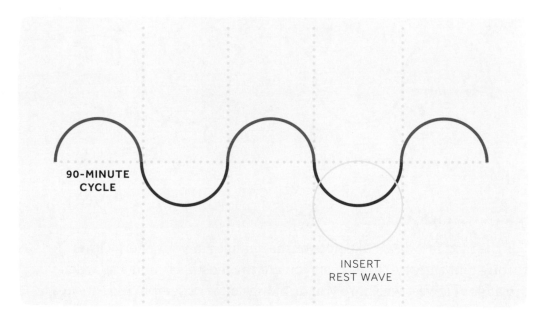

90-MINUTE CYCLE

INSERT REST WAVE

Passive Rest

These are true sleep naps and can be divided into two categories based on length and depth of sleep:

> *Power naps*
> *REM naps*

Power naps: These are 6–20 minute naps that are short and partially replenish our neurotransmitters. Because they are short and create quick recovery, they are ideal for your work day when time is usually limited. If they extend longer than 20 minutes, they can leave you in a groggy state.

REM naps: These are longer naps that actually place us in a complete sleep cycle, including the REM state. Because they need approximately 90-plus minutes, they are not practical for most during the working week. They are deeply restorative and, as long as they do not occur less than three hours before twilight hour, will not interfere with that night's sleep pattern and may help keep your energy high when it is needed.

Write down which ones are more helpful for you. Figure out what is the ideal amount of time for your power nap to restore your energy.

How are naps, especially REM naps, helping you to recover from sleep debt?

Active Rest

These are methods you can employ throughout the day that help boost your energy, calm your mind, and will also help you sleep better that night by keeping your mind from racing. There are four key areas that can help restore and balance your energy and alertness:

1. Physically: deep breathing, stretching,
2. Mentally: meditate, gratitude, listen to soothing music
3. Socially: family, friends
4. Spiritually: prayer

Write down which ones you are using and how they affect your energy levels:

Rest Waves Allow us to Recover

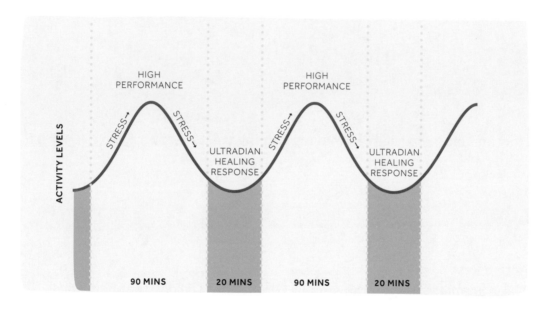

As a result of the insertion of either active or passive rest waves, you can see we are able to recover much quicker and be much more effective, alert, and productive, as well as take the stress burden and negative health consequences out of the equation. This is the true power of the Habits of Health Sleep and Energy restoration—taking suboptimal days and having them aligned with your health and wellbeing. Let's look at how we can assess and help make sure you are addressing any current gaps in how you are mastering both your sleep and energy.

Tracking your Sleep and Energy Level Log

We introduced the importance of tracking and measuring your progress towards a healthier and higher level of wellbeing back in Element 13, *Track Your Journey To A Healthy Weight And Beyond*. Here I am going to provide you with a way to evaluate your sleep and discover how we can use the Habits of Health Clock to help improve both the quality of your sleep and also track your energy level throughout the day.

In order to evaluate your current sleep habits, I would like you to answer these nine questions everyday for a week and enter them in the blank sleep log provided. Use the example for reference and, of course, you can download more at HabitsofHealth.com.

1. What time did you get into bed last night?

2. What time did you get out of bed in the morning?

3. What hours did you actually sleep?

4. Did you take a nap? For how long?

5. Did you consume alcohol? How much, and at what time?

6. Did you exercise? How long, and at what time?

7. Did you drink coffee or other caffeinated beverages? How much, and at what time?

8. How many hours did you watch television? At what time?

9. Did you take any medications? At what time?

TIME	SUN–MON	MON–TUE	TUE–WED	WED–THU	THU–FRI	FRI–SAT	SAT–SUN
6:00PM				Exercise			
7:00PM	Tv						
8:00PM		Tv	Caffeine		Alcohol	Alcohol	
9:00PM		Tv	Tv		Alcohol	Alcohol & Food	
10:00PM	Food	In Bed	Tv	Tv			
11:00PM	In Bed		In Bed	Tv	Alcohol		
MIDNIGHT				In Bed			In Bed
1:00AM	Asleep	Asleep			In Bed	In Bed	
2:00AM			Asleep	Asleep	Asleep	Asleep	
3:00AM					Awake		Asleep
4:00AM						Awake	
5:00AM							
6:00AM					Arise		
7:00AM	Arise	Arise	Arise	Arise	Caffeine		
8:00AM		Caffeine	Caffeine			Arise	
9:00AM	Caffeine			Caffeine		Caffeine	
10:00AM	Caffeine					Caffeine	Arise
11:00AM							
NOON							Caffeine
1:00PM							
2:00PM		Nap					
3:00PM						Exercise	Tv
4:00PM							Tv
5:00PM			Exercise				Tv
6:00PM							

TIME	SUN–MON	MON–TUE	TUE–WED	WED–THU	THU–FRI	FRI–SAT	SAT–SUN
6:00PM							
7:00PM							
8:00PM							
9:00PM							
10:00PM							
11:00PM							
MIDNIGHT							
1:00AM							
2:00AM							
3:00AM							
4:00AM							
5:00AM							
6:00AM							
7:00AM							
8:00AM							
9:00AM							
10:00AM							
11:00AM							
NOON							
1:00PM							
2:00PM							
3:00PM							
4:00PM							
5:00PM							
6:00PM							

Tracking Your Energy Level

Use the Energy Ruler as a measure of your energy and place the number on the chart which describes your level of energy in the morning and during our day.

Energy Ruler

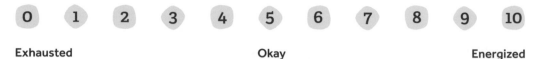

| 0 | 1 | 2 | 3 | 4 | 5 | 6 | 7 | 8 | 9 | 10 |

Exhausted   **Okay**   **Energized**

	SUN – MON	MON – TUE	TUE – WED	WED – THU	THU – FRI	FRI – SAT	SAT – SUN
HOW DID YOU FEEL WHEN YOU WOKE UP?							
HOW DID YOU FEEL DURING THE DAY?							
WERE YOU MORE ALERT IN THE MORNING OR EVENING?							

This chart is available to download at HabitsofHealth.com.

How can you use this information to track how your sleep and energy levels can be improved using all your new knowledge and tools?

YOUR PRIME TIME FOR PRODUCTIVITY

As we identify your problem areas and provide the rituals to assure a great night sleep, it is important to identify your biological prime time so you can complete the deep work that demands your attention and energy most.

Review the ways to find this prime time in the Part 2.13 in *Dr. A's Habits of Health, Healthy Sleep and Unlimited Energy,* and record below when that period occurs on your Habits of Health Clock.

If you can identify and use this time period to get your hardest work done, it will lower your anxiety and stress levels which will improve your overall sleep. Remember people say that anxiety and stress are the number one reason they do not sleep well.[6]

When is your biological prime time?

Record how you are using this time of highest energy and how it is affecting you and your work:

Hopefully you feel you are becoming the dominant force in determining your sleep and energy management. You will find that it will make all the difference in creating more optimal days while improving the quality of your work.

Now let's focus on how we can protect you from all of the ways the environment can harm you and learn how to maximize your anti-inflammatory strategy.

Notes to yourself:

Now that you have completed Element 19, *How Do You Create Healthy Sleep And Unlimited Energy?*, I encourage you to connect with your coach right away, so you can share your answers to the following questions:

What does this Element mean to you right now?

What does this Element give you the opportunity to reflect on?

What actions are you going to take as a result of this Element?

I encourage you to connect with your coach, so you can share your thoughts and actions as soon as possible.

Sharing your thoughts with your coach will help them become a reality.

Make sure you review all your notes and this Element often.

1 *Statement of the American Academy of Sleep Medicine and Sleep Research Society Current Issue* – Volume: 14, Number: 10.

2 *Sleep* – 1989 Feb;12(1):13 – 21. Sleep deprivation in the rat: III. Total sleep deprivation. Everson CA1, Bergmann BM, Rechtschaffen.

3 *Associations Between Sleep Loss and Increased Risk of Obesity and Diabetes* – Ann N Y Acad Sci. Author manuscript; available in PMC 2015 Apr 13. Published in final edited form as: Ann N Y Acad Sci. 2008; 1129: 287–304. doi: [10.1196/annals.1417.033] PMCID: PMC4394987 NIHMSID: NIHMS150220 PMID: 18591489 Kristen L. Knutsona and Eve Van Cauterb Obesity (Silver Spring). Author manuscript; available in PMC 2012 Feb 1. Published in final edited form as: Obesity (Silver Spring). 2011 Feb; 19(2): 324–331. Published online 2010 Oct 14. doi: [10.1038/oby.2010.242] PMCID: PMC3099473 NIHMSID: NIHMS296033 PMID: 20948522 The Relationship Between Sleep and Weight in a Sample of Adolescents Association between Reduced Sleep and Weight Gain in Women Sanjay R. Patel Atul Malhotra David P. White Daniel J. Gottlieb Frank B. Hu American Journal of Epidemiology, Volume 164, Issue 10, 15 November 2006.

4 2017-10-02 The Nobel Assembly at Karolinska Institutet has today decided to award the 2017 Nobel Prize in Physiology or Medicine jointly to Jeffrey C. Hall, Michael Rosbash, and Michael W. Young for their discovery that molecular mechanisms control the circadian rhythm.

5 According to The Cleveland Clinic, two-thirds of patients referred to sleep disorders centers have a psychiatric disorder. "Anxiety is an emotion that actually wakes us up," Dr. Steve Orma, author of Stop Worrying and Go to Sleep: How to Put Insomnia to Bed for Good, told The Huffington Post.

6 According to The Cleveland Clinic, two-thirds of patients referred to sleep disorders centers have a psychiatric disorder. "Anxiety is an emotion that actually wakes us up," Dr. Steve Orma, author of Stop Worrying and Go to Sleep: How to Put Insomnia to Bed for Good, told The Huffington Post.

ELEMENT 20:
MAXIMIZING YOUR ANTI-INFLAMMATION PROTECTION

Average time to complete: **1–2 weeks**

In Element 20, we will:

- Explore why your immune system is so important to optimal health.
- Identify where and how inflammation could be showing up in your life.
- Evaluate opportunities to reduce inflammation in your environment.

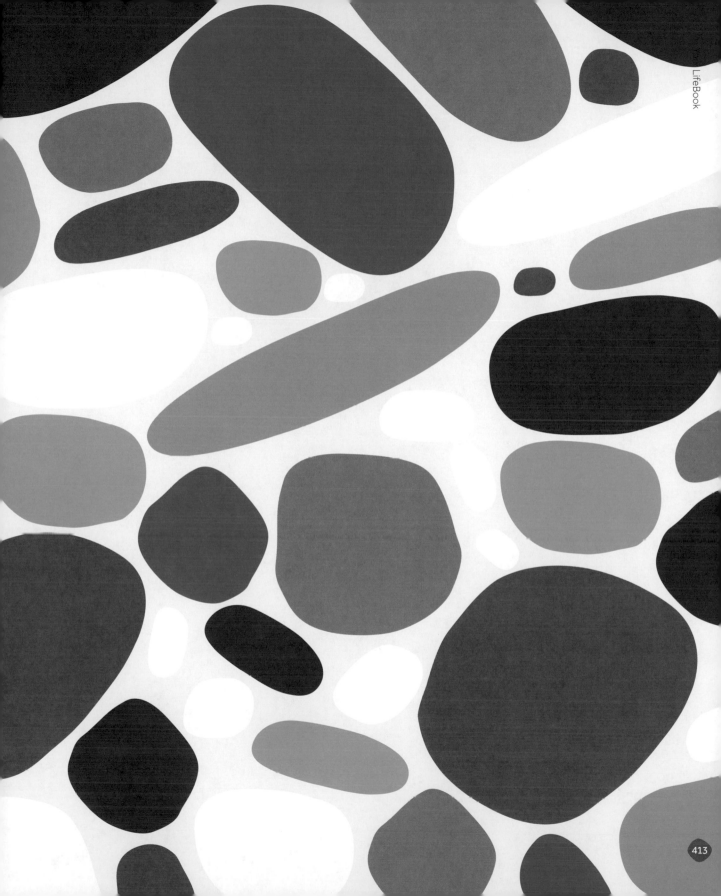

YOUR IMMUNE SYSTEM—BOTH A FRIEND AND A FOE.

It's your own personal 24/7 on-call emergency service and has an incredible ability to seek out intruders such as bacteria, viruses, and parasites. In fact, it's the most complex system in the body. It not only defends us but it remembers every battle it's ever fought so it can recognize repeated threats and avoid wasting time on the harmless ones. Its purpose is to restore balance to an unbalanced body, and once it's done its job it should settle down into its normal, vigilant state to await the next crisis.

Unfortunately, that's not always what happens. As medical science is beginning to discover, this benevolent protector has a darker side that can all too easily turn on its master—especially if we make the Habits of Disease our way of life.

In this Element I am going to ask to read Part 2.14 in *Dr. A's Habits of Health, Inflammation: Dousing the Flame*, to really get a handle on this critical area in your life, which is necessary to create overall health and wellbeing.

It will be essential when answering the questions and reflecting on how you approach your surroundings in terms of keeping your immune system from going dark!

Why is your immune system so important to your optimal health?

When does your immune system become a threat?

What three factors are the main cause of inflammation?

1.

2.

3.

What factors in your internal environment do you struggle with?

What factors in your external environment do you struggle with?

What inflammatory foods do you need to remove from your diet?

The illustration below can help you answer the above questions along with Part 2.14 in *Dr. A's Habits of Health, Inflammation: Dousing the Flame.*

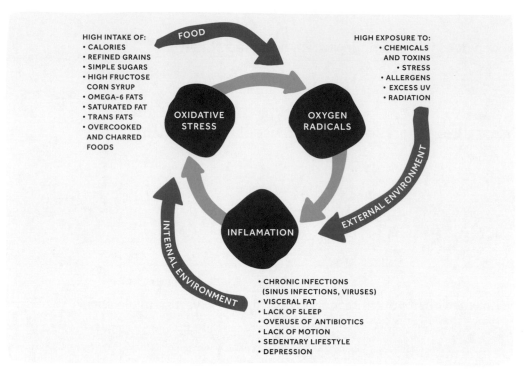

What test can you have to measure your current level of inflammation?

What does this mean and why should you do it?

What is your current level of inflammation?

Anti-Inflammatory Foods

What anti-inflammatory fats are you going to add to help protect yourself?

Inflammatory Omega-3 and Inflammatory Omega-6 Fats

ANTI INFLAMMATORY OMEGA-3	
Oils	Flaxseed, canola, walnut, olive
Fish	Mackerel, sardines, herring salmon, bluefish, cod scallops, tuna, lobster
Nuts/seeds	Flaxseed, walnuts, pecans
Greens/beans	Soybeans, tofu
Greens	Spinach, kale, collard greens
INFLAMMATORY OMEGA-6	
Oils	Corn, cottonseed, safflower, sesame, soybean
Margarine	
Ultra-processed foods or food with a long shelf life	

What other anti-inflammatory foods and cooking methods are you going to add to your diet to help protect you?

· · · · · · · · · · · · · · · · · ·

· · · · · · · · · · · · · · · · · ·

Make sure you have included all those in the green in the diagram below:

Pro-Inflammatory Components in the American Diet (Red)

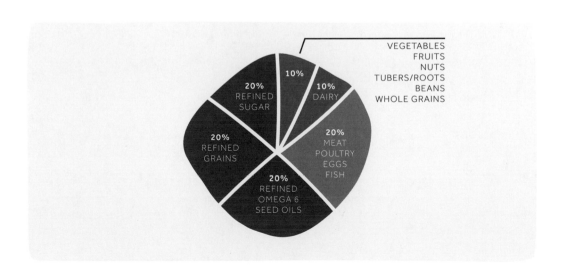

Beat Stress and Curb Inflammation with these Healthy Behaviors

No discussion of inflammation would be complete without addressing stress, which is one of the biggest contributors to a host of health complications. When our bodies are stressed—locked in fight or flight mode—we struggle to function at our best. Though much of the material we covered in this Element and in previous Elements can help you reduce stress—such as Stop. Challenge. Choose.™ or exercising more frequently—stress is best addressed in the context of your mind.

If stress is a significant challenge for you today, you might benefit from jumping ahead to Element 23, *Master Your Thoughts And Emotions*, to learn more about the MacroHabit of a Healthy Mind. In the meantime, begin to extinguish the flame of inflammation as you grow and improve your Habits of Health, thereby optimizing your life one choice at a time.

Notes to yourself:

Take a moment consider how your community is helping you along your journey to Optimal Health and check in with your coach right away to share your answers to the following three questions:

What does this Element mean to you right now?

What does this Element give you the opportunity to reflect on?

What actions are you going to take as a result of this Element?

Sharing your thoughts with your coach will help them become a reality.

Make sure you review all your notes and this Element often.

ELEMENT 21:
DO YOU NEED TO SUPPLEMENT?

Average time to complete: **1–2 weeks**

In Element 21, we will:

- Look at your body's changing needs to help you learn how to adapt as you follow your path to better and more vibrant health.
- Explore why supplementation is important and how it can work for you.
- Create an individualized, targeted plan that not only brings you into better balance but actually augments your health for optimal living.

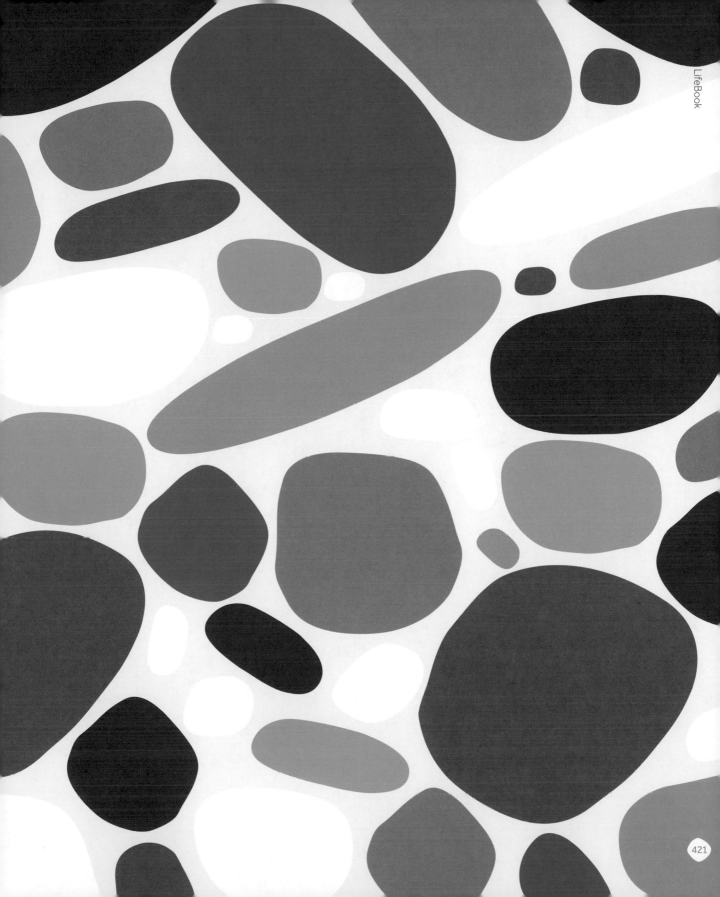

OPTIMIZING YOUR LIFE AT ANY AGE

As you continue on your journey to optimal health and wellbeing, there are a few more tools in our arsenal that can help optimize your current state and keep you in the best possible condition at any age. They could even extend your life.

Take a look at the illustration following which shows the Optimal
Health Journey.

The Optimal Health Journey

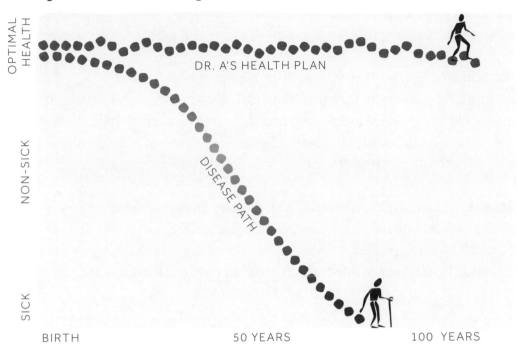

The line that turns orange and then red represents the lifeline of those
who remain passive to the daily insults and attacks of our obesigenic world.
Their optimal health quickly becomes a state of non-sickness—they are
overweight, have a poor diet, and are in a state of sarcopenia (flabby weak
muscles, insomnia, over stressed, and a higher state of inflammation) which
decays to disease over time. Medications may bring about some limited
improvement by decreasing the symptoms, but these folks never really
regain their health.

Contrast that with the new story you are creating as a graduate of the
Habits of Health (green line) who continue to enjoy optimal health for
life. It's worth taking note of something interesting—in order for you to
reach and maintain optimal health, you must continue to adjust to the
changing conditions of aging and their environment to remain in the
optimal health zone.

The upshot? Optimal health isn't static. It looks different at age 20 than at age 80, and it requires vigilance and constant adjustment to the changes your body undergoes as you mature.

It's now a good time to look at your body's changing needs to help you learn how to adapt as you follow your path to better and more vibrant health.

Medications Versus Nutritional Supplementation

For the first time in history, 55% of all insured Americans take prescription medications regularly for chronic health problems such as high blood pressure and cholesterol—problems often linked to heart disease, obesity, and diabetes. And, on average, they take four different medications![1]

These are the individuals tracking on the red line and the trajectory of their story and health is a losing battle against time.

You will supplement with vital nutrients as needed to make sure you are optimizing your intake of foods and supplements.

Nutrients aren't like medications. While medications are foreign intruders that work temporarily in acute situations (often with side effects), nutrients are already present in our body. By supplementing them in just the right amount, you're simply helping your body reach its optimal efficiency. In fact, nutrients are the very fuel of optimal health!

When it comes to the new specialty of creating optimal health and wellbeing, nutrients, not medications, are key.

REACHING THE SUMMIT

Up to this point, we've utilized your body's inherent capacity to heal itself, which has been accomplished by reaching a healthy weight, healthy eating and nutrition, increased daily movement, better sleep and energy habits, increasing your support, and creating healthy surroundings by removing the toxins from your internal and external environments.

Now we're going to augment these normal physiological processes with some valuable tools that can take you even farther up the summit of optimal health—namely vitamins, minerals, and other critical nutrients for enhanced vitality

It's important to reiterate the differences. Nutrients are very different from the medications that today's medical delivery system relies on to treat disease. Most medications become problematic—first, because they interrupt normal body function, and second, because they cause a large number of secondary side effects. Medications have their uses, but creating health isn't one of them.

Nutrients, on the other hand, are great facilitators. They may take a bit more time to create an effect but, since they're already present in the body, they're extremely safe. Nutrients can help you create a thriving, healthy life and augment the health of every cell and organ in your body. They're the very fuel of optimal health.

What supplementation are you now taking and why?

As a fellow consumer, I am sure you have been given varying advice on what or if you should supplement. Some experts say there is no reason to supplement and others, especially advertisements would have me take bottles of pills a day. What should I be doing? I would suggest you first read Mark Hyman's take on it in Part 2.15 in *Dr. A's Habits of Health, The Best You Can Be: Optimizing Your Life at Any Age*. Now write down if you should supplement and why. That way you are making an informed decision.

Renewing and Optimizing through Nutrients: Your Personal Guide (Part 2.15 in *Dr. A's Habits of Health*)

Why should you take fish oils (omega 3)? (Part 2.15 in *Dr. A's Habits of Health* and HabitsofHealth.com)

What vitamins, minerals, and amino acids should I take?
(Part 2.15 in *Dr. A's Habits of Health* and HabitsofHealth.com)

How can I get enough of each type of fiber? (Part 2.15 in *Dr. A's Habits of Health* and HabitsofHealth.com)

How can I optimize my microbiome? (Part 2.15 in *Dr. A's Habits of Health* and HabitsofHealth.com)

What are prebiotics versus probiotics? (Part 2.15 in *Dr. A's Habits of Health* and HabitsofHealth.com)

What are phytonutrients and how can I make sure I am getting them in my diet? (Part 2.15 in *Dr. A's Habits of Health* and HabitsofHealth.com)

Once you've identified your areas of deficiency and current health challenges, you'll be able to create an individualized, targeted plan that not only brings you into better balance but actually augments your health for optimal living. To do that, we'll first look at some general guidelines from the U.S. government and then at some of my own specific recommendations that you can use to guide your choices.

Your Optimal Health Guidelines
(Part 2.15 in *Dr. A's Habits of Health* **and HabitsofHealth.com to help guide you on these steps.)**

Now let's take a look at some guidelines that are based on you, rather that just a model calculated around deficiencies.

Step 1: *Add Fish Oil*

Make one of the following a part of your daily routine:
• 4 ounces of fatty fish three times a week (e.g., salmon, mackerel, sardines)
• 3–6 walnuts a day
• 1–3 grams of omega derived from a cold-water arctic fish, with EPA and DHA, and taken 30 minutes before meals (sprinkle flaxseed on your breakfast as well)

Long-chain omega-3 fatty acids are EPA (eicosapentaenoic acid) and DHA (docosahexaenoic acid). These are plentiful in fish and shellfish. Short-chain omega-3 fatty acids are ALA (alpha-linolenic acid). These are found in plants, such as flaxseed.

Remember, if you're pregnant or breastfeeding, limit your intake of fish to once a week.

Write down how you have acted on this step:

Step 2: *Take a Daily Multivitamin*

If you're not already taking a multivitamin, start today with a one-a-day multivitamin specifically designed for your sex and age. Make sure it's a high-quality bioavailable vitamin, not one from a wax matrix (some companies use a petroleum-based process that interferes with proper vitamin and mineral absorption).

Write down how you have acted on this step:

Step 3: *Add B Complex Vitamins*

The B complex vitamins work as a team. Unless you have specific needs, it's usually best to take them in the form of a high-potency B complex formula. If these aren't included in your one-a-day multivitamin, add them as needed to reach the following daily doses.

VITAMINS	FULL NAME	AMOUNT PER DAY
B1	THIAMINE	25MG
B2	RIBOFLAVIN	25MG
B3	NIACIN	30MG
B5	PANTOTHENIC ACID	100 – 300MG
B6	PYRIDOXINE	4 – 50MG
	FOLIC ACID	400MCG
B12	CYANOCOBALAMIN	100 – 400MCG
	BIOTIN	100 – 300MCG

If you're at high risk for heart disease, talk to your healthcare provider about increasing this amount.

Write down how you have acted on this step:

Step 4: *Augment with Other Key Vitamins*

Add any necessary vitamins and minerals that aren't part of your multivitamin and B complex.

VITAMINS	AMOUNT PER DAY
A	5,000IU
C	1,000MG
D	400 – 1,000
IU E (MIXED TOCOPHERALS)	100 – 400IU
K	20 – 100MCG

Red fruits and vegetables, like tomatoes and watermelon, are full of lycopene: an important antioxidant that may help protect against cardiovascular disease and certain types of cancer. Cooking tomatoes actually increases their lycopene content.

Write down how you have acted on this step:

Step 5: *Add Antioxidant Power*

To enhance vitamin C antioxidant capacity, combine it with one or both of the following:
- Quercetin. This includes compounds and is found in apples, onions, broccoli, and tea. Take 500 mg per day on an empty stomach.
- Pycnogenol. Part of a group of powerful antioxidants called proanthocyanidins. Take 50–300 mg per day as pycnogenol or grape seed extract.

For further antioxidant support, try these:
- Lutein. Obtained from kale, collard greens, spinach, and other green leafy vegetables, or take 40 mcg per day.
- Lycopenes. Found in high levels in cooked tomatoes. Eat ½ cup tomato sauce per week (500 mcg) or take 10–20 mg per day as a supplement.

Write down how you have acted on this step:

Step 6: *Add Key Minerals*

Take the following daily dose of these important minerals:
- Calcium. Check with your healthcare provider to find out more about cardiovascular risk research before starting. After menopause, women should take 1,200 mg, while men at risk of osteoporosis should take 1,000 mg.
- Magnesium. Supplement with 200–400 mg or take a warm Epsom salts bath.
- Selenium. Take 200 mcg as sodium selenite, selenomethionine, or, if you're not prone to yeast infections, yeast-derived selenium, or eat two Brazil nuts. Take with vitamin E to enhance its effectiveness.
- Zinc. Take 15–25 mg of zinc per day. If you can't taste it on your tongue, increase the dose until you do. A note of caution is that zinc competes with other minerals, especially copper, manganese, and iron. Don't exceed 200 mg per day.

Write down how you have acted on this step:

Step 7: *Take an Anti-Inflammatory Package*

Inflammation is an area that often goes unnoticed by both patients and healthcare providers, but as you've discovered throughout Phase III, extinguishing the inflammatory flame is a major part of our core strategic plan to optimize your health.

As we discussed in Part 2.14 in *Dr. A's Habits of Health, Inflammation: Dousing the Flame,* an hs-CRP (high-sensitivity C-reactive protein) test is a good way to determine your current level of inflammation. Here are some guidelines to follow once you know the results of that test:

- If your hs-CRP is over 3, we need to adopt an aggressive plan to lower it. Begin by reviewing the information in Part 2.14 and applying all possible techniques to reduce your immune activators. In addition to the Habits of Health, you should start on the following: at least 2 grams a day of vitamin C; 800 IU of mixed vitamin E; a mega B complex; 3 grams of fish oil; 1,000 units of vitamin D; chromium, magnesium, selenium, and zinc supplements; and increase your fiber to more than 40 grams per day.
- If your hs-CRP is 1–3, evaluate your risk factors, and in addition to applying the Habits of Health, make sure you're taking a multivitamin and fish oil.
- If your hs-CRP is less than 1, your immune system is in great shape! While this is a fine goal, you can actually do even better. In fact, our ultimate goal over time is to lower your hs-CRP to less than 0.5—a great marker that you've optimized your chances for long-term health!

Write down how you have acted on this step:

Step 8: *Bonus Round*

Ask your healthcare provider about these other key nutrients that can help you reach and maintain optimal health:

- Alpha lipoic acid. Take 100–300 mg per day. (Diabetics should note that this may lower your need for medications, but consult your healthcare provider before making any changes to your medication.)
- Coenzyme Q10. Yes, it's expensive, but by using a hydro-soluble form you can cut the dose to 100–200 mg per day.
- Chromium. Found in brewer's yeast, eggs, chicken, apples, bananas, and spinach, or supplement with 200–600 mg per day. (May cause mild insomnia. Diabetics should watch blood sugar closely with their healthcare provider, as levels will drop.)
- Probiotics. Take a dose that provides 4 billion lactobacillus per day, including acidophilus, bulgaricus, and bifido.

Write down how you have acted on this step:

You now have a great outline of the nutritional support you need, not only to correct any deficiencies that have resulted from our modern lifestyles, but to flourish and thrive at your best—today and for many years to come. Add this to the anti-inflammatory practices you learned in the last chapter, and you're nearly ready to take on the world!

But first, we're going to spend the next couple of chapters taking a closer look deep inside, where the seeds of health are planted. This is not the physical you that we've been optimizing through healthy foods and supplements, but the emotional you, whose ability to deal with stress and find happiness and fulfillment is a key component of the journey to optimal health.

Notes to yourself:

Your coach will be eager for you to share your thoughts and learning from this Element. Check in with them today to share your answers to the following questions:

What does this Element mean to you right now?

What does this Element give you the opportunity to reflect on?

What actions are you going to take as a result of this Element?

Sharing your thoughts with your coach will help them become a reality.

Make sure you review all your notes and this Element often.

1 *Americans Taking More Prescription Drugs Than Ever* – Survey August 3, 2017 (HealthDay)   A new survey finds 55% of Americans regularly take a prescription medicine—and they're taking more than ever.

ELEMENT 22:
CREATING OPTIMAL WELLBEING

Average time to complete: **1–2 weeks**

In Element 22, we will:

- Help you define what really matters to you.
- Explore where you are on the Fulfillment Success Continuum.
- Empower you to rewrite your story!

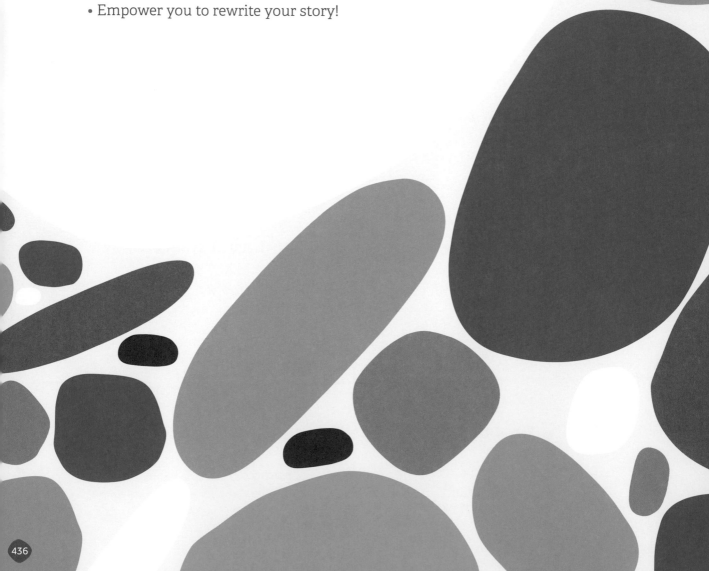

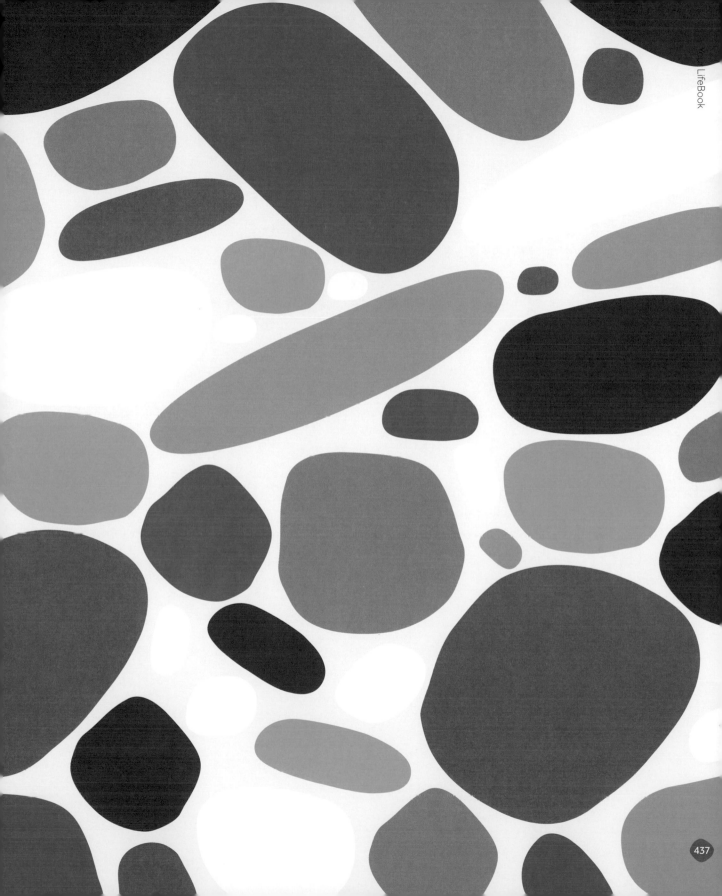

You haul yourself out of bed, drink a cup of coffee, rush to the car, get to work, turn on your computer, answer your emails, grab a quick lunch, struggle to focus all afternoon, drive to the dry cleaners, stop at the grocery store, go home, fix dinner, watch a little TV, and hit the bed to rest a few hours before getting up and doing it all again.

And then it's the weekend. You get home late Friday night, do chores on Saturday, sleep in on Sunday morning out of pure exhaustion, maybe spend some time at your place of worship, watch some afternoon TV but then, just about the time *60 Minutes* or your favorite series comes on, you get a sinking feeling in your gut because you know that in less than 12 hours you're going to launch yourself into another chaotic, energy-draining week of work.

Sound familiar?

The reality is that despite our material wealth, our generation ranks the quality of our lives lower than that of our parents—for the first time in history. Recall the story I've told again and again about our ancestors living 10,000 years ago under the stars in tribal communities. Think about their days of gathering food, resting when the sun is highest, and sharing stories around a campfire.

Now contrast that picture with today's overworked, overstressed, overweight, flabby, and sleepless society.

HOW DID THIS HAPPEN?

Well, here I go again with my familiar refrain. It comes down to our love affair with technology. We've become used to measuring success by our possessions, our house, our car, our income, and our status. As a result, our preoccupation with having the best "stuff" has taken us away from what really matters.

So, let's try and answer that question first.

Do you know what really matters to you? Sadly, many of us don't have any idea. We look to the Internet, the latest TV commercials, or our neighbor's driveway, as if someone else can answer that question for us.

And if we do try, what answer do we come up with? For many, it's financial security or the resources to be able to buy whatever they desire. But if you dig a little deeper and ask why they want those things, their answer is more fundamental. They believe that those things will make them feel better, happier, or more secure.

I have an important message for you.

First of all, money and material goods won't make you happy if you're unhappy to begin with.

Second, in our lives, there's no such thing as security.

I want to help you create not only optimal health but also optimal wellbeing for yourself and for the people who matter to you. As a physician, lifestyle professional, and agent of transformation, I've found that if an individual does not have purpose in their life, helping them create long-term health is an uphill battle. Conversely, aligning your mind with your heart's desire is a powerful force that can do much to support a lifetime of health.

The truth is that the modern world is a complicated, unsettling, and sometimes threatening place. Thanks to technology, we're more aware than ever of tragedies, political unrest, economic challenges, and climate change all around the globe. The chaos of modern life affects us all and our friends, families, and our neighbors may face challenges they want us to help them fix.

All of this means that if we're not in control of our intent, we can easily get caught in a vortex that feeds on stress and frustration—the vicious cycle of buying more things on credit, needing more vacations, working more hours in the hopes of a promotion. We search desperately for relief, hoping that the sleekest car, the most sophisticated possessions, or a new position will make us feel better, reduce our stress, or bring more meaning to our existence.

But there's a way to get back in touch with what's really important and a way to regain a sense of direction and create the life you really want, whatever that may be.

You've worked hard to learn and install new systems for healthy eating, movement, and sleep. Now I'm going to teach you a system to help build your life around what really matters to you.

Even if you're already happy on the whole, these techniques will teach you new ways to reduce stress and make your day-to-day life even more enjoyable. And if you feel you have lost touch with your guiding purpose, the lessons you learn will be just what the healthcare provider ordered.

In order to create and maintain optimal health, you need to organize your life around what matters most to you.

In *Dr. A's Habits of Health* we explored a study with end-of-life patients and their perspectives. If you have not read that section, do so now. What can we learn from those people who are at the end of their life about what is most important? (See Part 2.16 in *Dr. A's Habits of Health, Creating Optimal Wellbeing: Aligning Habits with what Matters Most*)

What brings purpose and value into your life currently?

FULFILLMENT AND SUCCESS

Are you happy? Are you doing what you really want? Are you financially successful? Can you do the things you want and have the things you want?

These are all important questions. In this Element, we want to put into perspective for you what it means to organize your life around what matters most. There are six types of life aspirations, three which are extrinsic aspirations—the stuff that American Dream is made of, the ones that define us, and what society says we need. This is whispered in our ear at an early age.

How do we define success? What are the three main categories? Refer to *Dr. A's Habits of Health* for an in-depth explanation if you need a refresher. Read Fulfillment and Success in Part 2.16 in *Dr. A's Habits of Health, Creating Optimal Wellbeing: Aligning Habits with what Matters Most.*

How do we define fulfillment? What are the three aspirations and intrinsic goals we want? Refer to *Dr. A's Habits of Health* for an in-depth explanation if you need a refresher. Read Fulfillment and Success in Part 2.16 in *Dr. A's Habits of Health, Creating Optimal Wellbeing: Aligning Habits with what Matters Most.*

Failure-Success Continuums: Where are you on a scale of 1–10?

Take a look at the illustration showing the Failure-Success Continuum below. Where would you say you are on this continuum? Actually put a mark where you think you are right now between one (a complete failure) to 10 (a complete success). Remember, success is defined primarily by external factors, like financial status, your place in the community, and your job. Are you comfortable with your current house, car, and professional position? What level of achievement would you say you enjoy now, compared to where you'd like to be?

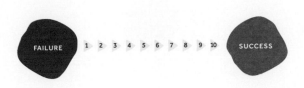

Depression-Fulfillment Continuums: Where are you on a scale of 1–10?

Now, let's look at the Depression-Fulfillment Continuum and determine where you would place yourself on this axis. Actually put a mark where you think you are right now between one (very depressed) to 10 (very happy and doing exactly what you want).

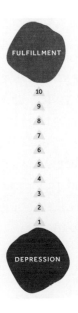

Now let's put these two parameters together to see how the external (Failure-Success) and internal (Depression-Fulfillment) determinants balance out. Take your position on the vertical axis and your position on the horizontal axis and see where they cross. This will tell you what quadrant you are in on the Wellbeing Chart. Looking at your current reality in two dimensions allows you to see if what you're doing with your life is in alignment with what matters most to you.

The Wellbeing Chart

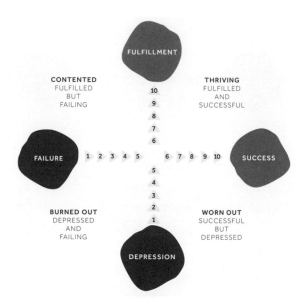

Which quadrant would you say you're in right now?

Comparing your success track to your degree of fulfillment can be an enlightening exercise. Think back to the elderly subjects in Leider's interviews (refer to *Dr. A's Habits of Health* for the full story). When asked what they'd do differently, they all responded with wishes from the Depression-Fulfillment axis—less focus on the daily grind, more meaningful work and relationships, making a difference. Not one of these people said they wish they'd had a better car, a bigger house, or more money.

What it comes down to is finding balance in order to create a comfortable life arranged around the things that matter most to you—whatever it is that puts you in that upper-right quadrant that signifies abundance.

Once you do, you'll find that when your life is guided by what really matters, the very way you respond to daily life and its inconveniences, complications and difficult relationships changes. When you're immersed in creating the things that are important to you, it suddenly all seems so much more tolerable. Whether you're working toward a new occupation, hobby, or relationship, having a purpose frees your mind from sweating the small stuff. You're too busy going after what really matters!

And even if over time things change and if what you thought mattered most turns out to be something else entirely, what's important is having the flexibility to recognize these changes and adjust accordingly. In fact, it's a fundamental Habit of Health. Without that flexibility, stress will return and, in time, you'll be back on your old path to non-sickness and disease. That's why being able to identify and reassess your position on the wellbeing chart is so important. It was for me.

Dr. A's Wellbeing Journey

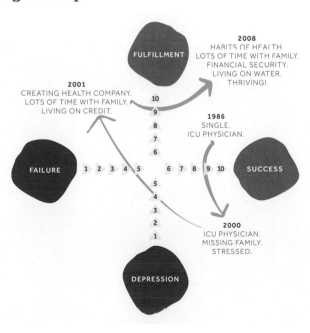

REWRITE YOUR STORY

So many people have written a story of how their life is, and they follow that routine like a playbook. They stay stuck and say everything is fine which is the biggest lie people hide behind in their lives. You can either be the victim or you can become the dominant force in your life.

Your LifeBook is guiding you along with your coach and the other parts of the Habits of Health Transformational System over the next 12 months to create a very different story: one in which we build your new set of habits that leads you up the trail to optimal health and wellbeing. This year of transformation will allow you to truly organize and live your life the way you want.

What I have seen so many times is that as someone really works on their inside and aligning their goals with what matters most, they grow and excel. I have seen them flourish in their occupations or leave them to find something brand new that aligns their heart and their head so that they are fully involved and satisfied, as well as no longer settling for less. Before we close and move on to our focus on your mind, list some things you can do right now to shift the alignment in your life.

How do we define fulfillment? The three aspirations and intrinsic goals you want are:

Finding What Really Matters: Some Final Tips

Most of us are familiar with the idea of reaching and setting goals for external things. However, it's important to ask yourself why you want what you do. Until you can honestly answer that question you will be searching for true meaning and fulfilment, and when you find what really matters it will directly satisfy a dynamic urge based on your most fundamental aspirations.

Here's an example: Sam has a very intense job. According to his wellbeing chart, he's successful but misses spending time with his children. Sam's boss has a Porsche that he's thinking of trading in, and Sam knows that if he takes on an extra account and works weekends, he can afford to buy it. If I were Sam, I would ask myself why I want that particular car. If it's for status, he might want to think twice. Having a Porsche might bring him some happiness while he's driving it (trust me, it will) and move him a couple of points forward on the success line, but the long-term effect—less time with the kids—will bring his already poor fulfillment score even lower (after all, they can't even fit in that two-seater!).

If you find you want a lot of external things, ask yourself why. Make sure that the reason is truly aligned with your fundamental aspirations and not just a short-term effort to feel successful at the cost of your long-term goals.

Knowing what's really going to fulfill us can be hard to figure out, especially for those of us who've been driven by today's success-at-all-costs mentality. I recommend you read *Your Life as Art* by Robert Fritz for a more detailed explanation of how to build the life you want but, for now, I'd like to give you a few concrete ideas for enjoying some areas of life that are too often neglected in our drive for success.

Follow your passion.

In an unforgettable scene from the movie *American Beauty*, the main character asks his wife what happened to the passion in their lives. "When did you become so. . . joyless?" he asks.

Find something or someone to be passionate about. You want something that has you jumping out of the bed in the morning, and love is one of nature's greatest healers. If you had it before, you can get it back! It can be restored, rediscovered, renewed. Take a word of wisdom from the elders in Richard Leider's interviews: If you're struggling in a relationship, be courageous enough to reach out and call a truce. Let your loved ones know how much you care, then sit down and rediscover each other. If your paths have diverged so far that they can't realign, you need to accept that too, and move on to find your true love.

Instead of going through the motions of living our life day in and day out and then recognizing 20 years later, "Yes, I drive a nice car, but it's actually not the car that I wanted. Well, I live in a nice house, but this isn't the life that I wanted", by creating optimal wellbeing, we're able to develop a greater lifelong correspondence with our own hearts, with our own understanding, and with who we want to be in the world and what matters most to us.

Rekindle your romance in large or small ways, perhaps by leaving love notes. On a past visit to the Ronald Reagan Museum, I found myself fascinated by the handwritten notes the former president would leave his wife, Nancy, before departing on Air Force One. Even as he led the free world, he made time to pay attention to the person who was most important to him.

Remember, kindness and love can bridge any chasm.

Here are some other ideas:

- Take up a new hobby. Find a craft, sport, or adventure that you've always wanted to do, and do it.
- Enjoy the arts. Learn an instrument, act with a local theater company, or take up dancing.
- Reconnecting with nature by breathing fresh air on your daily walks while strolling on the beach or in the woods, or just by spending time in your backyard, can do wonders for your stress levels.
- Get in touch with your spiritual side. If matters of the spirit are important to you, join a church, synagogue, or other place of worship or spiritual growth.
- Spend time with others. Join a special interest group in an area that appeals to you, whether you're an advocate for peace, environmentalist, animal lover, or political junkie.

Increase your wellbeing with simple but meaningful activities like making time to see a friend, starting a scrapbook of happy memories, or helping others by giving blood.

And since most of us have to work, here's a final guideline:
Do what you love or love what you do. It really is that simple.

This may require you to quit your job, go to school, enter a new line of work, or invent what it is you want to do, or it may simply mean finding new ways to bring meaning to what you're doing right now. Whatever you do, it should bring you passion, spur your interest, and tap into your talents. Get out and live to the fullest every day, and your body will respond with glee. You might want to explore joining us to help others obtain optimal health and wellbeing!

Becoming the dominant force in your life is a big opportunity for your wellbeing, and I hope that this Element becomes the spark that ignites an entirely new beginning for you. There is a lot of work for us to do in this area, so don't forget to keep opening *Your LifeBook* and working through the exercises and material here to continue building your momentum into action.

Living a fulfilling life not only satisfies us emotionally, it also has the power to make us more physically vibrant. In fact, without fulfillment, we can't achieve optimal health.

In the next Element, we are going to unpack your ability to manage your emotions in a way that allows you to experience life to the fullest.

Notes to yourself:

Take a moment to check in with your coach and discuss your answers to the following 3 questions:

What does this Element mean to you right now?

What does this Element give you the opportunity to reflect on?

What actions are you going to take as a result of this Element?

I encourage you to connect with your coach, so you can share your thoughts and actions as soon as possible.

Sharing your thoughts with your coach will help them become a reality.

Make sure you review all your notes and this Element often.

ELEMENT 23:
MASTER YOUR THOUGHTS AND EMOTIONS

Average time to complete: **2–4 weeks**

In Element 23, we will:

- Determine your readiness to step onto a conscious path that will move you from a state of ego or self-orientation to one of being more social and in service of mankind: from me to we.
- Learn how to create a window of tolerance that will allow you to maintain internal stability despite what the world throws at you.
- Explore the role of our emotions and learn to manage and master how they can be channeled to help us create optimal health and wellbeing.

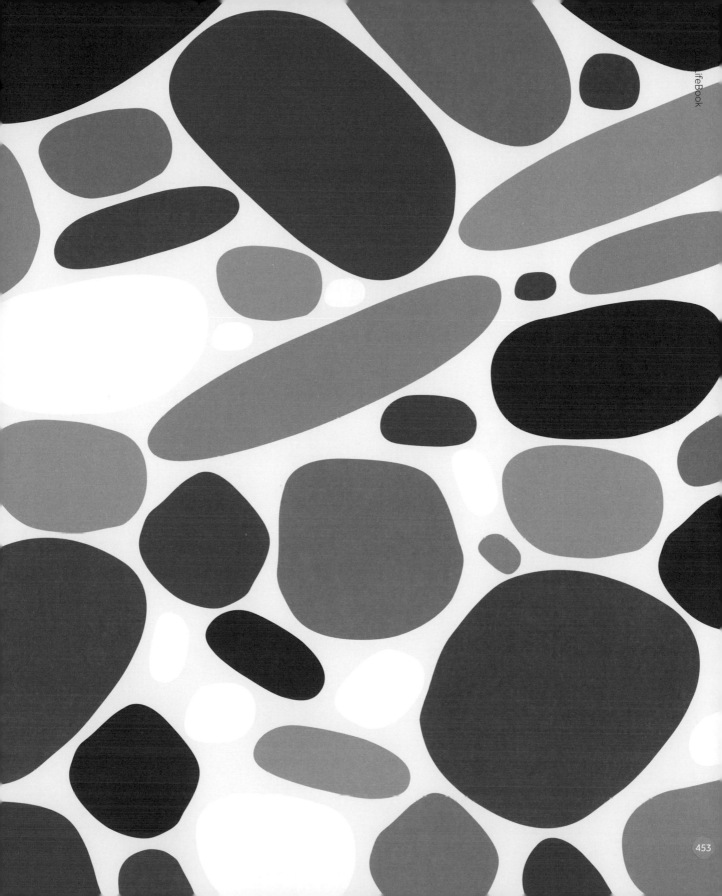

We have spent the first 22 Elements focused on how you can create optimal health and wellbeing.

You now have knowledge, techniques, and a system, and you're steadily developing the skills through practice and experience to install and master the fundamentals necessary to improve your health and wellbeing. Hopefully, you're far enough down the track in improving and transforming your life that you'll need a telescope to look back and see where you started from.

I have brought you to this point with the intention of helping you become as healthy and happy as you can at your current level of development. Using *Your Lifebook* book with both the App and the main book gives you the operating manual to predictably create better health and a better life.

But there is more if you are ready for it. You are? Good. Then let me explain why I would like to go and play in the deep end of the pool.

I want to refer back to Part 1.1 in *Dr. A's Habits of Health, It's Not Your Fault That You're Struggling*. You may recall we addressed how technology is impacting our health and wellbeing. I referred to best-selling author Thomas Friedman's new book in which he talks about how everything is accelerating. "Today," he says, "is the slowest change will ever be." He states that our ability to adapt to change is lagging behind the speed of technological developments.

The world around us is volatile, uncertain, and becoming more complex. The only way we can assure our continued wellbeing is if we have the flexibility and resilience to adapt to changing conditions.

If we are too rigid, we get stuck, and as the conditions change, we rely on the past to guide us which can lead to frustration and a temptation to avoid the issues.

However, if we just react to change without much thought, we create chaos which leads to anxiety and sometimes anger.

A state of rigidity or chaos is not a recipe for a vibrant, healthy, living system, especially as everything around us is in a constant state of flux.

I have another option.

Imagine creating a window of tolerance that would allow you to maintain internal stability despite what the world throws at you, so that you are in equilibrium with your external world, your relationships, and your ability to perform whatever the conditions.

It means taking the Habits of Health we have developed so far and turning your mind and body into a coherent duo that allows you to thrive and set an example to help others in your social circle do the same.

We want to integrate your physiologic and emotional self with your thinking and doing through a series of microHabits and exercises designed to increase your awareness, improve your responses, and give you control of your life. It's about being able to navigate the river of life and to enjoy challenges as opportunities to grow and get better, rather than see them as threats.

To do this will take both desire and a decision.

WHAT AM I ASKING YOU TO DO?

By the time we reach 14 years-old most of us have the skills and capabilities required to function in an adult world. There is no burning need to develop further. We graduate from high school and either get a job or move on to college and then start our career.

We feel we have all we need and believe we have finished our development. We continue to learn our trade or career skills but, for most, school is out on any real internal work. And yet, it is this invisible work that holds the key to unlocking our immense potential.

This Element will expose you to a different way of looking at the world and will perhaps equip you with more effective ways of managing your life.

Stated quite frankly, I am going to help you *wake up* and *grow up*!

I started down this path a few years ago, and it has made all the difference.

If I can help you awaken and expand your awareness so you are less attached to any one perspective of how life should be, your window of flexibility to whatever life throws at you can improve. And because you are developing a progressively deeper understanding of yourself and the world around you, it will give you the freedom to choose the responses that support your optimal health and wellbeing.

The truth is that most people are oblivious to the fact that they look through their lens with a very rigid perspective based on their level of maturity.

If I can help you understand where you are and help you become a student of reality to expand and grow in perspective and consciousness, you will be capable of improving your ability to adapt to both your own internal world and also the world of those that surround you.

In order for you to truly benefit from this work, it is important that you are ready to take this next step.

Until now, I have been helping to equip you with a comprehensive system to create optimal health and wellbeing. This is like filling an overnight bag.

What I am proposing is to swap your overnight bag for a suitcase so that you can increase your capacity to step up to the challenges of modern life. This conscious path will also move you from an ego or self-orientation state to one of being more social and in service of mankind: from me to we. This path is one that will help you build emotional agility. This will help you approach your inner world with an orientation that is curious, courageous, and compassionate but which also chooses actions that are highly supportive of your values.

Are you ready?

It's a big step because we're about to leave your comfort zone.

And discomfort is the price of a meaningful life.

A. Are you open-minded? Curious? Have a burning desire to grow?

B. Are you close-minded? Defensive ? Have a desperate need to be right?

If you answered A, you are currently in a creative or growth mindset which means that the material we will now cover will appeal to your increasing awareness of yourself and your world.

You are ready to move from wanting to change to now being willing to change.

If you answered B, it will be important to use some of the insights you have been learning throughout this book to become more open and less protective of your current position. We have been using a great tool throughout the book, which may soften up your tendency to react rather than respond. I have found that utilizing Stop. Challenge. Choose.™ can be very helpful in creating a pause for reflection and an opportunity to widen your perspective. This may help develop your openness, desire, and reinforce the importance of growing in order to be able to adapt to the changing world.

It takes moving into the present state and knowing where you are in relation to your desire to grow versus being right.

This emotional resiliency or ability will allow you to deal with any number of troubling thoughts, emotions, or stories and yet manifest in a way that is the highest version of yourself.

Take my word for it. It's a lot more fun to learn and grow than hold on to the old thinking that may have served you in the past. In fact, now when my old ego based thinking tries to take over I just laugh at how much energy I would expend needing to be right.

A couple of ground rules before we carry on. It's important that you go at your own speed and make sure you are using *Your LifeBook* to help guide you. Practice the exercises and start to document your progress as you are better able to recognize and manage your emotions and your response. Also, you read Element 4 at the beginning of your journey, and the first thing I want you to do is go back and read it again.

Also, read all of your responses and notes and reflect on what has changed in terms of your perspective and perceptions.

Write down how your understanding, perspective, and the way you view yourself and others has changed since you completed Element 4.

. . . .
. . . .
. . . .

As you reflect on how you have grown, learned, and installed new habits, recognize that your transformation is underway. Your growing self-awareness is a powerful tool because without it we have a tendency to contract with fear. It has been said that we have almost 70,000 thoughts during a day, and most of them are the same thoughts we had yesterday. Often they are difficult (negative) and critical of ourselves or others.[1]

We are going to teach you how to move out of that level of thinking and instead integrate your thoughts, emotions, feelings, and actions to support your optimal wellbeing.

This emotional agility and how we deal with our inner world drives everything in our lives.

It's going to be a bit scary, but it will be worth it. Think of it as a series of lab experiments to open up your thinking and start exploring all of the cool stuff you are capable of doing.

So before we start, I want to offer you congratulations on having the courage to step out of your comfort zone.

Let's start increasing your capacity and your capabilities and prepare you for our new world!

. . . .
. . . .
. . . .

HOW IMPORTANT IS IT TO DEVELOP YOUR MIND AND GROW BEYOND?

" We are coming to understand health not as the absence of disease, but rather as the process by which individuals maintain their sense of coherence or a sense that life is comprehensible, manageable, and meaningful and the ability to function in the face of changes in themselves and their relationships with their environment." [2]

Aaron Antonovsky

Normally when we think of our health, we think of our body. And throughout this book we have addressed pretty much every aspect of your physical health. We have focused on reaching a healthy weight and how you can install great eating habits that allow you to fuel your body and optimize your performance.

We have also addressed motion and exercise and how you can become a perpetual motion machine to keep both your body, your brain, and mind healthy. High-quality sleep of course is the key Element of nightly restoration and—along with naps – provides the energy and attention to allow your mind to put you in the best possible state of health and wellbeing. We've also unpacked the importance of minimizing our self-judgement so we can conduct ourselves in a compassionate way and pursue our job, career, or profession with passion.

If we can understand, learn, and apply all those applications, our body, mind, and relationships create a strong powerful set of MacroHabits that in reality act as the power behind our optimal health and wellbeing.

Unfortunately, there is an invisible force that prevents so many from reaching this state and a growing body of scientific research suggests that the root of disease and low wellbeing is different from what you have been taught.

What determines how much, how often, and how healthy we really eat?

What determines how active and how often you really exercise?

Our emotions.

Our emotions affect us every second of every day. They are the energy that directs every aspect of our life. Their deep, ancient, and central role in directing our brain and mind is only just unfolding as our understanding of our interpersonal neurobiology grows.

When functioning as designed, our emotions connect our biology and our behavior into a beautiful resonating song that flows through our body and creates a sense of wellbeing. We have all felt it at times, and it is a beautiful thing. We wish those moments would last forever. Unfortunately, less than five percent of people have developed mastery of their emotions so that they truly have the calm and focus that allows them to be the dominant force in their lives.[3]

The inability to successfully navigate our emotions is now thought to be the central cause of almost all disease and lack of wellbeing. That's a bold statement, and I plan on exploring it in detail.[4]

How well would you say you manage your emotions currently?

Which areas do you struggle with the most?

MISMANAGED EMOTIONS

Mismanaged emotions not only determine whether you will become sick but also whether you will be happy, fulfilled, and successful in your life.

Your management of your emotions will determine how effective you will be in installing and sustaining the Habits of Health and how healthy your relationships will be with the people who you interact with on a day-to-day basis.

And yet, mismanaged emotions, such as worry, hopelessness, anxiety, and depression, are as significant a risk factor as smoking a pack of cigarettes a day![5] In addition, these difficult emotions have considerable affect in our ability to be happy, fulfilled, and successful.

As kids, we didn't learn how to differentiate between our emotions and manage them. As a result most believe that emotions are to be avoided or to be kept buried deep inside of us.

As a result, we reach adulthood with a level of emotional illiteracy that can detect little more than feeling good or feeling bad. Because we were programmed 10,000 years ago to be acutely aware of any threats, negative emotions can dominate our lives. Those emotions create long-term negative loops that play over and over, day in and day out like a stuck record, until it becomes an ingrained habit of disease.

Yet our emotions have existed to help us survive and adapt and are still critical, as we can learn and uncover much about what we value by analyzing our difficult or negative emotional experiences.

For instance when we are angry, we think of it as a bad emotion and that we should not feel this way.

We actually usually only tend to get angry about stuff that we care about. Now, it doesn't mean that because you feel angry, you've got permission to act on the anger, and that you are right and the other person is wrong. But what it does indicate is that you are feeling angry and that this is something that you care about. So, this difficult emotion showing up is signal or signpost to a reaction that is important to us.

It can help us appreciate what we are feeling. Then we can adapt our surroundings and actions in a way that actually supports or values what is important to us.

Can you think of a time when you avoided an emotional situation by stopping or repressing it. What was the outcome?

Was there a time when you actually understood why you were feeling a certain way and responded appropriately? What was the outcome?

WHO IS IN CONTROL?

Our ability to control our lives is also very important in managing the state of our emotional wellbeing. We know that people who are in control of their lives are healthier, more cheerful, and more active.

A study by Langer and Rodin in the 70s carried out on nursing home residents split senior citizens into two groups. The first group was encouraged to make more decisions for themselves (even simple things like picking a house plant for their room). The second group was told what to do.

The results were astounding.

The group given more control were much more active and healthy. Even better, they were still alive. Less than half as many had died in the next two years.[6]

The message is clear: When the locus of control is within us and we feel we are dictating the conditions of our life, we are emotionally much better off, healthier, and our wellbeing is in a stronger state.

In the last Element, we talked about intrinsic motivation being important for creating wellbeing.

The good news is that in this Element we are going to provide several ways for you to develop your emotional literacy, emotional coherence, and self-management to align your emotions with your goals of reaching and maintaining optimal health and wellbeing.

I am not saying we are going to use positive thinking to suddenly create a happy-ever-after story because life itself is not that easy. In fact, it is downright intrinsically unstable. Something will get in the way. It always does. But what you will soon learn is that it is not the events or situations that impact the outcome but rather what happens emotionally as a result of those events.

And your response and management of the outcomes will either help buffer you if you manage them effectively, or you will fall into a reactive state that can send a toxic wave through your biology.

If we ignore how we feel about ourselves and allow these emotions to run our lives, we can find ourselves in trouble.

Over the last 17 years, I have helped so many people transform their lives, and one of the most common feelings that people have when I meet them is that they think they are not enough. They believe they are deficient in some way or there is something lacking in their surroundings or the world that surrounds them.

Women feel bad about the way they look. Men feel inadequate about their strengths, physical ability, or ability to provide.

This self-guilt, self-disgust, and remorse is what is doing the damage. Emotional mismanagement is harming people's biology by releasing cortisol and suppressing the immune system, thereby wreaking havoc on our metabolic and inflammatory pathways.

Emotions are the active ingredient coursing through our life. Adjusting our actions can give us a powerful advantage in daily life, both now and in the future.

So, if emotions are at the center of our world, let's dive in and explore what they are and how they have such influence over our minds, our bodies, and our relationships.

Feelings are the observation of our emotions. How we manage our emotions and use feelings to become aware is the key to taking control of our lives and developing emotional literacy, agility, and resilience.

Why is this so important?

The purpose of our 10,000 year-old design was survival and responding to threats in a rapid and successful way. It is not a very sophisticated system, but it is very effective.

The motor that drives the system is emotions. The emotional tune drove you to fight, run, freeze, and faint with instant recognition of which strategy was the optimum one.

It powered your autonomic nervous system, provided information to your cortex once you were safe, and adjusted your endocrine system and hormones to pump up the levels to minimize swelling or bleeding or any other consequences of miscalculations in strategy.

With that much power, no wonder emotions are the most important contributor to either radiant health and wellbeing or destructive disease and depression.

In ancient times, we always erred on overkill. Potential threat recognition kept us alive.

Almost everything was a threat, and avoiding threat was performed at a subconscious level. As a consequence, vast amounts of information or cues can trigger emotions, as well as change our behavior and decision-making and we have no idea why.

So, we have this emotional programming stored deep in our brain that determines how we respond to the world.

As we discussed in Part 1.6 of *Dr. A's Habits of Health, You in Charge of Yourself: Setting Up for Success*, the brain's emotional early warning system is the amygdala. We have two of them (one for each side of the brain).

As you can see, the external or internal stimulus triggers a response without it ever reaching the thinking brain.

Our Lower Brains

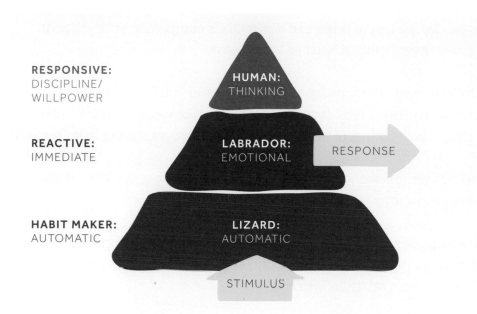

RESPONSIVE:
DISCIPLINE/
WILLPOWER

HUMAN:
THINKING

REACTIVE:
IMMEDIATE

LABRADOR:
EMOTIONAL

RESPONSE

HABIT MAKER:
AUTOMATIC

LIZARD:
AUTOMATIC

STIMULUS

Since we are born with only two fears (falling and loud noises), everything else we fear is learned by experience or from someone else. Fear of success, failure, death, spiders, snakes, heights, and sharks have been conditioned in us.

It does not have to be a logical reason—just a conditioned reflex. When I was a child, we had planned to go on a picnic up in the mountains. I was thirsty, and I remember drinking a whole thermos of lemonade on the drive up to the campsite. Shortly after arriving, I became violently ill and have a vivid memory of tossing my cookies into a clear mountain stream overlooking one of the Rocky Mountain ranges. To this day, I have an aversion to lemonade. The smell alone conjures up a feeling of nausea 60 years on. Once conditioned, our emotions are very powerful things.

If the event is sufficiently painful, then the conditioning is immediate. Usually, it is a slower process that requires repeated experiences to ingrain it in our memory, but the point is we have thousands of emotional responses that don't match the situation.

From the day you were born, the amygdala is comparing your current reality with everything it learned in the past.

It's why you meet someone for the first time and you feel anxious or worried and you have no idea why. It could be what they're wearing or the color of their shirt which connects to your unconscious programming from the past.

Sometimes we remember the conditioning and sometimes it is buried deep in our subconscious.

All of which goes to suggest that if we go around interacting with our world and our relationships on an unconscious level we are going to have a lot of emotional mismanagement.

That doesn't mean we have to suppress our emotions.

A key skill you will learn is to observe and release your emotions. This happens naturally if we do not interfere. It is like any normal biological process. Eating, drinking, and breathing have a natural course of in and out. The same is true for our emotions and our feelings.

When we repress an emotion, it becomes bottled up inside and may actually prevent the release of other more helpful emotions. Then we start thinking about it, our minds become involved, and we create an endless loop that adds up to anxiety, frustration, and emotional mismanagement.

Unfortunately, we have a tendency to repress and deny to both others and ourselves that we are feeling things. Men are particularly susceptible to hiding their emotions based on peers and work.

As kids, we were told that some emotions were acceptable and others were taboo. They are simply feelings we sense from emotions that should be experienced and then released naturally. And because emotions are energy where the feeling is an accompanying sensation moving through our body, they are neither good or bad and not who we are. They are just what we are feeling! So, it makes a lot more sense to call them difficult or tough rather than negative, which creates an immediate judgement that this is a bad thing. The reality is that we are experiencing something tough or we are going through a hard time.

So, we need to become aware of our emotions and learn to observe them in a more curious, investigative way. That way we can learn, grow, manage, and master how they can be channeled to help us create optimal health and wellbeing.

Emotional Awareness

Intelligence is awareness and, in recent years, "emotional intelligence" as a phrase has been thrown around a lot. What it really means is that you are aware of your emotions, can identify them, and know how they affect you. Once you are self-aware, you are in position to take command and use them for proper management in an emotionally agile way.

So how many emotional states are there? Walsch says there are two opposing emotional states:[7] They are love and fear.

Other researchers have come to a consensus that there are eight primary emotions:

- Anger
- Fear
- Joy
- Sadness
- Acceptance
- Anticipation
- Surprise
- Disgust

Like primary colors, when we combine primary emotions, we can create secondary ones. You will find an expanded chart on the website (HabitsofHealth.com) which shows over 70 positive and negative derivatives.

LEVEL OF CONSCIOUSNESS:
YOUR AWARENESS AND YOUR ABILITY TO KNOW WHERE
YOU ARE AT ANY MOMENT

Our first step is to start becoming aware of the different emotions you are feeling, and simply sense whether they are directly supportive of your values (positive) or difficult and unsupportive (negative).

In this section, you will learn to use a chart to track your emotions.

It will allow you to become more curious about your emotions and feelings, and help you become more conscious as well as able to build familiarity with how you are operating in your world. It gives you more practical support, as well as a system to record and evaluate your emotions.

Most of us are not aware of the multitude of emotions we experience throughout our day, so an important first step is to be able to identify them.

It will be very helpful if you use it to track what emotions you are feeling over the next couple of weeks. It may sound goofy, but ask yourself if your emotions are the key player in your health, your relationships, and your life.

You will want to:
- Note any emotional states you feel during your day.
- Identify whether you detected these emotions as a result of feelings.
- Consider how many of them directly support what is important to you.
- Question how many are difficult or tough and not serving you directly in a helpful way.

To start with, you may notice that many of them are difficult (negative). This is because that is our natural default in design to pick out the perceived (or real) threats. Many feelings also come from a scarcity mindset—the feeling that there is not enough. We are designed to move away from conflict and threat, rather than move towards opportunity. So, this first exercise is to improve the awareness or intelligence of your emotions. This means that we can then develop the skills to distinguish between them and learn how to label them.

It starts by understanding the emotion we have uncovered so we can use it if it is helpful or manage it if it is not. Remember that emotions drive action and this can be a very powerful tool if we can direct them towards our health and wellbeing.

Second, knowing where we feel the emotion can help us develop maturity when dealing with that emotion. Certain emotions show up in certain regions of the body and express themselves as sensations or feelings. Anger has a tendency to show up in the jaw, neck, shoulders, or back. Fear has a tendency to hit us right in the gut and sadness hits the eyes, throat, or heart area of our chest.

In this way, the location of the sensation or feeling in the body can act as an indicator of what emotion may be involved and lead you to rapid awareness.

Let me give you an exercise to help move you from awakening to managing your emotions.

Sit in a chair or comfortable couch, and simply bring you attention to your breathing. Once you have taken a few deep centering breaths, scan your body for any feelings or emotion that may be present.

If you cannot detect any, create one through a recent memory or event.

Once one appears, identify it, and then write it in your emotions chart in as much detail as possible.

This will help you to start seeing patterns and trends in how you handle your world. It also creates the opportunity to have a real dialogue with your coach.

Your Emotions Chart
Describe it in as much detail as you can. You want to get really detailed in your understanding: the location and intensity, and if it has sound, color, or temperature. Where is it moving in your body? How does it leave your body? How long does it last?

Emotion Checklist
What am I feeling?

Anger		Fear	
Joy		Sadness	
Acceptance		Anticipation	
Surprise		Disgust	
Other			

Are you sure?

What other two options could it be?   or

Where is it moving in your body?

How does it leave your body?

How long does it last?

Is there anything else special about it?

Write down your insights:
I am feeling
Why am I feeling this?
What is this emotion telling me?
What is at stake?
How is this affecting what is important to me?

You will want to repeat this for several days. Patterns will start to emerge and you will have an objective way of evaluating something that, until this point, was totally subjective. You will gain control and be able to watch emotions take their natural course. Once we recognize and harness the flow of energy and its release, it will feel like a great weight lifted.

On average, an emotion last 90 seconds if you do not interfere with it. They also come in waves. They rise, crest, and abate. By releasing the feelings that come with them, you will feel a period of calm as they leave your body. And because you are aware and in control they will yield great information if you allow them to.[8]

If an emotion arrives with great intensity and you feel the sensation rising, you can quickly get control of it by using Stop. Challenge. Choose.™

Over time, as you come to recognize and become familiar with your emotions, their location, and why they are triggered, you will evolve emotional mastery.

If you practice this daily you will know what a specific emotion means and—like a detective—it will give you insight into whether the emotion is appropriate or not and you will be able to manage it in a way that builds health and wellbeing.

The following questions will allow you to become a keen observer and take you out of becoming immersed and stuck in a loop.

Write down your insights:
I am feeling
Why am I feeling this and why am I feeling this?

What is this emotion telling me?

What is at stake?

How is this affecting what is important to me?

As an example: if you are feeling conscious anger (which is appropriate to the situation), the feeling helps to give you feedback that something is not working and needs to be addressed (as opposed to allowing the conversation to go below the line into the Drama Triangle).

If you find that the anger you are feeling is unconscious, it is usually some previously conditioned response where you are feeling threatened and is probably coming out as a need to blame (someone or something) or the need to be right.

If you take the time to examine these feelings, you will start to build a deeper understanding of what makes you do what you do. And you will become better at recognizing when you are below the line and you can regain control and produce the outcome that is in your own and others' best interests. Fully experiencing emotions that are a pure response to changing conditions is important.

In your old story, you may have been bottling your emotions, pushing them aside, or brooding on those emotions until they become fact, which lowers your state of wellbeing as you get stuck in this loop. There's a lot of talk that goes on in the loop and there's a lot of playing things out in our minds, but it's from the position of the emotion. You're swamped and you're seeing the world from the perspective of your emotion. It also affects your relationships because when you push your emotions aside it is hard to connect with others in an authentic way.

Also, if you are commiserating with a friend and co-brooding on a situation, it really does not let you focus on what you can learn but, instead, validates why you are upset with your mother-in-law. This also makes your friend an enabler.

Now you are an observer with a courageous, curious perspective that allows you to figure out what this emotion is telling you. This attitude helps us to contemplate why we are feeling this and what value it holds for us. It means we can question what we need to do to use our thinking brain in this situation and to consider what makes sense in terms of our health and wellbeing.

Stop. Challenge. Choose.™ creates a space between stimulus and response. And in that space is the power to choose growth and freedom.

When we are hooked by an emotion, whether you bottle it or brood on it, there is no space between stimulus and response.

It shows up as :
"I am upset, so I am going to tell them what I really think by telling them off". Creating that space is what allows you to become emotionally agile.

Pick a difficult situation, reoccuring emotion, or area where you are currently stuck in your life and work through it using these questions. Do it from a place of curiosity, compassion, and courage, as well as one of self-acceptance and self-love. Act as if a dear and trusted friend was giving you advice from their perspective.

What are you feeling?

What's going on here?

What do you need to do?

What aligns with your values?

What serves you?

What serves the outcome here?

Our values are what guide our decision making and determine what secondary choices we make in any difficult situation. We will choose to act in a manner that supports our values.

They determine what secondary choices or actions we make. So, I may feel guilty that I was unable to take my daughter out to dinner tonight because I have a writing deadline for this Element, but it doesn't mean I am a bad parent.

By the way, life is not all about being happy all the time. When people only want happiness, it can actually slow down their development because the quest for happiness can suppress emotions and other aspects of our experiences. When someone dies it is important to be sad and grieve; when you are in peril it is paramount that you sense fear. The true meaning of being alive is not just to feel happy. It is to sense and feel the full range of human emotions (which helps explain why we like scary movies and roller coasters). What we want to do is eliminate the negative destructive emotions like disgust, shame, guilt, rage, and so on.

Once emotions and their resulting feelings are managed correctly, they become a rich tapestry that allows you to experience life in all its aspects. Emotional mastery and agility is about feeling all the emotions and then deciding what to do with them.

The basic emotions that are central to our humanity are pure in nature. We have a tendency to overthink and add our own stuff to them. Sadness is a pure emotion. Depression is not. While sadness can almost be nourishing, depression is filled with anxiety, self-guilt, and doubt. It is maladaptive and so, by studying our feelings, we can stop repressing emotions that end up hurting us.

Using emotions to fuel your day.
Some of the more recent work on how to use emotions in a positive way recognizes that we do not make that many conscious decisions during our day. We are creatures of habit, which means that our emotional levels throughout the day may actually be relatively flat.

We can actually add energy to our routines to improve our efficacy.

Imagine that instead of experiencing the post alarm-clock dread you add 30 seconds of appreciation for the fact that you are alive, it's a beautiful day, and you have control over your life. Waking up focusing on our values and what brings meaning to our lives can charge and set the right tone for the day.

Just a 15-second addition of feeling connected and thinking about what you are going to do today can dramatically increase our satisfaction.

Emotional mastery can significantly improve our health, relationships, and our wellbeing. It improves our ability to learn and focus, elevates the quality of our decisions, improves our working conditions and can bring resilience when adjusting to change. Our motivation and quality of life will all improve.

So, think about whether you spend as much time in the mental gym working on your emotional literacy as you do in the physical gym working on your physical body.

Invest in this critical area of emotional development and your journey to better health and wellbeing will get easier and you will have great personal satisfaction as you develop more control over your world.

In the next Element we are going to set your path to increase your level of consciousness using many of the tools and things you have been learning and practicing to date.

Although the circumstances of life will continue to have their ups and downs, you will change your world by the responses and outcomes you will now masterfully create.

Notes to yourself:

**Take a moment to check in with your coach to share your answers
to the following questions:**

What does this Element mean to you right now?

What does this Element give you the opportunity to reflect on?

What actions are you going to take as a result of this Element?

I encourage you to connect with your coach, so you can share your
thoughts and actions as soon as possible. Sharing your thoughts with your
coach will help them become a reality.

Make sure you review all your notes and this Element often.

1 This is still an open question but LONI faculty have done some very preliminary studies using undergraduate student volunteers and have estimated that one may expect around 60 – 70K thoughts per day. These results are not peer-reviewed/published. There is no generally accepted definition of what a "thought" is or how it is created. In our study, we have assumed that a "thought" is a sporadic single-idea cognitive concept resulting from the act of thinking, or produced by spontaneous systems-level cognitive brain activations.

2 *Antonovsky's Sense of Coherence Scale and its Relation with Quality of Life: A Systematic Review* – J Epidemiol Community Health. 2007 Nov; 61(11): 938 – 944. doi: 10.1136/jech.2006.056028.

3 *Coherence* – Dr Alan Watkins, Kogan Page Limited.

4 *Depression and The Course of Coronary Artery Disease, American journal of Psychiatry* – Glassman, A H and Shapiro, PA (1998),155,(1)p. 4 – 11.

5 *Hopelessness And Progression Of Heart Disease, Arteriosclerosis Thrombosis Vascular Biology* – Everson, S A, Kaplan, G A, Goldberg, D E, Salon, R,17,(8) pages 1490 – 1495.

6 *The Effects Of Choice And Enhanced Personal Reponsibility For The Aged: A Field Experiment In An Institutional Setting* – Langer, E., & Rodin, J., JPSP, 1976, 191 – 198.

7 *Conversation with God* – Book 3, Walsch ND (1998), Hampton Road Publishing Company.

8 In brain researcher Jill Bolte Taylor's book, A Brain Scientist's Personal Journey, Taylor describes the 90-second rule as, "Once triggered, the chemical released by my brain surges through my body and I have a physiological experience. Within 90 seconds from the initial trigger, the chemical component of my anger has completely dissipated from my blood and my automatic response is over. If, however, I remain angry after those 90 seconds have passed, then it is because I have chosen to let that circuit continue to run."

ELEMENT 24:
YOUR JOURNEY TO HIGHER CONSCIOUSNESS

Average time to complete: **1–2 weeks**

In Element 24, we will:
- Explore how to grow, learn, and develop your consciousness.
- Learn about the four levels of consciousness.
- Decide what is truly important to you and then bring that into being.

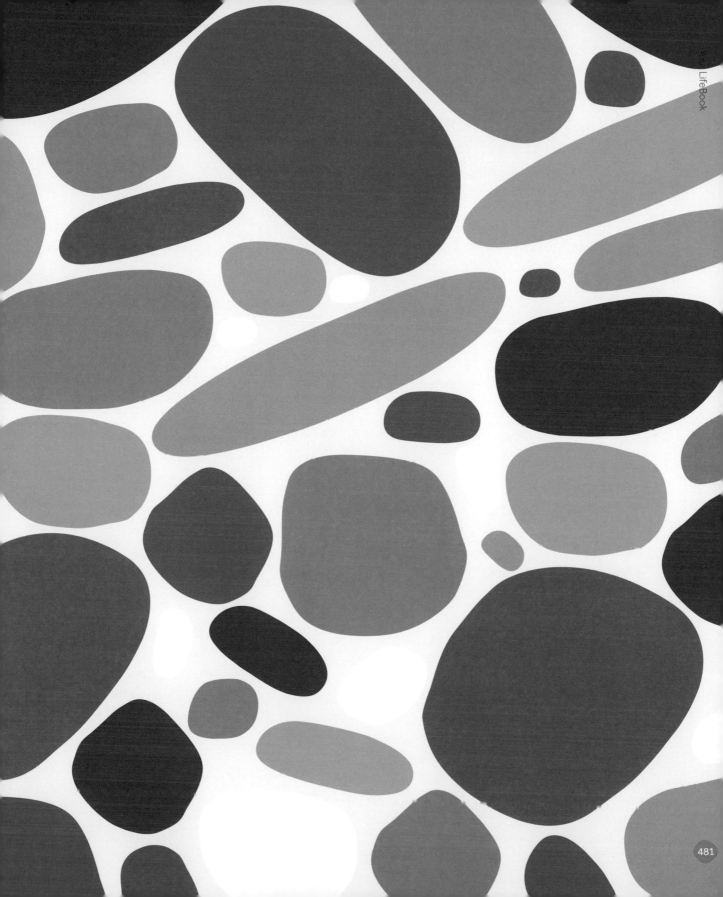

YOUR LEVEL OF CONSCIOUSNESS

As you develop emotional coherence or mastery, you are adding the keystone on which all adult psychological maturity is based. This skillset puts you firmly in the driving seat of your life. It puts you in control and really sets the stage for all future growth. Your level of awareness and self-awareness will continue to expand as you become a higher version of yourself.

Most of us settle in at a rather fixed level of awareness and maturity because it is all our world was asking of us 30 years ago. It's because everything is changing so rapidly that the need to progress our awareness and advance our level of consciousness has never been more important.

It's like a fish swimming in water. It has no idea that it is swimming in water even though its whole life and very existence is determined by water. We, as humans, are swimming along in our own river of consciousness. We have a tendency to think that everyone else is swimming in the same pool, seeing the same things, feeling the same, thinking the same, and looking at the world in the same way and it is just not true.

As we decide to grow, learn, and develop our consciousness, we will expand to a bigger and bigger river, then our experiences and thoughts will become wider and deeper.

Our reality will become clearer and our depth, perception, and insight will grow. There are several books written on the progressive level of consciousness. For the moment, let's limit it to four progressive states that are specific to reaching optimal health and wellbeing, which will serve you well in your social world.

Each of these levels builds on the previous level, so as we grow from one level to the next the landscapes become more complex. We will begin to add contrast to how we think, which will also add potential challenges. As we discuss each of these levels of consciousness write down at which level you currently sit and what has to happen for you to progress to the next level. Since it's all about consciousness all of the lessons from Element 4, Part 1.6 in *Dr. A's Habits of Health, You in Charge of Yourself: Setting Up for Success*, and the material in this Element and the previous Element will help you determine your current level and also give you some insights on how to progress.

LEVEL ONE: SELF-INTEREST

Survival, belonging, feeding our self-esteem—this is the normal level of development that we all go through from our birth until we leave parental authority. It is very much about our ego and making sure that we are being looked after. We look at life through our own eyes and everyone else is secondary.

By the time we finish high school, we have learned a skill set that allows us to negotiate our world; this is much like a cookbook. While we are in this phase, it is common to have the orientation that it's us against the world. We have a tendency to blame everything either on ourselves or someone else. We are very much about our identity and may feel separate to society. Many people unfortunately get caught in this level for their whole life and never work on growing out of it.

They become a victim and never rise above the struggles of everyday life, and many people live comfortably at this level.

Are you at this level? When you are at this level, you will find yourself below the line a lot. There usually is a feeling of scarcity, that there is not enough love, money, friends, and that there is a threat to your security, approval, control. You will have a tendency to blame and find fault and your ego is in charge and wants to be right all the time.

Your personal comments:

The way to progress at this level is knowing where you are and shift back above the line. That means when you are contracted with fear or sense some sort of threat you *Stop* before responding and recognise that you have slipped below-the-line. You become fully aware of the emotions and shift your consciousness back to your thinking brain. Then you *Challenge* why you are feeling this way and *Choose* to shift back into a state of being open, curious, and willing to learn by taking some deep centering breaths, changing your body posture, and feeling love and acceptance. Stop taking yourself so serious and laugh at yourself and have some fun.

And be open to letting your coach help you!

LEVEL TWO: ACTUALIZED SELF

We are now moving beyond what was taught to us and are ready to explore what really matters to us as an individual. We need to figure out what works best for us in the world. We may even change our orientation and identity as we find out what is important to us, thereby moving beyond the cookbook we learned growing up.

Discomfort is the price of a meaningful life. It means you will have to get out of your comfort zone in order to grow and learn.

Your personal comments:

At this level, we take responsibility for our life and make the decision to be in charge. Once we take this position we start growing and everything becomes possible. This is the breakout that starts to change everything. At this level you define what you want and can move toward making it a reality.

In terms of your health and wellbeing, the Habits of Health is your operating manual with the strategies, tactics, and guidance to help you become a higher version of yourself. This will lead to optimal healthier and wellbeing and, most probably, a more successful life as defined in the last chapter.

In the structural tension chart below, you can see that you can now create the life you choose, as long as you pay attention to the secondary choices that set you free and if you are open and curious with a desire to grow. In addition, if you are open, coachable and teachable, open to applying feedback, and you are willing to do the work, this level of your development will be exciting and fun. You will begin to expand your consciousness beyond that of most others.

Taking Responsibility

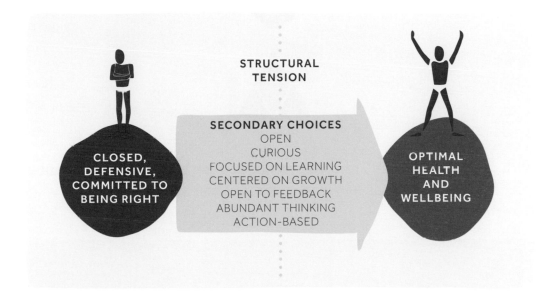

During this phase you will still have plenty of moments when you are going to go below the line. Your increasing awareness will help you see that you have gone below the line and you can quickly decide to shift back to the responsible vantage point and not descend into the Drama Triangle, which will create a better outcome in support of both your desires and those belonging to other people.

Healthy Mind Shift

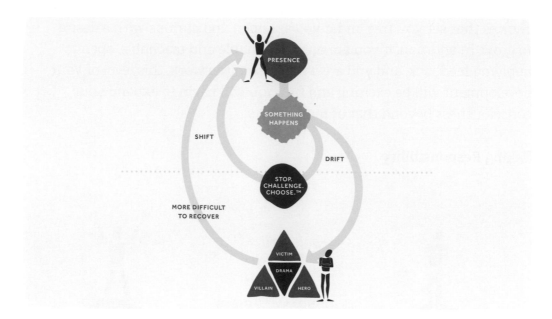

With desire, decision, and focused practice, you can become the dominant force in your life. And, of course, your coach remains integral to your growth and progress.

LEVEL THREE: INTEGRATED SELF

This level of development requires you to have mastered emotional literacy and to have done the work on the areas of your thinking that have not served your best interests.

This is the level where you are beginning to master both how you operate internally but also how you interact with others and your surroundings in a highly effective way.

By the time you have mastered this level, you will have completed most of your major development work and you should have resolved any emotional baggage. You now are integrated—no longer rigid or chaotic in any of your interactions.

You can handle pretty much anything.

You are internally stable, flexible, adaptable, and can see only confidence and energy in your future. You are fully capable of making choices and creating change.

This is the goal for everyone that starts this journey to optimal health and wellbeing. We welcome you to continue on with us in our journey to become higher versions of ourselves.

Your personal comments:

At this level, having a conscious mentor that is more advanced than you is important. It is, of course, also essential to have lots of deliberate practice.

LEVEL FOUR: SELFLESSNESS SELF

At this level, life really has no struggles. We are no longer frustrated, judgemental, and negative emotions are gone from our days. We are compassionate all the time. Life is happening through us and we feel very connected to something bigger than us. This state continues to grow as we develop our spirituality and connect to a higher level of consciousness, either through our religion or our own spirituality.

My reason for describing these four arbitrary levels of development is to make the point that beyond our current perspective there is always the possibility to grow and learn more. And when it comes to real transformation, to be able to change and widen our perspective is much more powerful than just giving you more knowledge, skills, and experience. When we can see the world through new eyes, everything changes, and we are equipped to fully embrace the world.

Your personal comments:

Here you are contributing, along with other conscious leaders, to be at the service of mankind.

Expanding our awareness and our level of consciousness is a lifelong journey.

THE LAST PIECE OF THE PUZZLE

One of the keys to becoming the dominant force in your life and having a healthy mind is to really organize your life around what matters most to you.

In other words, decide what is truly important to you and then bring that into being by deciding and putting your focus, energy, and time into creating and bringing it into your life.

You become the creator and your intrinsic motivation, increasing competency, and desire to relate and share fuels your progressive ability to accomplish your goals.

It looks like this:

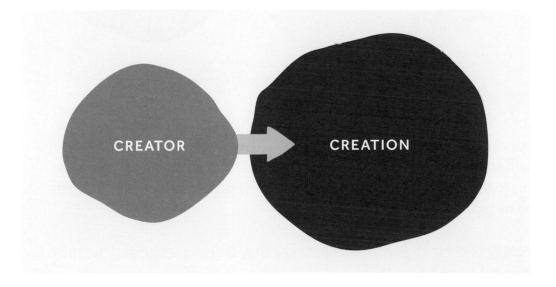

What you are creating for yourself is not a reflection of who you are, what you are feeling, and what you are thinking about yourself. You recognize that all those things do not matter in the lifebuilding process.

As demonstrated in the diagram you are the creator and the focused individual that is creating something separate and magnificent because you are open, curious, and have a growth mindset. You are not limited by what you or others think about you.

Unfortunately most people that have not learned to focus on the desired outcome as the organizing principle for all that they are creating have a tendency to make it about themselves as the diagram below illustrates:

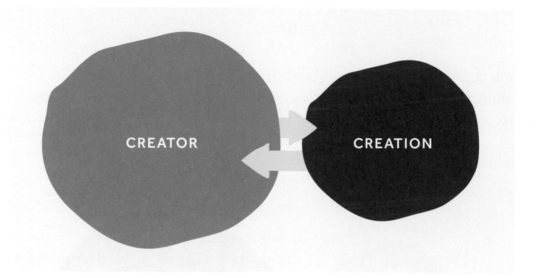

As a result, how they feel, how they act, what they are creating directly speaks about who they are as a person. Their success or failure is personal and so people who make what they are creating about them are much more likely to be closed minded, defensive, and much more likely to want to be right.

And because it all becomes about how they feel about themselves, they become more hesitant to act without being sure and, as a result, are usually less successful.

In our book, *Identity*, Robert Fritz and I go into much more depth but for now the point is use your thinking brain to determine what you want and keep yourself and your emotions out of the equation.

You will be amazed at how much you can create once you realize that what you think about yourself has nothing to do with what you can create in your life in terms of your health, wellbeing, and overall success.

How are you going to improve your ability to remove what you feel about yourself from what you want to build in your life?

Hopefully you are as excited as I am for you as you increase your self-awareness, master your emotions, and learn to separate what you are creating for yourself from yourself. You are well on your way to becoming the dominant force in your life.

Being able to focus your mind where and when you want is a talent that separates those that are fully conscious and thriving from the rest.

Now that you are aware of what is available, I hope you accept the challenge to become a higher version of yourself. I will include some books on my website, HabitsofHealth.com, that can help assist you as you continue this journey. As we end this section, you should feel confident that you have the operating manual that will allow you to reach optimal health and wellbeing.

In the next Element, we will shift gears and address living longer in a healthier state. This will help to understand that the most important foundation for the next section is to apply and live by the Habits of Health you have been developing throughout this last year.

Notes to yourself:

It is crucial that you stay close to your community and your coach as you continue to develop along this path. In fact, now is a great time to check in with your coach to share your answers to these three questions:

What does this Element mean to you right now?

What does this Element give you the opportunity to reflect on?

What actions are you going to take as a result of this Element?

I encourage you to connect with your coach, so you can share your thoughts and actions as soon as possible.

Sharing your thoughts with your coach will help them become a reality.

Make sure you review all your notes and this Element often.

ELEMENT 25:
HABITS OF LONGEVITY

Average time to complete: **2–4 weeks**

In Element 25, we will:

- Focus on what will enhance your chances of living longer by adopting certain key behaviors.
- Explore the habits of those who have lived longer, healthier lives.
- Understand the importance of a Healthy Mind and how it relates to overall longevity.
- Devise an action plan of what you can do today to make Dr. A's Longevity Plan work for you.

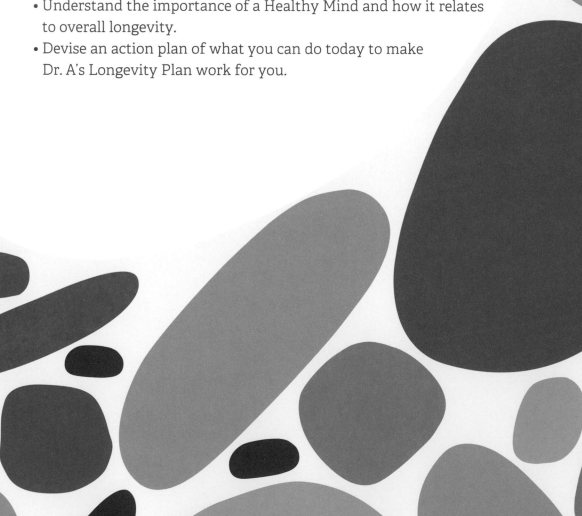

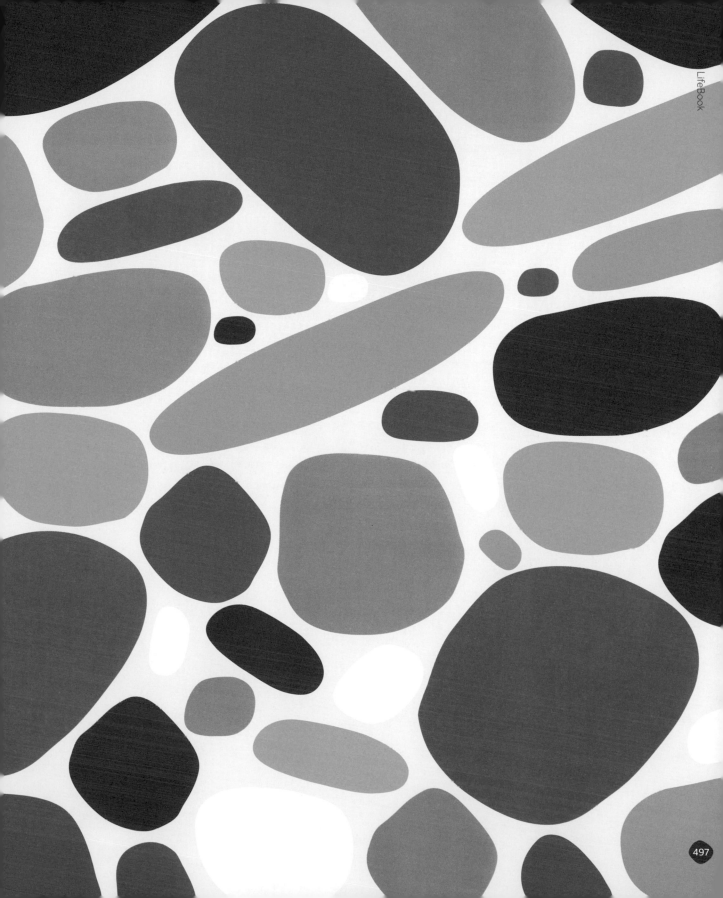

The last two Elements in *Your LifeBook* are a preview of what you will be doing to continue your journey beyond the first year. They will give you some guidance on how you can live longer in a healthy state. My take on longevity is that it only makes sense when you have thriving health. And, in fact, the best way to do that is to keep doing the things I've already taught you. Practice the Habits of Health forever. They're your guarantee that you're giving your body the best possible chance to live out your genetic programming which, based on our current understanding of the aging process, means you could live 100 years or more.

So, most of you will have filled your mason jar with great understanding and you are well on your way to mastery of the six MacroHabits.

I selected a year as that is what it will take to create this next level of optimal health and wellbeing. And the Element of a Healthy Mind and the level of consciousness which you are working on now will also help determine how long and what quality your life will be moving forward. For those of you who are anxious to move on to Ultrahealth™ you will want to read all of Section 3 in *Dr. A's Habits of Health*.

We will outline some of the key Habits of Ultrahealth™ in Element 26, *Ultrahealth™: Living Longer Full Out*.

In this Element, we will focus on what the key behaviors that will enhance your chances of living longer.

What is the first principle of longevity? Is aging reversible? How fast can we start potentially improving your life expectancy using the Habits of Health? What part does genetics play? What part does lifestyle play?

How long do you want to live? What factors matter?

Note that we say potentially as we have no way of predicting how long ou will actually live. We know that as you adopt *Dr. A's Habits of Health* and other healthy behaviors your statistical chances improve based on the research.

What can I learn from the centenarians described in *Dr. A's Habits of Health* and the Blue Zones. How will I incorporate this into my own life?

The Blue Zones: Lessons for Living Longer from the People Who've Lived the Longest by Buettner

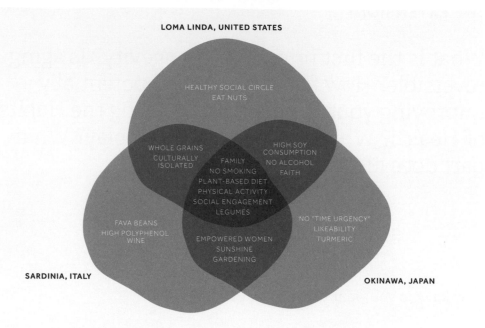

LOMA LINDA, UNITED STATES

HEALTHY SOCIAL CIRCLE
EAT NUTS

WHOLE GRAINS
CULTURALLY
ISOLATED

HIGH SOY
CONSUMPTION
NO ALCOHOL
FAITH

FAMILY
NO SMOKING
PLANT-BASED DIET
PHYSICAL ACTIVITY
SOCIAL ENGAGEMENT
LEGUMES

FAVA BEANS
HIGH POLYPHENOL
WINE

EMPOWERED WOMEN
SUNSHINE
GARDENING

NO "TIME URGENCY"
LIKEABILITY
TURMERIC

SARDINIA, ITALY

OKINAWA, JAPAN

Habits of Longevity

Jeanne Louise Calment, who was 122 years old at the time of her death, holds the record for human maximum life span, but I predict that within a few years, science will be able to extend the life of a healthy individual—probably someone who's mastered the Habits of Health Transformational System and are living an optimally healthy lifestyle—to closer to 150 years. Most humans will not see the century mark because of the profound effect our obesigenic world and unhealthy lifestyle has on the principle of secondary aging.

How long do you want to live?

I bet you said that "I only want to live longer if my brain and mind are operating at a normal level." This is a concern for most people as they age.

Secondary aging affects all our organ systems, but one that's of particular concern is the brain. While genetics certainly play an important role in memory loss and Alzheimer's, an unhealthy lifestyle and environment make these conditions much more likely to occur. Fortunately, the Habits of Longevity can actually reverse decreases in vital brain chemicals.[1]

Why so much discussion on brain aging? Well, if you make it past 100, we want to make sure you have a fully functioning CPU! That's why in Part 3.5 in *Dr. A's Habits of Health, Reaching a State of Ultrahealth™: Living the Future of Wellbeing*, as we look at brain longevity, we'll spend time focusing on specific strategies you can use to keep your brain humming. When we combine the work you are doing to improve your emotional management, you are setting your brain and mind up for optimization.

How long do you want to live if you are able to maintain a Healthy Mind?

Okay we are going to start putting the odds in favor of you living a longer healthier life with my longevity plan. It will outline the tangible things you can do right now to improve your chances.

DR. A'S LONGEVITY PLAN

Here's my plan for a longer life, broken down into simple steps that you can start taking today. These steps include a number of basic actions and behaviors that will reduce your likelihood of falling prey to preventable diseases, accidents, and the ravages of an unhealthy lifestyle.

They culminate in optimal health, but that's not the end of my longevity plan. In fact, these steps are really a prelude for a lifestyle that can take you even further, to cutting-edge techniques that many scientists and medical researchers believe can extend your life well into a second century. We call it Ultrahealth™.

The Habits of Longevity
Step 1: Right Now
- Eliminate tobacco.
- Eliminate all recreational drugs.
- Wear a passenger restraint system any time you're in a car, and purchase a vehicle with front and side airbags as soon as possible. And when possible an auto-drive car as currently the prototypes are twice as safe as a human driver.
- Drive at the speed limit: I don't want you dying age 100 because you're showing off!
- Limit your intake of alcoholic beverages to less than two drinks a day, and never drink while driving or operating machinery. For more information on red wine and longevity, see HabitsofHealth.com.
- Avoid situations that put you at risk of contracting a sexually transmitted disease (such as having multiple partners).
- Avoid sunburn at all costs.
- Don't exercise on roads used by motor vehicles.

What else can you do right now to optimize your choices?

Step 2: Create a Healthy Environment
• Eliminate toxic foods, cleaning supplies, and other poisons, such as radon.
• Ensure that your water is clean.
• Ensure that your air is clean.
• Check your smoke detectors to make sure they're working.
• Cover or fence swimming pools.
• Eliminate potential hazards that could cause falls.
• Lock all doors when you're home.
• Lock up firearms.

What else can you do right now to optimize your surroundings?

Step 3: Get a Yearly Check-Up
If you didn't see your healthcare provider before you began your weight-loss and movement program, do so now. You're in the process of a whole-body makeover, and it's important to make sure your blood, heart, and general physical health are all in order. Tell your healthcare provider you're taking part in a program that includes a healthy diet, regular movement, better sleep, and stress reduction and see what they say! After they recover from fainting, have them check the following:

- Record your weight, waist measurement, height, blood pressure, heart rate, and body mass index so you can track your progress. (When you've reached a state of Ultrahealth™, go back for another check-up so you can watch them faint again).
- See if you should lower any of your medications as you lose weight.
- Review the full list of medications you're currently putting in your body. Drug interactions can cause serious side effects, erode our health, and increase the likelihood of falls, motor vehicle accidents, and even cellular aging. And because records aren't always complete—not to mention the fact that many of us have multiple healthcare providers—it's really your responsibility to talk with your primary healthcare provider about lowering or eliminating medications. Remember, prescription medications are one of the top five causes of death.
- Ask for a full lipid profile to assess your cardio-metabolic risk and an hs-CRP test to assess your current inflammatory state to ensure you're staying in control of your immune system; it's also a good idea to continue with follow-up tests for life. If you're 50 or older, a baseline echocardiogram and stress test are in order as well.
- Have appropriate cancer screenings.
- Make sure you're up to date on your immunizations, including:
    - Pneumovax if you're over 50 (repeat at 65)
    - Tetanus (every ten years)
    - Whooping cough (once for adults)
    - Influenza (yearly)
- Get a baseline TSH to assess thyroid function if you're over 35.
- Have a mineral density scan if you're perimenopausal. Repeat every five years.
- Test sensory systems, including eyes, hearing, and balance. Repeat yearly.

What else can you do to optimize your health and prevent disease?

Your Cancer-Screening Guide for Lifelong Health
- Breast: self-examine monthly; healthcare provider exam once or twice a year; first mammogram at age 40, then yearly after 40.
- Cervical: first pap smear at age 21 or within three years of sexual activity
- Colon: first colonoscopy at age 50, then every ten years; hemoccult test every five years.
- Prostate: digital exam and PSA pros and cons considered with counsel from your physician.
- Skin: self-examine regularly for unusual or quick-growing lesions.

What else can you do to detect any potential cancer?

Oral Health and Inflammation: Pathways to Disease

Gum recession and medication-induced dry mouth—two common complaints related to aging—set us up for cavities and gum disease by creating an environment where bacteria can flourish. As plaque infects the tissues around the teeth, the gums become swollen and red and slowly begin to pull away, resulting in loose teeth and bad breath. But that's not all. This process also sets up an inflammatory state that can lead to heart disease and diabetes.

Step 4: Go to Your Dentist

It may surprise you to know that dental health is critical for optimal health and longevity. Keeping your own teeth and maintaining excellent gum and oral health minimizes inflammation and is an important part of our plan.

As a whole, baby boomers, the nation's first fluoride generation, enjoy extraordinary oral health. But this may come to a halt as boomers enter their retirement years and come face-to-face with gum disease. In fact, if recent trends continue, three out of four boomers will develop gum disease as they age.[2]

Why is that the case? As we get older, we're more prone to certain conditions that put our teeth and gums at peril, including hormonal changes, medical conditions such as diabetes, receding gums that leave roots exposed and vulnerable, and medication-induced dry mouth, which can cause bacteria to proliferate. In addition, the elderly are more likely to have poor dental hygiene and make fewer visits to the dentist.[3]

What can you do about it?

For starters:
• Brush at least twice a day with fluoride toothpaste.
• Floss daily.
• Get a yearly check-up from your dentist.
• Have your teeth cleaned twice a year.
• Don't use tobacco products, including cigarettes, chewing tobacco, snuff, pipes, and cigars.
• Drink alcohol in moderation, if at all.
• Use lip balm that contains sunscreen.
• Avoid lipsticks that don't contain sunscreen (recent research has shown that the pigment in lipstick can actually intensify UV damage).
• Combat dry mouth and keep your oral cavity moist by taking sips of water or chewing sugar-free gum.

What else can you do to optimize your oral health?

Dental health is often neglected (until it's too late!) but it's an important part of optimal health and longevity. After all, you want to be able to continue to enjoy healthy fresh foods into your 100s!

Step 5: Reach and Maintain Your Healthy Weight

Reaching a healthy weight not only lowers your risk for disease but actually lengthens your life by several years. If you haven't yet begun the healthy meal plan introduced in Phase I, then there's no better time. In *Your LifeBook* and your App you will want to continue to optimize your weight management. It is not something you reach and then back off. It requires weekly monitoring for the rest of your life![4]

Step 6: Incorporate all the Habits of Health

From learning to eat right, reaching a healthy weight, incorporating movement into your daily schedule, to making better sleep a priority, learning to reduce stress, and manage your world through a healthy mind, the Habits of Health Macro Habits take you on a complete journey from surviving to thriving.

Step 7: Obtain Optimal Health

No matter what your age, optimizing your health is a fundamental principle of living longer. Not only is it necessary, it makes sense. After all, if you're going to have a longer life, why not be able to fully enjoy everything this big adventure has to offer?

Now, if you stop right here at this step and focus on being at the height of health for your whole life, you may live longer. But there's even more you can do. Remember, just as there are no shortcuts to health, there are no shortcuts to longevity. It takes discipline. And just as you made a fundamental choice to be healthy, you can make a fundamental choice to be Ultrahealthy, and take your place among an exciting new generation— the New Centenarians. We will give you guidance in the next Element on how to add the next chapter 2 in your lifelong transformation.

Notes to yourself:

**Make sure you go over the details of Longevity in Habits of Health.
Also sit down with you coach and let them know all the changes you are
making to improve your self-care. Be sure to share the answers to the
following questions:**

What does this Element mean to you right now?

What does this Element give you the opportunity to reflect on?

What actions are you going to take as a result of this Element?

What role does community have in helping you create longevity
in your life?

I encourage you to connect with your coach, so you can share your
thoughts and actions as soon as possible. This will help your thoughts
become a reality.

Make sure you review all your notes and this Element often.

1 Cleveland Clinic Healthy Brain Initiative Research and key lifestyle changes.

2 A study titled Prevalence of Periodontitis in Adults in the United States: 2009 and 2010 estimates that 47.2%, or 64.7 million American adults have mild, moderate or severe periodontitis, which is the more advanced form of periodontal disease. In adults aged 65 and older, prevalence rates increase to 70.1%.Sep 4, 2012.

3 *Burden of Oral Disease Among Older Adults and Implications for Public Health Priorities* – Susan O. Griffin, Ph.D., Judith A. Jones, DDS, MPH, DScD, Diane Brunson, RDH, MPH, Paul M. Griffin, Ph.D., Am J Public Health. 2012 March; 102(3): 411–418. Published online 2012 March. doi: [10.2105/AJPH.2011.300362] PMCID: PMC3487659 PMID: 22390504.

4 *How Much Should We Weigh for a Long and Healthy Life Span? The Need to Reconcile Caloric Restriction versus Longevity with Body Mass Index versus Mortality Data* – www.hsph.harvard.edu/healthy weight Front Endocrinol (Lausanne). 2014; 5: 121. Published online 2014 Jul 30. Prepublished online 2014 Jun 3. doi: [10.3389/fendo.2014.00121] PMCID: PMC4115619 PMID: 25126085.

ELEMENT 26:
ULTRAHEALTH™: LIVING LONGER FULL OUT

Average time to complete: **2–4 weeks**

In Element 26, we will:

- Outline some of the key Habits of Ultrahealth™.
- Define your Progressive Plan for Ultrahealth™.
- Explore how you can optimize your brain health.

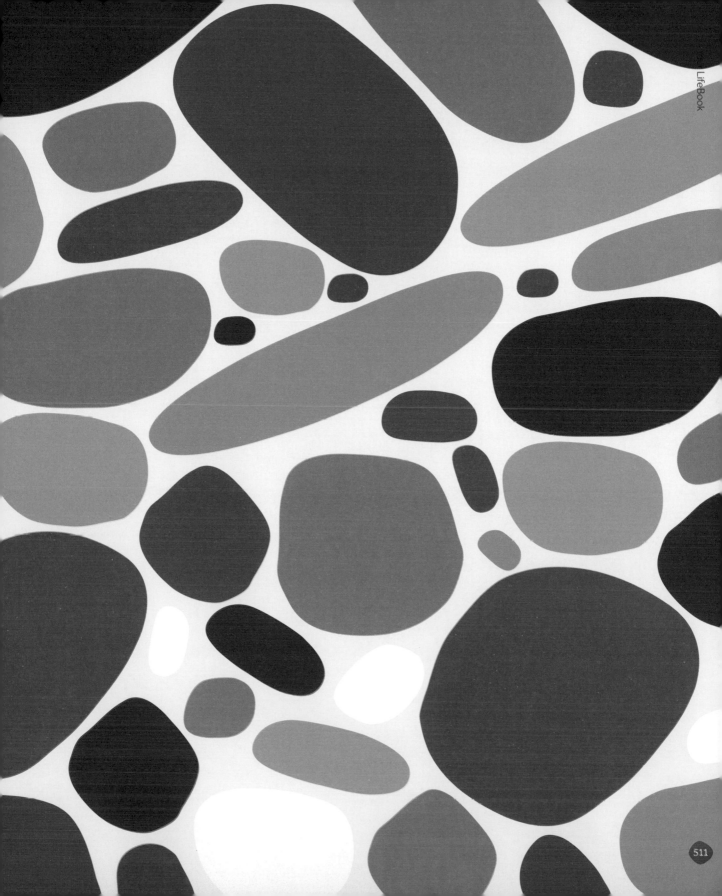

ULTRAHEALTH™: GOING BEYOND WHAT MOST WILL DO

The Ultrahealth™ system you're about to discover uses principles drawn from the cutting edge of scientific research.

Once you've reached a state of optimal health by adopting the Habits of Health, you can use it to go to the next level and attain your maximum life span. The goals in your weight management system at the longevity level are:

Phase IV Longevity[1]
BMI 21–24.9

| Waist Circumference: | Male <32 | Female <29 |
| Body Fat (optional) | Male ~10% | Female <17–22% |

In the third part of *Dr. A's Habits of Health*, we will explore in detail the things you can do to create Ultrahealth™ and potentially live a longer healthier life. Let's look at the components that determine just who achieves this ultimate state. Basically, your maximum life span is determined by these three factors, in the following proportion:

• Genetic programming (20%–30%)
• Position on the health continuum (70%–80%)
• Luck (<0.1%)

Lifestyle versus genetics—the cards you're dealt in terms of longevity—actually play a much smaller role in determining life span than your lifestyle. And fortunately, lifestyle is a factor you can control.

Your Progressive Plan for Ultrahealth™
1. Apply the Habits of Health Transformational System and lifestyle.
2. Reach and maintain optimal health.
3. Add Ultrahealth™ practices as an additional level of vigilance that focuses on increasing your resilience to aging and disease.

Adopting a lifestyle that supports optimal health is by far the biggest factor in longevity. This means that the Habits of Health—which are all about moving forward on the health continuum—are a great way to position yourself for a long and healthy life.

In fact, I believe you can potentially add 10 to 20 years to your life just by adopting the optimal health lifestyle I've been teaching you. If you're a woman, this means extending your life from potentially 80 to 100 years, or, if you're a man, from potentially 75 to 95—simply by living the Habits of Health. Studies show an extension of seven years just by maintaining a normal weight, not smoking, and drinking alcohol at moderate levels. Our focus on emotional management, stress reduction, and healthy sleeping can all potentially help us live longer.[2]

What I propose is a state of health that pushes you to be the very best you can be and in a state where your body operates at optimal efficiency. A state of living a robust and thriving life, eating only the freshest, nutrient-rich foods, becoming lean and strong with terrific stamina—kind of like our prehistoric ancestors 10,000 years ago (just without the risk of saber-toothed tigers).

It's a state called Ultrahealth™, and it's really an augmentation of the Habits of Health lifestyle through dietary optimization, intensified weekly workouts, and a focus on brain health. And it has the potential to add another 10 to 20 years to your life beyond the extra years that optimal health can give you.

That potential is becoming a reality in the research as they have used these techniques on monkeys and they are living much longer. Whether this will translate to humans is too soon to know. But what I do know is the strategies we use in Ultrahealth™ will keep you healthier.[3]

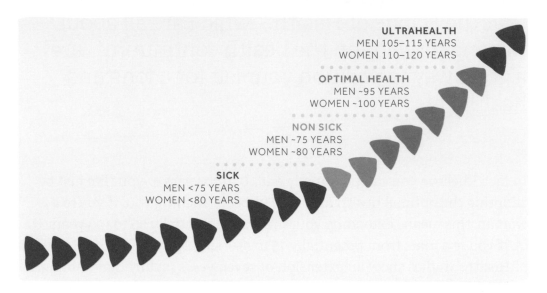

ULTRAHEALTH
MEN 105–115 YEARS
WOMEN 110–120 YEARS

OPTIMAL HEALTH
MEN ~95 YEARS
WOMEN ~100 YEARS

NON SICK
MEN ~75 YEARS
WOMEN ~80 YEARS

SICK
MEN <75 YEARS
WOMEN <80 YEARS

Ultrahealth™ by the Numbers

The ultimate state of health—one that can take you well into your second century of life—is an entirely new standard for health optimization. Here are the key parameters we're aiming for:

Systolic blood pressure	110–95 or less
Diastolic blood pressure	75–60 or less
Body mass index	24.9–20 21–23 is ideal; no less than 20
Body fat	<12% for men; 17–22% for women
HDI (good cholesterol)	50–70 mg/dl
Fasting blood sugar	75 mg/dl
hs-CRP	0.5

The Ultrahealth™ Plan: Extend and Thrive

Up to this point, you've learned a practical system to integrate all of ways medical science has to help us stay healthy and protect against disease. Now, the Ultrahealth™ plan will take all that and add yet another level of daily choices. Think of it as your postdoctorate degree in health optimization.

This state of Ultrahealth™ is obtained by making the decision to play full-out with all you have and to organize your life and your daily choices around what's best for your physical, mental, and social wellbeing.

Now before we go on, let me emphasize that if you haven't learned the Habits of Health and applied them to your daily life, and if you haven't reached a healthy weight and aren't currently living an active lifestyle, you aren't going to be able to apply the Ultrahealth™ program to your life.

Why? Well, it will simply be too hard for you. First, it would be like trying to perform jumps on a double black diamond ski run when you haven't even learned how to snowplow on the bunny slopes. And second, it won't work. If you're still eating a tub of ice cream at bedtime, your high-sugar, high-fat intake is creating an inflammatory state that totally negates the Ultrahealth™ activation of cellular protection activation and signaling of longevity.

However, if you've already reached and are maintaining optimal health, Ultrahealth™ really won't seem like much of a stretch. Let's break it down and see why.

The Ultrahealth™ plan has three major areas of focus:
• Dietary optimization (Part 3.4 in *Dr. A's Habits of Health, Brain and Mind Longevity: Protecting and Enhancing Your Future*)
• Movement enhancement (Part 3.4 in *Dr. A's Habits of Health, Brain and Mind Longevity: Protecting and Enhancing Your Future*)
• Brain-health optimization (Part 3.5 in *Dr. A's Habits of Health, Reaching a State of Ultrahealth™: Living the Future of Wellbeing*)

In *Dr. A's Habits of Health* I'll show you specific strategies to enhance your energy management and optimize your brainpower. We will start by focusing on adjusting your dietary intake to improve your body's functioning, reinvigorate you on a cellular level, and set you up with the lowest possible risk for disease as you continue your extended journey through life.

Here we will create the space for you to start working on the next step in your story.

When can you start the Ultrahealth™ longevity program?
Are you ready? What do you need to do?

Eating for Ultrahealth™: Adjusting Your Daily Intake
First let's calculate your Ultrahealth™ daily energy intake.
Use the example in Part 3.4 in *Dr. A's Habits of Health, Brain and Mind Longevity: Protecting and Enhancing Your Future* to do this.

What does your dietary optimization look like?

Does yours include:
• Optimal Health TEE x 0.85 kcal/day
• No processed foods
• Lowest-glycemic carbohydrates
• Increased soy intake (based on Okinawan longevity studies; see Part 3.2 in *Dr. A's Habits of Health, The Habits of Longevity: Living Longer in Ultrahealth*)
• Healthy fats, especially olive oil, fish oils, walnuts, and flaxseed
• Eating every three hours
• Drinking 64 ounces of water a day

Note that while the Ultrahealth™ plan involves reduced caloric intake, it still requires you to fuel every three hours. To make this doable, I recommend you take another look at the fueling strategies, in the healthy eating section in Part 2 of *Dr. A's Habits of Health*. It's worth noting that OPTAVIA®, as a pioneer and leader in restrictive-calorie meal plans, provides an excellent method to help you implement a regimen of dietary restriction. Scientifically formulated portion-controlled meals are particularly effective in delivering a nutrient-rich, low-calorie diet that also provides plenty of health-supporting soy!

Exercise Enhancement: The Other Half of the Equation

It starts with increasing your Your Ultrahealth™ Movement Plan

• NEAT
• EAT Walking
• EAT Resistance

The idea is to not just increase your energy expenditure but to also push your cardiovascular and strength training by designing an enhancement program that's sustainable, provides just the right intensity, and is minimally intrusive to your busy schedule. These additional movements complete our EAT System, which enhances your energy expenditure and cardiovascular fitness to help support maximum functional longevity.

Intensifying Your Workouts: Options for Enhancement

I've developed several options for increasing your energy output. First, let's look at some ways to boost your current resistance workouts. Second, we'll explore high intensity interval training again, which is an option you can use to enhance the intensity of two of your 30-minute walks per week.

Six Options to Boost Your EAT Resistance Workouts (Part 3.4 in *Dr. A's Habits of Health, Brain and Mind Longevity: Protecting and Enhancing Your Future*)

Pick which ones you are using and review how you are using it

1. Increase Repetitions
2. Increase Resistance
3. Increase Sets or Rotations
4. Decrease Recovery Time
5. Increase Your Speed
6. Maintain Muscular Contraction

Intensifying Your EAT Walking Workouts through Interval Training (Refer back to Element 18 as well as Part 3.4 in *Dr. A's Habits of Health, Brain and Mind Longevity: Protecting and Enhancing Your Future*).

High intensity interval training is a time-efficient way to train your aerobic (cardiovascular) and anaerobic (muscle) energy-burning systems. It's called interval training because it consists of short periods, or intervals, of high-intensity cardiovascular activity followed by short periods of lower-intensity cardiovascular activity. By alternating high- and low-intensity intervals, you intensify the metabolic challenge to your muscles, increasing the amount of calories burned in each twenty-minute session, which can help prevent injury by keeping exercise time shorter and saving muscles from overuse.

How are you using HIIT?

Protecting and Enhancing Your Future

The brain and the mind are the source of all health and the master controller of aging. Its most fundamental function is to control all the movement of the body. Without it we would quickly go down the path to disease and death. In fact, our brain is one of the first organs to suffer if our daily movement is impeded. And if we don't protect our master controller, we may lose our memory and our ability to think. At which point it really wouldn't make sense to extend our life anyway.

I've singled out the brain for special attention not only because of its central role in health and longevity but also because it's become particularly vulnerable to injury in our rapidly advancing, technologically driven society. Our Western lifestyle, with a diet high in animal fats and high-glycemic carbohydrates, a lack of exercise, and excessive stress is pounding away at our brains as well as our hearts. Fortunately, reaching optimal health and wellbeing through the Habits of Health eliminates most of these negative factors.

Our goal is for you to become laser-focused on the specific habits that will protect and enhance your brain and enable it to continue directing you toward a state of ever-increasing health.

Our strategy concentrates on three major areas essential for brain health and longevity
• Brain exercise (including physical exercise)
• Stress reduction
• Brain food (nutritional enhancement)

We can maintain optimal levels of cognition in our brain and mind if we:
• Use it
• Keep enough blood flowing to provide the oxygen it needs to flourish
• Feed it enough of the right nutrients

Brain exercise (including physical exercise)

Describe what brain exercises you are adding to optimize your brain health

Stress reduction

Most of us rarely experience true relaxation (outside of vacation, that is). Yet this state—being relaxed, creative, intuitive, vibrant, intelligent—should be our brain's normal default state. It's how we're supposed to be. In Part 3.5 in *Dr. A's Habits of Health, Reaching a State of Ultrahealth™: Living the Future of Wellbeing*, in the Progressive Relaxation and Mind section we discuss some ideas of how to relax.

Describe what methods of stress reduction you are adding to optimize your brain health

Brain food (nutritional enhancement) (See HabitsofHealth.com)

The brain is a fatty organ. In fact, your neurons are about 60% fat.[4]
This high fat content makes your brain especially vulnerable to attack by destructive oxygen radicals. When you eat saturated fats in particular, you bathe your brain in oxygen radicals from saturated and polyunsaturated oils. If you were to pour these oils into an open container, they would oxidize quickly, becoming cloudy and rancid as they filled with damaging oxygen radicals. That same scenario takes place in your body as oxygen-rich blood mixes with unhealthy fats and rushes to your brain.

In addition, excess dietary fat can impair cerebral circulation and clog your arteries with LDLs (bad cholesterol), thereby decreasing the elasticity of your brain's blood vessels. That's why it's so important to avoid saturated and polyunsaturated fats such as margarine, as well as all sources of trans-fat.

Fat and oil intake

To protect your brain, confine your fat and oil intake to these healthy choices:
• Extra virgin olive oil
• Flaxseed oil
• Canola oil
• Fatty fish and fish oils, including eicosapentaenoic acid (EPA)
  and docosahexaenoic acid (DHA)

To further decrease oxygen radical formation, reduce the total number of calories you eat and choose only the lowest-glycemic carbohydrates. When it comes to your daily intake, be sure to include the full antioxidant supplement battery you learned about in the optimization program in Part 2.15 in *Dr. A's Habits of Health, The Best You Can Be: Optimizing Your Life at Any Age*, including vitamins E and C, beta-carotene, zinc, selenium, and CoQ10. These will help your body create an environment that is rich in radical scavengers to protect your brain.

Herbs and Spices

The following choices are especially useful in helping the brain replenish its neurotransmitters and remove the dangerous presence of beta-amyloid:

• Turmeric (curcumin)

• Basil

• Lemon balm

• Black pepper

• Sage

• Mint

• Salvia

• Lemon rosemary

Foods for Better Blood Flow

• Chocolate—in the form of pure cocoa or 70% dark chocolate—contains flavonoids that help keep your cerebral blood vessels open, which is something that's particularly important when we're over 55.

• Other flavonoid-rich foods include wine (especially red wine), grape juice, and black tea.

• Avoid foods that are high-glycemic!

Supplements for Your Brain

The supplements you added as part of your optimization program are a great start, but there are a few more that are particularly important for brain health. For a serious boost to brain longevity, try the following:

• Vitamin E (400 IU mixed tocopherols and gram [1,000 mg] of vitamin C)

• Vitamin B6 (40 mg), vitamin B12 (800 mcg), folic acid (100 mg), niacin (100 mg) in the form of a mega B complex

• Acetyl-L-carnitine (100 mg)

• Alpha lipoic acid (200 mg)

• Phosphatidylserine (100–300 mg)

• Coenzyme Q10 (100 mg)

• Zinc (20 mg)

• Selenium (200 mcg)

• Magnesium (400 mg)

• Vitamin A (2,500–5,000 IU)

And, although conclusive research is still pending, you might want to consider these:
• Ginkgo biloba (90 mg)
• Lecithin (1,500 mg)
• Green juice products and green tea (1–2 servings per day)

As always, check with your healthcare provider before beginning any supplement protocol.

With the addition of these brain-boosting nutritional supplements, a regular course of brain and body exercises, and some healthy stress-reducing techniques, you now have a whole new additional set of Habits of Health for your brain! Use them to protect this most important organ from harm and ensure that you stay in the best possible shape to enjoy the longer life that's now within your grasp.

Reaching a State of Ultrahealth™

Once you settle into your Ultrahealth™ program, you'll want to track your progress closely, especially for the first year. I suggest quarterly visits to your healthcare provider to make sure your body is responding properly. Your healthcare provider will be very interested in your progress because you will represent a new type of patient with potentially these outstanding health parameters:
• You'll be coming off most or all of your medication.
• Your lab results will be to the far left (low normal) of the reporting range.
• Your lipid profile may fall into the 50–70 range for LDLs (bad cholesterol).
• Your fasting blood sugar may drop into the low 70s.

Let's focus on three critical parameters that together really serve to define your Ultrahealth™ state:

• Your hs-CRP
• Your body mass index (BMI)
• Your percentage of body fat (body composition)

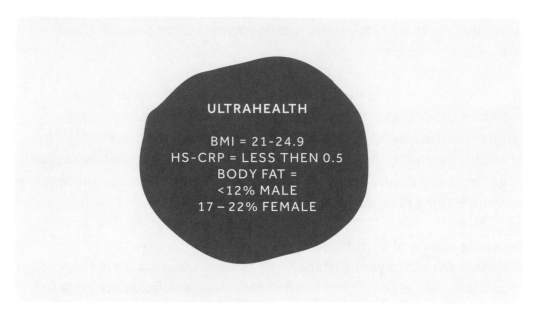

ULTRAHEALTH

BMI = 21-24.9
HS-CRP = LESS THEN 0.5
BODY FAT =
<12% MALE
17 – 22% FEMALE

What About Dietary (Calorie) Restriction?

Throughout this year, we've discussed the importance of gaining control over your calorie intake, and have used that control as an essential Element to guide you on this journey.

First, we used it to help you reach a healthy weight. Then, as your body became able to move more freely, we found a balance between energy in and energy out. And then we set our sights on helping you reach optimal health. At each of these levels, we've also added many Habits of Health, thereby building a foundation of behaviors that will last you a lifetime.

Now, through the Habits of Longevity, we've taken your newfound mastery of energy intake, as well as those important supporting habits, and given you access to a state of health that few adults have ever experienced, or ever will. The final verdict on dietary (calorie) restriction as a longevity enhancer isn't in, nor do we yet know the absolute optimal intake needed to slow the aging process. But what we do know is this—dietary restriction, when accompanied by a balanced, nutrient-dense diet, should provide the same benefits of disease reduction and metabolic adaptation in humans as it does in animal studies.[5]

Even if it turns out that dietary restriction doesn't extend mankind's maximum lifespan, its ability to help us spend more time in a healthier state is enough to be excited about. After all, who knows what possibilities are about to unfold? By living and thriving in Ultrahealth™, you'll be in a great position to take advantage of all the new advancements that science will gradually reveal.

A number of other opportunities for longevity show promise on the level calorie restriction. For example, red wine might be part of the reason why we see consistently higher rates of longevity in the Mediterranean. I'm following this research closely, and you can go online to read the latest insights (my guide to wine and longevity included) by visiting HabitsofHealth.com.

A FINAL WORD FROM DR. A

One of the leading cultural anthropologists of our time, a woman named Inga Treitler, evaluated a group of individuals who had mastered successful weight loss by losing at least 60 lbs and keeping it off for at least five years.

Although the subjects had lost weight in many different ways, these long-term success stories had one thing in common—every one of them had changed the way they lived their lives. They made a 180-degree change in orientation and in the way they experience the world. In fact, Treitler describes this phenomenon as a "rite of passage". For some, this meant leaving their old jobs to become coaches, teachers, and mentors. They went from being passive to active participants in their own lives.[6]

They had undergone a transformation that would last them for a lifetime.

As you know, the Habits of Health Transformational System is a compilation of the lessons I've learned from people who've been successful at losing weight, reaching optimal health, and creating wellbeing in their lives and the lives of others. By studying their successes—and the failures of others—the Habits of Health provides a path that many are following in order to reach and maintain optimal health. We have created a predictable system to help transformation become a reality for you.

Your coach, like many of the people who are living the Habits of Health, is now helping others which, as Treitler observes, also helps them maintain optimal health and wellbeing. Working together, as well as staying connected through an environment that inspires and creates long-term success, is a great way to give yourself the gift of comprehensive support and a lifetime of personal health and fulfillment.

Now that you recognize the importance of support as you install and master the MacroHabits you have learned to date, you're hopefully seeking more support and a community of kindred spirits.

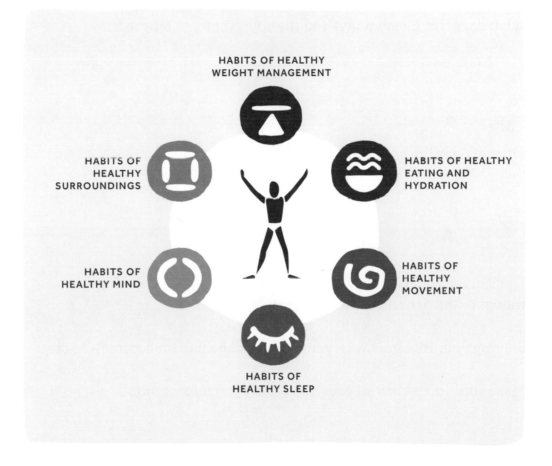

Notes to yourself:

Your coach and community will be thrilled to celebrate the creation of your new story. Please reach out to your coach right away and share your answers to the following 3 questions:

What does this Element mean to you right now?

What does this Element give you the opportunity to reflect on?

What actions are you going to take as a result of this Element?

I encourage you to connect with your coach, so you can share your thoughts and actions as soon as possible.

Sharing your thoughts with your coach will help them become a reality.

Make sure you review all your notes and this Element often.

1 *Selected Health Conditions and Risk Factors, by Age: United States, Selected Years 1988–1994 Through 2015–2016* – www.cdc.gov/nchs/hus/contents2017.htm Table 53, 1. J.R. Cerhan, et al. A pooled analysis of waist circumference and mortality in 650,000 adults. Mayo Clinic Proceedings. 2014;89:335.2.Healthy weight: Assessing your weight. Centers for Disease Control and Prevention. www.cdc.gov/healthyweight/assessing/Index.html. Accessed May 10, 2017.3. J.P. Despres. Waist circumference as a vital sign in cardiology 20 years after its initial publication in the American Journal of Cardiology. American Journal of Cardiology. 2014;114:320.

2 *A Healthy Lifestyle Increases Life Expectancy by up to Seven Years* – July 20, 2017 Source: Max-Planck-Gesellschaft Summary: Maintaining a normal weight, not smoking, and drinking alcohol at moderate levels are factors that add healthy years to life.

3 *Healthcare Provider Caloric Restriction Improves Health and Survival of Rhesus Monkeys* – Nat Commun. 2017 Jan 17;8:14063. doi: 10.1038/ncomms14063. J.A. Mattison, R.J. Colman, T.M. Beasley, D.B. Allison, J.W. Kemnitz, G.S. Roth, D.K. Ingram, R. Weindruch, R. de Cabo, R.M. Anderson.

4 *Essential Fatty Acids and Human Brain* – Acta Neurol Taiwan. 2009 Dec;18(4):231-41. C.Y. Chang, D.S. Ke, J.Y. Chen.

5 *Healthcare Provider Caloric Restriction Improves Health and Survival of Rhesus Monkeys* – Nat Commun. 2017 Jan 17;8:14063. doi: 10.1038/ncomms14063. J.A. Mattison, R.J. Colman, T.M. Beasley, D.B. J.W. Allison, Kemnitz, G.S. Roth, D.K. Ingram, R. Weindruch, R. de Cabo, R.M. Anderson. Nat Commun. 2017 Jan 17;8:14063. doi: 10.1038/ncomms14063.healthcare provider Caloric restriction improves health and survival of rhesus monkeys. J.A. Mattison, R.J. Colman, T.M. Beasley, D.B. Allison, J.W. Kemnitz, G.S. Roth, D.K. Ingram, R. Weindruch, R. de Cabo, R.M. Anderson.

EPILOGUE:
YOUR NEW STORY

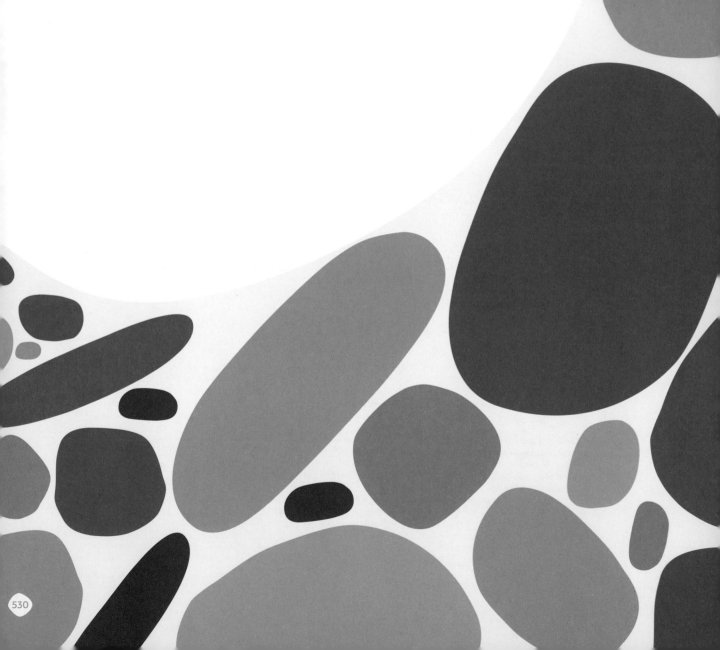

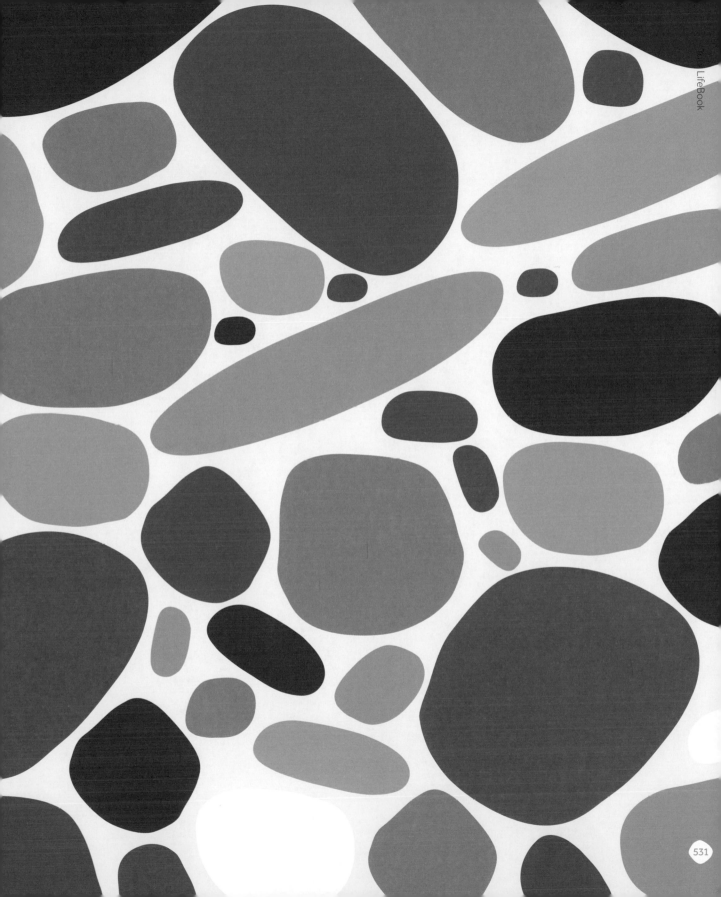

Congratulations!

You have just gone through 26 Elements which are fundamental to building optimal health and wellbeing in your life. If you have spent two weeks, on average, on each Element, you will be coming up to your one year anniversary of starting your journey to lifelong transformation.

The time may have gone fast or slow but no matter as you will have progressed a considerable way on your journey since that first day.

The story you are writing may have changed everything for you.

You may not totally recognize how much you have developed so I would like you to retake the wellbeing evaluation and compare your scores.

Once you have compared your two scores and reviewed your original notes from the current reality section spend some time reflecting on how far you have come. Also note what areas you still need to improve on and go back to those Elements for a refresher. Also, discuss this with your coach.

Your Original Scores – Date taken

	Bad	Poor	Fair	Good	Great	Optimum
Physical Health	10	20	30	40	50	60
Mental Health	10	20	30	40	50	60
Financial Health	10	20	30	40	50	60

	Failing	Poor	Surviving	Above Average	Thriving	Optimum
Overall Wellbeing	30	60	90	120	150	180

Your Scores Now – Date now

	Bad	Poor	Fair	Good	Great	Optimum
Physical Health	10	20	30	40	50	60
Mental Health	10	20	30	40	50	60
Financial Health	10	20	30	40	50	60

	Failing	Poor	Surviving	Above Average	Thriving	Optimum
Overall Wellbeing	30	60	90	120	150	180

How have your physical health and scores changed this year?

How have your thoughts, emotions, actions, and scores changed this year?

How have your level of success, fulfilment, and scores changed this year?

Have you changed quadrants in your Wellbeing Chart? (See Element 22, *Creating Optimal Wellbeing*).

Look how far you have come in just a year. Using the creative process that is embedded in our system, now imagine how your life is going to grow from here.

MY INVITATION

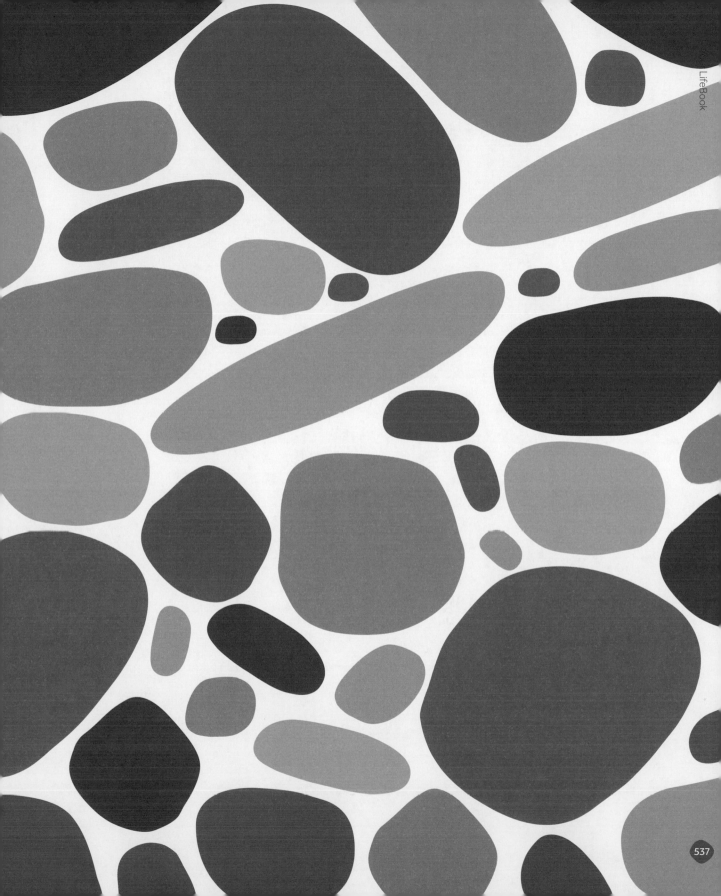

Hopefully by now you are fully immersed in our community and you are building powerful connections and bonds that are serving you well on your journey.

You may have already made connections, joined our coaching team, and helped others on their transformational journey.

If not, this is something you might want to explore as a potential catalyst to help you advance to the next level of your development. Our coaches live and breath the Habits of Health and are taking full advantage of living optimal health and wellbeing, as well as helping others do the same.

The meaning and purpose created by helping others organize their lives around what matters most can be a powerful engine to accelerating your personal growth. Our community is especially well equipped to handle the constant change that is the reality of our modern lives. We provide a platform and the support necessary for you to become the highest version of yourself. That purpose provides the passion to awaken the energy you need to jump out of bed in the morning ready to create another optimal day.

It's not a utopia that I am describing because a perfect world does not exist. A world without discomfort and challenges is a utopia but even if it was possible it would be stagnant and quite boring without problems to solve.

Unlike utopia, which is a destination we seek, protopia is a state we strive to become.

It is a process where each day you are excited about getting just a little better than you were yesterday. You have just experienced a year of slow progress and incremental improvement.

It is not always easy but being present and enjoying today's work is a wonderful state to live in. It's focused on becoming fully conscious moment to moment doing something that is important to you.

Protopia

If you have not heard this word before, the "pro" in protopia describes the notion of process and progress. And "topia", is an imagined place or state of things. Protopia has been used in the technology world to describe the continual changes in a world that is forever in a state of flux.

And for most of us who grew up before this revolution in the speed of innovation of technology, movies like *Back to the Future* and its flying car opened our imagination and introduced us to future possibilities. Today the luster has worn off, and just the thought of ever advancing technology brings dread to most who are not prepared to change any faster as the current pace has already turned their world upside down. It is the realization that we will all need to be perpetual newbies in learning as continuous innovation allows nothing to remain the same.

My approach to technology protopia is quite simple. We need to create a parallel human protopian approach which embraces change as inevitable and use the process to progress and help us grow at a rate that can keep up with technology. I mentioned at the beginning of both *Dr. A's Habits of Health* and in the beginning of *Your Lifebook* that Thomas Friedman's new book sadly reveals that human adaptability is lagging behind tech innovation. The unfortunate outcome is a poorer quality of life for those who are not flexible enough to keep up with change.

Yet, this challenge has created great opportunities.

For those that are joining our community and fully engaging in our protopian model, we are providing a safe place to organize your life around what matters. This is what we are doing and what I can offer you moving forward on your journey of transformation.

It is not idle theory but evidence based fact that those that have joined our community are becoming more and are developing the skills to lead the mission to provide optimal health and wellbeing for the world. We have always led innovations that could help assist in creating optimal health. For example, Dr. A's system for healthy eating featured the plate system for portion control and the color-coded system of healthy eating.

That simple plate system was later adopted by the USDA system in their similar My Plate method which eliminated the obsolete food pyramid. My low-glycemic colorized system, which simplified choosing healthy food with the simple adage "stay in the green to be lean" has recently been validated by experts such as Harvard's head of nutrition, Dr. Ludwig.[1] Previously the use of the glycemic index was dismissed as being too difficult. Our Habits of Healthy Motion's NEAT system pioneered the idea of perpetual motion as far more important than exercise for preventing poor health. In the last few years, the research has proven that living a sedentary lifestyle, despite active exercise, is responsible for the unprecedented levels of disease globally.

This was recently coined the sitting disease and the recommended treatment is to dramatically increase our daily NEAT activity. Almost two decades ago, we introduced and placed emphasis on the importance of health coaches as guides that assist individuals to create health for themselves. This has since gained momentum and now there is a whole movement of health coaches. This is helpful and has good intentions but they still have not been able to replicate what we have created.

Why?
Because people want be supported to become autonomous just like you have experienced during your journey. It is imperative that we help the individual be the key determinant of their health and wellbeing. People do not want to be told what to do anymore. They want to be heard, validated, and put in a position to win. That is why the Habits of Health in its evolution is now a transformational system that, when guided by a coach, creates real change. We will lead that change while medicine tries to catch up as because they focus on only reacting to and treating disease, rather than preventing it, their pace will be slow.

In the meantime, we are growing this mission daily and while we are realizing our dream of thinking big I offer you an opportunity to do the same. I invite you to join our mission and become part of our journey as you continue with yours. Together, we will create tremendous success for ourselves and for all of those that raise their hand and are ready to take responsibility for their health and their life. In fact, who do you know right now that could use our help to regain their hope and a way to better health and wellbeing. It could be really cool to bring them with you! This is only the beginning of your story and there are many chapters yet to come!

I would write down what you envision for your future in the next few pages and allow that future to inform you what you will do each day as you continue to become healthier and improve your wellbeing.

Make the decision that you are going to pursue Ultrahealth™ for yourself and help others improve their health and wellbeing. In fact, write down all the people you would like to help. This is a gift that is certainly worth sharing with people you love and care about!

Our goal is to make the world a better place to bring up our kids and for all to live in.

Let's grow to serve ourselves as humans and use technology as our partner to enhance the human experience. This will create a thriving period of awakening in mankind, as well as a kinder and more compassionate place to live.

Once again, congratulations on creating better health and wellbeing for you and the people around you.

I wish you continual health and growth in your life and hopefully you are now fully utilizing our community to advance your life and wellbeing for many, many, more years to come.

In Health,
Dr. A

Describe what your future life looks like and what date it will become real.

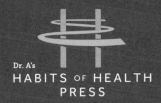

Dr. A's
HABITS of HEALTH
PRESS

P.O. Box 3301
Annapolis, Maryland 21403
www.drwayneandersen.com

Copyright © 2019 by Dr. Wayne Scott Andersen

What are the three main areas you are going to work on now based on that future?

1 *Always Hungry? Conquer Cravings, Retrain Your Fat Cells, and Lose Weight Permanently* Hardcover – January 5, 2016, David Ludwig, M.D., Ph.D.